PRAISE FOR
CHASING THE WIDOWMAKER

"Though at first I was scanning only, I soon became engrossed, reading more deeply the history of medicine, the history of my chosen field of cardiac surgery/cardiology, and the personal stories of the great individuals whose discoveries have advanced our field which have been so expertly intertwined with patient and personal experiences of training and practice over [Meshkov's] career. . . . A very readable, hugely informative book that will be of immense interest to all cardiovascular physicians as well as to any physician or layman who wants to learn more about the most common cause of death worldwide—coronary artery disease—and the great advances that have been made in its understanding and treatment."

—**MICHAEL ACKER, MD,** Chair and Professor Cardiothoracic Surgery University of Pennsylvania School of Medicine

"Finally, a comprehensive and compelling treatise about the complex disease that kills more Americans than any other. Intertwining his own vast experience in the field with the well-researched and fascinating lives of the pioneers of heart disease research and treatment, Dr. Meshkov has crafted a book that splendidly entertains while effectively teaching. A must-read for anyone who treats or suffers from coronary artery disease."

—**PETER KOWEY, MD,** Emeritus Chief of Cardiology, Lankenau Heart Institute; William Wykoff Smith Chair, Cardiovascular Research, Lankenau Institute for Medical Research; Professor of Medicine and Clinical Pharmacology, Thomas Jefferson University, Philadelphia, PA

"Dr. Meshkov's book, *Chasing the Widowmaker: The History of the Heart Attack Pandemic*, is a must-read for heart patients like myself. Presented in non-technical terms, it reads like a sensitive physician taking extra time to educate his or her patients. Based on years of clinical experience, *Chasing the Widowmaker* also provides important lessons in modern medical history in a felicitous fashion."

—**LANCE J. SUSSMAN, PHD,** Senior Rabbi, Reform Congregation, Keneseth Israel, Elkins Park

"For thousands of years the 'widowmaker' has plagued mankind as a stealthy, shadowy figure who suddenly appears and wreaks havoc and death on the human heart and soul. This highly engaging book chronicles the life and impending death of this relentless killer, through the heroic efforts of many brave souls committed to defeating him. His voice is brought to life in a frightening fashion, yet the reader will eventually delight in his (soon-to-be) demise, and also discover how to keep him at bay."

—**BRUCE ALAN KEHR, MD,** Author of *Becoming Whole: A Healing Companion to Ease Emotional Pain and Find Self-Love*, and International Award-Winning Psychiatrist and Blogger

"The widowmaker is a term familiar to most cardiology trainees—a single word that conjures up a host of severe clinical events, such as heart attack and sudden cardiac death, that result from a specific narrowing in one coronary artery. In *Chasing the Widowmaker*, Dr. Arnold Meshkov describes the history behind the understanding and modern treatment of coronary artery disease and acute myocardial infarction (heart attacks). This is a remarkably reader-friendly volume. In the historical text the author artfully intersperses personal experiences as physician and cardiologist, as well as imagined views of a humanized widowmaker. The book transports the reader from the early discoveries of basic cardiac physiology and pathology to more recent advances and discoveries that opened the door to modern diagnosis and therapy. The end result of these efforts has been a marked improvement in the current survival of cardiac patients. Dr. Meshkov profiles the physicians and scientists whose discoveries changed the course of the widowmaker's outcomes. We learn about interesting aspects of their personal lives and how these impacted on their work. The book is well written, keeping the reader's attention throughout, while providing a substantial volume of relevant and meaningful information. I highly recommend this book to laypeople, patients with heart disease, as well as physicians—both cardiologists and those who practice other disciplines."

—**BARRY L. ZARET, MD,** Robert W. Berliner Professor Emeritus of Medicine, Yale University; Former Chief of Cardiology, Yale-New Haven Medical Center

Chasing the Widowmaker:
The History of the Heart Attack Pandemic

by Arnold B. Meshkov

© Copyright 2021 Arnold B. Meshkov

ISBN 978-1-64663-338-8

All rights reserved. No part of this publication may be reproduced, stored in a retrieval system, or transmitted in any form or by any means—electronic, mechanical, photocopy, recording, or any other—except for brief quotations in printed reviews, without the prior written permission of the author.

Published by

◤ köehlerbooks™

3705 Shore Drive
Virginia Beach, VA 23455
800-435-4811
www.koehlerbooks.com

CHASING THE WIDOWMAKER

THE HISTORY OF THE HEART ATTACK PANDEMIC

ARNOLD B. MESHKOV, MD

VIRGINIA BEACH
CAPE CHARLES

> "It is not incumbent on you to finish the task, but neither are you free to absolve yourself from it."
>
> **Ethics of the Fathers, 2:21**
> Pirkei Avot (190-230 CE)

This book is dedicated to many people: my professors and so many colleagues at the University of Pennsylvania, Temple University, and Yale University who taught me to love science and the art of medicine, and the patients who over many years have entrusted me with their care.

To my family: my best friend and love Norma for over fifty years, to my children Adam and Karen, who too often wondered where their father was for so many hours, and my grandchildren Harriet, Madeleine, Samuel, and Asa, with the hope that at least one of them will follow in the footsteps of their grandfather and be blessed with the opportunity to join the community of the world's most gratifying profession: Medical Doctor.

TABLE OF CONTENTS

Author's Note xi

The Timeline of the Chase xiv

Prologue: Joining the Chase 1

1. Generation After Generation: The Gathering Epidemic 3

2. The Early Observers: How Long Has This Been Going On? 13

3. The Explosion of Chemistry: Amyl Nitrite and Nitroglycerin 27

4. The Days of the Dutchman: Engineering the
   Electrocardiogram Machine 40

5. The Russian and His Rabbits: Cholesterol
   and Atherosclerosis 55

6. Divining the Signals: The Creation of the Stress Test 67

7. Destroying the First Shibboleth: The Premier
   Heart Catheterization 86

8. Tracking an Epidemic: The Framingham Heart Study 101

9. Spinning Into Control: Lipoproteins and Cholesterol 114

10. An Out-of-Body Experience: The Heart-Lung Machine 124

11. It's Alive!: The Shocking Invention of Defibrillators
    and Pacemakers. 140

12. Preloading and Afterloading: Helping the
    Heart Fight Back 157

13. Dispelling the Second Shibboleth:
    The Coronary Artery Catheter 170

14. Back from the Brink: The Invention of
    the Coronary Care Unit 185

15. Slow Down, You Move Too Fast: Harnessing the
    Power of Beta-Blockers 201

16. The Dressmaker's Son and the Gift of the CABG 216

17. Metabolism Men: Unlocking the Cholesterol Code 234

18. Stopping Time: The Radioactive Heart Images 252

19. The German Icarus: Andreas Grüntzig and
    the Angioplasty Revolution 270

20. Who Ya Gonna Call?: Heralding the Age of Clot Busters 296

21. The Fungus Among Us: Cultivating the Rise of Statins 315

22. Keeping the Beat: The Personal Defibrillator 329

23. Shattering the Third Shibboleth: Heart Disease
    in Women 345

24. The Fire Inside: Tamping the Flames of Coronary
    Artery Disease 360

25. Apprehending the Widowmaker: How Close Are We? 382

Glossary 404

Bibliography 412

Index 451

Acknowledgements 490

About the Author 492

AUTHOR'S NOTE
MARCH 2020

I first heard the term "Widowmaker" when I was a medical student and came face to face with death, struggling to learn how to deal with the loss of too many of my cardiac patients. Widowmaker is a harsh and, unfortunately, accurate word to describe what was occurring.

No one knows for certain who coined the term, but it was in common usage in the 1970s when I was in training and the fight against heart attacks intensified. Many of the cardiac patients who died were men who had developed a severe blockage in the major artery to the heart. Their condition was often unrecognized until the artery was completely blocked and destroyed the heart muscle, sometimes in a matter of minutes. The result was a heart attack, or what we medically call a myocardial infarction, often resulting in sudden death.

Hidden from most doctors at the time was that the heart attack affected many women as well, but usually at an older age than the men, often leading to the belief that the death of these older people was just a natural consequence of aging. But the term Widowmaker has persisted and in recent decades describes a particular form of heart disease rather than a gender or socially specific designation as a problem of married men.

I've spent my career chasing the Widowmaker, driven by the desire to help people prevent and recover from that most dreaded form of heart disease. My life as a cardiologist was the right choice for me. I'm satisfied that my work on the frontlines has helped thousands of people survive their heart attacks and prevented many more in recent years. I also had the great satisfaction of teaching the next generation of medical students, residents, and cardiology trainees. Then one day I received inspiration from an unexpected source about the next contribution I could make to the chase.

Some friends recommended that I read a book about the history of cancer called *The Emperor of All Maladies* by Siddhartha Mukherjee MD, and a few pages in, I was hooked. Fancying myself as both a cardiologist and scientist, I was struck by how Mukherjee was able to weave together the medical facts and the science, the triumphs and the failures, with his personal experiences and patient interactions. He brought the book to life resulting in a tremendously satisfying read. Somewhere in the middle of his book, I realized that in my field there is no similar book that explains the remarkable history of the most important form of heart disease: the heart attack. There are very few of us whose own lives, families, or friends have not been affected by this condition. Heart disease is still the most common cause of death in the world, and most of those deaths are from disease of the heart's arteries.

The audacious notion that I could write such a book became more and more real to me. After all, I mused, I have been in this field for over forty years and have experienced firsthand the incredible evolution that has occurred since I finished my fellowship training in 1981. I remembered back to my third year as a medical student when I did a cardiology elective and my long interest in the heart accelerated. At the end of my clinical rotation, I spoke to my faculty instructor and told him how interested I was in this subject.

"It's a great field—there's only one problem," he said.

"What's that?" I asked.

"You see a lot of people die."

That was the reality at the time.

Thankfully, over the last five decades, this perspective has been turned upside down. Early treatment of a heart attack has improved the outcomes for millions worldwide, and the understanding of the process has given life to the greatest change for us all: the prevention that is now possible. The data from 2018 indicates that cancer will likely replace heart disease as the leading cause of death in the near future.

This is a great story to tell, not just from the intellectual interest of medical history, but to explore how the knowledge of the cause and the treatment of this disease has evolved. The data are without question: people who understand how they can prevent a heart attack live longer and happier lives.

This book is a story about the people whose insight and diligence changed the world of medicine forever. Their diverse ideas span the ivory towers of academia to the insights of a country doctor. Thanks to them, we are now armed with many weapons to prevent and combat the disease. We owe them a great debt of gratitude, and we will continue their quest of chasing the Widowmaker. I am convinced the future is bright.

TIMELINE OF THE CHASE

Ancients describe patients with chest pain
2000 BCE – 500 CE

W. Heberden describes angina pectoris
1768

A. Sobrero synthesizes nitroglycerin
1830

T. Brunton uses amyl nitrite to treat angina pectoris
1870's

W. Murrell uses nitroglycerin to great angina
1879

Nitroglycerin becomes commercially available
1885

W. Einthoven invents the electrocardiogram
1901

N. Anichkov proves that cholesterol causes atherosclerosis
1912

W. Forssmann performs self-heart catheterization
1929

F. Wood and C. Wolferth perform the first stress tests of the heart
1931

A. Master invents the "Two-step" stress test
1942

The Framingham Heart Study begins
1947

J. Gofman identifies low-density lipoprotein as the specific cause of atherosclerosis
1949

J. Gibbon uses the "heart-lung" machine in cardiac surgery
1952

P. Zoll uses a defibrillator to restore a normal heart rhythm
1956

M. Sones performs the first coronary artery angiogram
1959

First Coronary Care Unit opens
1964

Lidocaine used to treat cardiac arrhythmias after heart attacks
1965

J. Black invents the first "Beta-Blocker" medication	R. Favaloro performs first coronary artery bypass surgery	Johns Hopkins researchers produce the first nuclear images of cardiac muscle function and blood flow
1966	**1967**	**1971**
M. Brown and J. Goldstein discover the molecular receptor controlling cholesterol metabolism	A. Grüntzig performs the first coronary artery angioplasty	M. Dewood discovers that blood clots cause many heart attacks
1973	**1977**	**1980**
"Clot-buster" drugs used widely to treat heart attacks	Coronary artery stents with medication used to reduce the risk of restenosis after coronary angioplasty	N. Wenger organizes research identifying the nature of coronary artery disease in women
1980 – 1993	**1992**	**1992**
US FDA approves use of new medication to lower cholesterol levels and risk of heart attack		
2015		

PROLOGUE

JOINING THE CHASE

UNANSWERED QUESTIONS: A FRIDAY NIGHT IN DECEMBER 1965

A MURMUR SWEPT THROUGH the crowd, softly and slowly at first, then louder and faster. Someone was listening to a transistor radio, and something happened outside of our little world of a couple hundred students at a high school basketball game in suburban Philadelphia. I strained to hear the news, as a little shudder of fear and increased heart rate built in me. I remembered the assassination of President Kennedy just two years earlier. Judging from the facial expressions of the people talking, I knew that the news story was not going to be good. I was just fifteen years old.

After only a minute or two, I had the news: my friend David's father was dead—suddenly. His dad was a famous man, a civic leader. Ike Richman was a successful lawyer and the owner of the Philadelphia 76ers, the city's professional basketball team. Mr. Richman had flown with his team that night to watch the 76ers play the Boston Celtics. Early in the first half of the game, he collapsed in his seat at courtside. He could not be resuscitated. He was a man at the peak of his life, with all the success in the world—he was fifty-two years old, and he was gone in an instant.

My friends and I were stunned, and Mr. Richman's family was devastated. The adults said that Mr. Richman had died from a heart attack, and while I had heard that term before, I did not know what it meant. To a teenager, it just sounded terrifying.

Growing up, my best friend, Bob, lived in the house next door, and my bedroom window overlooked his home's driveway. In the middle of the night, I had sometimes been awakened by the sound of a garage door opening. The lights in the garage would go on, a car engine would rev up, and Bob's dad would drive off. A few years earlier, I asked Bob what kind of a doctor his father was, and he told me he was a cardiologist. That was another term I didn't understand. He said he took care of people having heart attacks, that these events sometimes happened at night, and that he needed to drive to the hospital to see the person. I remember vividly him adding, "Sometimes people die from those things." Bob's comment frightened me, but it didn't fully sink in until that night in 1965.

I had so many questions. How come the doctors weren't able to save Mr. Richman? Why had a doctor not known this might happen, and wasn't there anything to do to prevent it? What in the world was a heart attack, and what caused someone's heart to just stop working so suddenly? I didn't realize at my tender age that America was living through an epidemic of a disease that was claiming thousands of lives of both men and women—the heart attack. I was perplexed when frequently my parents would say that someone they knew had suffered a "coronary." But with this personal event, I became fascinated with the human heart. There had to be more to do to help people like Mr. Richman.

Even though I thought about many other choices, once I made it to medical school, it was the heart that drove my passion. It would take fifteen years to become a member of the posse chasing the Widowmaker. Only years later did I realize how this deadly disease, the myocardial infarction, became a modern plague, with its origins stretching back centuries but spreading so much faster and wider in the lifetime of my parents and myself.

CHAPTER 1

GENERATION AFTER GENERATION: THE GATHERING EPIDEMIC

I am a moment in time.

You may be sound asleep spooning with your loved one, or chasing your granddaughter up the hill, maybe finishing off that last piece of dripping roast. Most often, I arrive without knock or notice, your look one of shock.

I see you there clutching and grasping,
trying to pull in air and a second chance.
Many of you will beg, and I will hear you,
like a whisper in the wind.

They call me the Widowmaker.

CHRISTMAS DAY, 1944—BASTOGNE, BELGIUM

All his long life, the memories were fresh and vivid. My father Stanley Meshkov, a twenty-year-old kid from Philadelphia, was a battlefield sergeant in the 101st Airborne Division, the "Screaming Eagles" paratroopers. A week after a surprise attack in mid-December 1944 known as "The Battle of the Bulge," the 101st was surrounded by the Nazi Army in the crucial road intersection town of Bastogne, and my father and his buddies dug the deepest "foxholes" they could in the frozen earth. It was a terrible Christmas for the 101st as they huddled together against the fear, the darkness, and the biting cold, praying their nest would not be blown to bits by the deadly 88-millimeter mortars of the Wehrmacht.

Hungry all of the time and fearing lighting a fire to cook something would attract the attention of the German artillery gunners only a few hundreds yards away from them, their only option was to reach for their government-issued cold food—the K-ration. The United States military, with the advice of Ancel Keys MD (1904-2004), a nutritionist from the University of Minnesota, had devised a set of breakfast, lunch, and dinner rations in small boxes to provide about three thousand calories a day. There were high-carbohydrate items like biscuits, malted milk tablets, chocolate bars, sugar, and chewing gum, and high-energy components like canned meats, usually veal and ham, full of animal fat, enormous amounts of salt, and some protein. K-rations were intended to prevent starvation, not to be eaten on a regular basis, but by 1944, the government had produced 105 million of these boxed meals.

The K-rations included something of a different nature, though equally harmful over time. The meals were finished off with the typical soldier ritual of cigarettes, with four in each and every K-ration package, twelve a day, more than half of a standard pack of twenty.

Millions of U.S. soldiers, including men and women,[1] lived for weeks on K-rations with cigarettes and developed habits that would continue to plague them. Coming home from the war in 1946, my

---

[1] Over sixteen million Americans served in the United States military during World War II, including 350,000 women. When not eating K-rations on the front lines, many of the women who joined the Women's Army Corp (WAC) ate the same diet as the men and gained excess weight from foods like pastry, lard, syrup, mayonnaise, potatoes, and pork.

dad was a full-time cigarette smoker and a dedicated carnivore. As many of the fifties' housewives did, my mom began catering to my father's new tastes, and our meals were loaded with fat and salt. By 1955, my father was fifty pounds overweight, smoking heavily, and working long hours in his dental practice. Then an event woke him up: his father died at age fifty-nine from a stroke.

There and then, my father had an epiphany; he needed to take better care of himself. He stopped smoking immediately (never to return to the habit), pared down his diet to powdered decaffeinated coffee, ate only "rye crisps" for breakfast, cans of tuna fish, and a late-night dinner of a lean steak, a baked potato without butter, and a salad with Russian dressing. He would only indulge in a more sumptuous meal if he and my mother went to a restaurant on a Saturday night with friends. I never saw him drink alcohol.

Though he still didn't exercise (I don't think he owned a pair of sneakers), the weight came off, and his blood sugar and blood pressure were normal for many years. For over fifty years, my father maintained his weight and watched his diet meticulously, passing away at age ninety-one from kidney problems and a heart valve problem—not atherosclerosis. My mother was not nearly as careful with her diet as my father. She died of complications of atherosclerosis, diabetes, and kidney disease at age seventy-four.

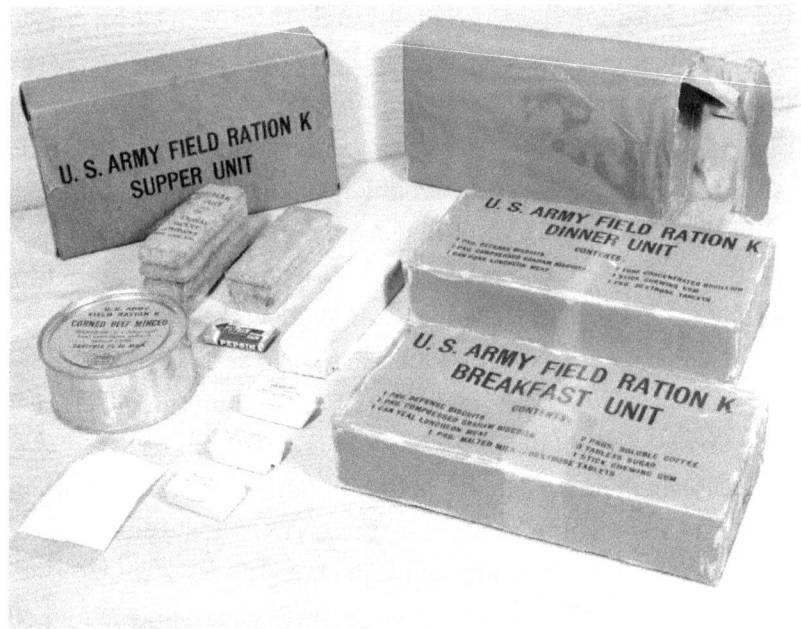

Figure 1. Typical K-rations eaten regularly by the US military during World War II. (copyright Shutterstock)

THE EPIDEMIC BLOOMS

Not many people were as disciplined as my father. By 1930, even before WWII, death from heart and coronary artery disease had already become a common form of death for men and women in the United States; in 1900, it ranked as the fourth leading cause behind infectious diseases. But the greatest increase came in the decade after the end of World War II in 1945, when the United States mortality began sharply rising from approximately 250/100,000 people per year (just over 300,000 for a population of 123 million) in 1930 to over 300/100,000 (456,000 for a population of 152 million) in 1950.

Many of the victims from "The Greatest Generation," male and female, learned the seductive allures of a high animal fat diet, fried foods, lots of carbohydrates and salt, and the pleasure of cigarette smoking during their military service, and American companies responded to fill the burgeoning desire. Burger King opened in 1954, with the arrival of McDonald's just a year later. The tobacco industry followed suit with major marketing efforts after World War II, like the "Marlboro Man," introduced in 1954 and Virginia Slims' "You've come a long way, baby" in 1968. Even as early as the 1950s, companies like Philip Morris helped bring the number of cigarettes manufactured in the US each year to 350-450 billion and the per-capita consumption to roughly 3,500 to 4,500 cigarettes a year.

The results were devastating to the human heart. The nasty molecules in cigarettes didn't just damage the lungs; they injured the blood vessels throughout the body and increased the development of atherosclerosis. Hypertension and high blood pressure, often caused by genetics but exacerbated by salt intake, was detected more commonly, and this disease damaged blood vessels and made them more likely to develop atherosclerosis. A new type of diabetes mellitus, "Type II," caused by obesity, rose in incidence and together with hypertension and smoking created the *milieu* for atherosclerosis of the heart's arteries, followed by a devastating foe. The Widowmaker, the heart attack or myocardial infarction, began to strike down thousands of men and women in the prime of their lives. Among those who did survive the first strike, many were left with severe damage to their heart muscle, leading to a slow death from congestive heart failure or sudden death from a lethal electrical heart disturbance.

And it would seem that no one was immune, as the epidemic played havoc with not only the lives of the everyday citizen, but the most famous as well. In 1961, at age fifty-nine, Clark Gable, the greatest male movie star of his time, died of a heart attack complication. Three US Presidents since the 1940s have died from cardiovascular disease: Franklin Roosevelt at age sixty-four from stroke, high blood pressure, and heart failure in 1945; Dwight Eisenhower at age seventy-nine from multiple heart attacks and heart failure in 1969; and Lyndon Johnson suddenly at age sixty-five after four heart attacks in 1973. All three were heavy cigarette smokers. Their habits were not exceptional. They were consistent with the culture. Women were not immune. Mother Teresa (1910-1997), the Nobel Peace Prize–winning missionary of Calcutta, India, had her first heart attack at age seventy-three, a second six years later, and died of heart failure as a result of atherosclerosis and damage to her heart muscle.

The epidemic of the heart attack was in full bloom, growing in incidence in not just the United States but all of the countries of Europe, Russia, India, and the Far East[2]. The children of the World War II veterans, the "Baby Boomers" born after 1945, also became victims of atherosclerosis. Fortunately, for many of them, the doctors working on the revolutionary science and treatment of heart attacks in the later part of the twentieth century would make life-saving discoveries. Because of their hard work, many would be spared from the Widowmaker.

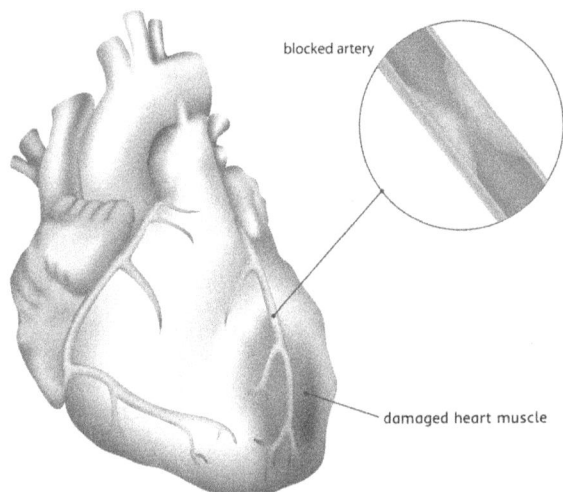

Figure 2. MYOCARDIAL INFARCTION—The coronary arteries and image of atherosclerosis leading to blockage of blood flow and heart muscle damage. (Copyright Shutterstock)

---

[2] In China, the problem would take until the 1980s for the epidemic to surface.

BORN AT THE RIGHT TIME: SAVING BILL CLINTON

To many, his charisma was irresistible: tall, brilliant, striking, with a Southern accent that just oozed charm. William Jefferson Clinton, born in 1946, was in his early thirties when he was elected governor of Arkansas and became a two-term president of the United States. He loved being president. But like so many of his generation, atherosclerosis disease was lurking inside President Clinton's heart arteries, and he was not aware of it. While he did jog several times a week, he was overweight and had a famous fondness for "fast food."

Bill Clinton was only fifty-four when he became a private citizen again, traveling and lecturing extensively, but also trying to take better care of himself. After all, there was a history of heart disease in his mother's family, and his blood tests in 2001 revealed a mild elevation of his "bad" blood cholesterol—the low-density lipoprotein or "LDL." He began exercising two to three times a week with a trainer and lost thirty pounds on the "South Beach Diet." Based on his "risk factor" profile at the time, the medical history that predisposes to early coronary atherosclerosis, Clinton was not a "high risk" patient.

But in the summer of 2004, working on John Kerry's presidential campaign and maintaining a hectic schedule, Clinton began noticing shortness of breath with physical exertion and periodic chest pressure. He thought that he was having indigestion, however as all cardiologists know, that assumption can be fatal. In spite of his efforts to improve his health habits, what the President didn't know was that his atherosclerosis had been developing since he was in his twenties and the progress, although slow, was persistent. When the symptoms just wouldn't go away, the President told his family and, since he was living in Chappaqua, New York, took himself to the local hospital, Northern WestChester Hospital. I suspect his emergency room waiting time was very short.

The doctors at Northern WestChester quickly determined that the symptoms were angina pectoris, the shortness of breath and chest pain due to atherosclerosis of the coronary arteries. Clinton had symptoms that are often the prelude to a heart attack. Angina was first described accurately by an Englishman at the time of the American Revolution in the eighteenth century.

Fortunately, blood tests and the electrocardiogram revealed that Mr. Clinton had not already had a myocardial infarction, but a procedure needed to happen. Since there was time to act to prevent the final work of the Widowmaker, the doctors recommended that a cardiologist perform a catheterization to closely examine his heart arteries. The catheterization findings were alarming. The human heart has three coronary arteries, and in President Clinton's case, all three of them had over ninety percent blockage from cholesterol buildup over many years. The next step was clear: he required coronary artery bypass surgery.

At Columbia in New York City, Craig R. Smith MD, the chairman of Cardiothoracic Surgery, saw a grateful Clinton. Dr. Smith agreed the bypass surgery was indicated, and while awaiting surgery in the hospital, the former President called the *Larry King Live* broadcast on CNN. He said, "I've got a chance to deal with this," and noted, "Let me just say this, Republicans aren't the only people who want four more years here." With great insight, he also said, "I feel really blessed, you know, because a lot of people who have a heart attack never get any advance warning." Any cardiologist can vouch for that statement.

On September 7, 2004, Mr. Clinton had his surgery, and Dr. Smith and his team used two arteries from the underside of his chest wall, the sternum, to bypass two of the blockages, and a piece of a vein from his leg to bypass the third blockage. Blood would now flow from his aorta, the largest blood vessel in the body, into his coronary arteries beyond the point of the cholesterol blockages. Bill Clinton left Columbia only a few days later. Allan Schwartz MD, the Chairman of Cardiology at the hospital, said that Mr. Clinton would, in two to three months, be able to again live an "extraordinarily active lifestyle."

But like with so many other men and women, the Widowmaker was not done with Clinton. The former President did resume his vigorous life, but in 2010, he began to have chest pain again. Another catheterization revealed that one of the bypass grafts was blocked. But with angioplasty, first introduced in the 1970s, his cardiologist dilated (increased the size of) his right coronary artery that the blocked bypass was sewn in to, with a balloon imbedded in a catheter, and then placed two metal stents in the artery to improve the blood flow to that specific area of his heart.

This second wake-up call brought further impactful changes. Bill Clinton has taken responsibility for his lifestyle and diet; he is a vegetarian and walks long distances several times a week, maintaining his weight loss over the years. In 2008, he appeared on *The Late Show with David Letterman*, and significantly, both Clinton and Letterman have had life-saving coronary artery bypass surgery. Like millions of others, they had been the beneficiaries of the advances in treatment of atherosclerosis of the heart's arteries. How did this happen? Magic? Good luck? Imagination? Or was it something else?

Before the latter half of the twentieth century, there was no treatment for a heart attack, but this quest to understand and then treat an illness did not happen just because of the intuition of some doctors who thought this drug or therapy would work. The magic came from science, driven by the philosophical concept of empiricism. The "scientific method" largely deserves the credit for being able to effectively pursue the Widowmaker. The logic behind an experiment starts with an idea, really a conjecture, based on observations, the work of others, and intuition. A good scientist is a *skeptic*; he or she is always concerned that the prediction will not be confirmed by the observations. Francis Bacon (1561-1626), the famous English philosopher, described The Scientific Method in this way: "If a man begins with certainties, he shall end in doubts; but if he will be content to begin with doubts, he shall end in certainties."

How did science save Bill Clinton and countless other men and women? Through decades of work by those dedicated to understanding the causes and potential treatments of the heart attack. Fortunately for him and so many others, for over a century, there are those who have dedicated their lives to chasing this pernicious killer. What follows is the story of those brave souls and the amazing discoveries they made.

CHAPTER 2

THE EARLY OBSERVERS: HOW LONG HAS THIS BEEN GOING ON?

Though I am as old as the hills, my name was given to me by a
young researcher, trying to make sense of the havoc I wreak.
But it is a misnomer, for I as often make widowers of men.

Silencing such exquisite beauty has never been my intention,
but ever so slowly the groundwork is laid, the orders given,
and I respond, like a soldier.
Still, in those fleeting microseconds between
the million calls to action there is a past that haunts me.

RECOGNIZING THE WIDOWMAKER

While disease of the heart and chest pain were reported millennia ago, little progress was made for many centuries. There were accounts of sudden death in ancient Egypt from cessation of the pulse, but there was no further insight in the thousands of years during which infant deaths, infections, trauma, and war caused most deaths. Reports of people with chronic intermittent chest pain, often leading to death, were sometimes documented but not explained, let alone treated.

The Roman philosopher and medical writer Lucius Annaeus Seneca (a. 65 CE) described his own chest pain in this way: "To have any other malady is to be sick; to have this is to be dying."

Even by the early Renaissance, it was still unclear what made the heart function and beat properly. The first astounding breakthrough was the discovery of William Harvey MD (1578-1657), the English anatomist, that the left side of the heart was a pump that pushes blood out to the arteries and the tissues of the body, and then the veins return blood to the right side of the heart, and a second propulsion of blood from that chamber pushes blood into the lungs to acquire oxygen. Harvey proved that there was a "circulation" of blood. But what gave the heart its own energy supply, its unique source of blood and oxygen? Finally, by the eighteenth century, anatomists recognized that the two very small tubes embedded on the surface of the heart muscle, the coronary arteries, carried the blood that drove the heart pump and that occluding them in animals resulted in rapid death.

In 1768, a general practitioner in England, William Heberden[3] MD (1710-1801), introduced new observations about chest pain. Heberden's detailed description of a particular type of chest pain caught the attention of his colleagues, a disorder that he named Angina Pectoris, angina derived from the Latin verb *angere*, "to choke or throttle," and the Latin *pectus* meaning "chest." His lecture at the Royal College of Physicians in London entitled "Some Account of the Disorder of the Breast" described his observations of this problem in twenty patients and remarkably included most of the typical aspects of angina pectoris that have stood the test of time. At the end of his talk, he commented, "What the particular mischief is, is not easy to guess and I have had no opportunity of knowing with certainty." Heberden didn't understand the problem, but he knew its characteristics.

Heberden went on to compile a book entitled *Commentaries*

---

[3] Heberden is best known for describing the swollen joints of patients with osteoarthritis, abnormalities known as "Heberden's nodes."

on the History and Cure of Disease of his long observations as a physician, including one in Chapter 70 of "Pectoris Delor," Latin for "chest pain," just another name for angina pectoris. This description is worth recounting for its detail and importance to understanding the nature of this disease. In an era where the history from the patient was paramount, Heberden was a master of eliciting and documenting such narratives. His conclusions were drawn from the observations of one hundred patients with Pectoris Delor—one woman, one twelve-year-old boy, and ninety-eight men, all over the age of fifty. The paucity of women may reflect a very low incidence of angina in women at the time but more likely that women were believed just not to suffer from the disorder, a bias that lasted for over two centuries.

Heberden wrote, "Here is a disorder of the breast marked with strong and peculiar symptoms, considerable for the kind of danger belonging to it, and not extremely rare, which deserves to be mentioned more at length . . . They who are afflicted with it are seized while they are walking, (more especially if it be up hill, and soon after eating) with a painful and most disagreeable sensation in the breast, which seems as if it would extinguish life, if it were to increase or to continue; but the moment they stand still, all this uneasiness vanishes."

Heberden called this particular description " . . . the most usual appearance of this disease." But there were variations. Sometimes the pain was not situated on the left side but the right, sometimes it occurred while awakening from sleep, and sometimes the pain went down the arm, associated with numbness and swelling. Rarely the pain lasted for hours or days. The astute doctor also noted what happened as the "natural history" of the disease progressed. "The termination of the angina pectoris is remarkable. For if no accident intervene, but the disease go on to its height, the patients all suddenly fall down, and perish almost immediately." Heberden had witnessed Sudden Cardiac Death.

While Heberden's observations captured the essence of angina pectoris and the heart attack, at least in men, there was little he could do to ameliorate the disease. Likely with remorse, he wrote, "With respect to the treatment of this complaint, I have little or nothing to advance."

A contemporary of Heberden, Edward Jenner MD (1749-1823), the developer of the smallpox vaccine and another Englishman, was making interesting observations of his own. In 1776, Jenner wrote a letter to Heberden and described the hearts of two patients he had autopsied who had died from angina pectoris. In the coronary arteries of both people, Jenner identified "a kind of fleshy tube formed within the vessels with a considerable quantity of ossific material dispersed irregularly through it." Decades later, Jenner's findings would be recognized as those of atherosclerosis, a combination of cholesterol plaque, white blood cells, blood clots, and eventually calcification of the arteries. Jenner's observations provided a suitable explanation for angina: the heart was malfunctioning because there was not enough blood getting to the heart muscle. This was a start to understanding the "mischief" that perplexed Heberden.

A RISKY BUSINESS

Over the next several decades, more physicians recognized Heberden's "disorder of the breast" in their own practices, and one of these was to fall victim to this malady.

The greatest surgeon of the time in England was Mr.[4] John Hunter[5] (1728-1793). Hunter was a multi-talented surgeon, scientist, a naturalist and anatomist, and referred to as "the Father of modern surgery." He

---

4 Surgeons are still proudly referred to as "Mr." in Great Britain, a vestige of the origin of their profession in barbershops, where primitive surgery was performed by men without general medical training.
5 Hunter was not only a famous surgeon (eventually the surgeon of King George III of Great Britain) but an obsessive collector who built a museum of hundreds of plant and animal specimens on the grounds of his home, including the body of a giant man with a tumor of the pituitary gland of his brain that made him grow to seven feet seven inches tall.

was hard-working and driven to a pathologic extreme and was aware that his behavior and terrible temper resulted in his sometimes having little self control. Nonetheless, his obsessive behavior allowed him to go further than others of his day. Fascinated by "inflammation," the response of body tissues to injury or infection, specifically pain, swelling, redness, and warmth, Hunter was also a very adventurous surgeon and the first to repair aneurysms, diseased outpouchings of traumatized arteries in the leg. His exploits with blood vessels would serve as a key clue to the conclusions of an American physician 150 years later trying to understand the nature of the Widowmaker's work.

Ironically, Hunter was struck by the very disease for which he would later contribute so much understanding. By 1775, when he was forty-seven years old, Hunter began to have angina pectoris. Just as Heberden noted, the symptoms came and went, without any apparent long-term damage, and Hunter continued his hyperactive life and work. But by 1789, Hunter's condition had worsened. His personal medical doctor, John Conkley Lettsom MD, reported, "He can scarcely go up stairs so much is he affected by dyspnea (*shortness of breath*) on the least motion." On October 16, 1793, Hunter was attending a board meeting at St. George's Hospital in London, and after having another one of his arguments with a member of the hospital board, Hunter "immediately ceased speaking and left the room." Trying to calm the "tumult of his passion," Hunter walked into an adjoining room, where "with a deep groan he fell lifeless into the arms of a colleague." John Hunter was dead at age sixty-six. Hunter's brother-in-law, Sir Edward Home, performed an autopsy on the famous man and found thickened and ossified arteries throughout Hunter's body and in particular the arteries of his heart, just as Edward Jenner had found in his two patients. John Hunter suffered from atherosclerosis and was ultimately another victim of the Widowmaker.

In addition to Hunter's work, however, the story of his temperament would add to our understanding of the causes of heart attacks. According to an 1839 article in the English medical journal *The Lancet*, Thomas

Pettigrew reported that Hunter was "remarkable for his irascibility through life and it probably served to shorten the duration of his existence." The man had "no command over his temper." Since that time, scientists have developed an understanding that these reactions are due to the brain and the adrenal glands, those two tiny organs in the abdomen just above the kidneys, pouring out powerful molecules into the circulation. These organic chemicals include adrenaline, a powerful constrictor of blood vessels and a stimulant of the heart rate, and cortisol, the major steroid of the body. For the practicing cardiologist, there is little doubt that the "mind-heart" interaction is a profound one in many patients. Mental stress influences the frequency and severity of chest pain in a patient with known coronary artery disease. Who among us has not felt the surge of adrenaline and the racing of our heart under stress?

The story of John Hunter and his angina pectoris was a slow awakening into the idea of the "risk factors" for atherosclerosis. Did the mind and one's personality influence the development and outcome of this increasingly recognized disease? They surely seemed to have a great effect on the life of Mr. Hunter. Future research into one's mental outlook and stress levels, with their effects on the hormones and clotting system of the body, would uncover such potentially important relationships.[6] In her publication "John Hunter's Heart" in 2013, Fay Bound Alberti summarized well the impact of this famous man's life and death on the future ideas about

---

[6] It was not until the mid-portion of the twentieth century that the possibility that one's mind could influence atherosclerosis of the coronary arteries would reach the world of clinical research. Two cardiologists, Meyer Friedman MD (1910-2001) and his partner Raymond Rosenman MD (1920-2013) had a problem with the furniture in their office waiting room. The front edge of the seats and the armrests were being worn down by some of their patients with angina pectoris and coronary artery disease. These patients, almost all men, were always inpatient and frequently jumped up from their seats to ask how much longer they would need to wait to see the doctor. Friedman and Rosenman's work led to the concept of the "Type A" personality; driven, impatient, easily angered, hostile, and ultra-competitive people, usually but not exclusively men. Their research in the 1970s identified the Type A personality as a risk factor for coronary artery disease, although their conclusions have been challenged in more recent decades.

atherosclerosis and heart disease: "Hunter possessed the passionate temperament, commitment to overwork, lack of self-control, and psychological tendencies that made him an archetype and touchstone for work on angina pectoris for the following century."

In the early nineteenth century, the problem of heart attacks became more common. More and more people were living longer, and many reached the age of over fifty, as did all but one of the cases Heberden described in the late eighteenth century. The "prime time" for angina was now a dangerous decade for many. There was also no understanding of how the problem could cause such severe symptoms randomly. Patients would report chest pain while shaving in the morning but be able to walk several miles later in the day.

The progression of the disease seemed inevitable. When there is little one can do to treat a condition, at least a doctor could try to understand what happens to the unfortunate victims, recording their stories and publishing them for the world to see. In the pursuit of the Widowmaker, some exceptional observers found effective and sometimes unusual ways to document what they found.

A NEW WAVE OF CHRONICLERS

In 1888, Chicago was an emerging hub of American entrepreneurship as well as a site for the increasing phenomenon of heart disease. The stockyards were bursting with cattle, ready to be shipped by rail all over the United States, and businesses brought thousands of new people to the city. With this urban civilization came a greater number of people living longer and developing the Widowmaker's malady. James Bryan Herrick[7] MD (1861-1954) was there to try to treat them.

---

7   Herrick was from Illinois and a graduate of the University of Michigan. He taught school for several years before enrolling in the Rush School of Medicine in Chicago, graduating in 1888 and entering practice in Chicago. In addition to his office and hospital work, Herrick was a teacher of medical residents at Presbyterian Hospital in Chicago, where he and one of his residents were the first to identify a young man from the Caribbean with a peculiar blood disorder that became known as Sickle Cell Anemia.

What was known about Heberden's "mischief" of the heart was that it was lethal, and while Herrick agreed that this was usually true, he was the first one to say not always. He described four distinct forms of the same basic disease, angina. First, Herrick recognized that angina could cause sudden death—"instantaneous, perhaps painless, death." Secondly, a patient could suffer a severe attack of angina, followed minutes later by first shock (*low blood pressure*) and then death. But the last two varieties of angina were different. In the third case, angina could cause death but not immediately. Finally, there were patients with mild angina who could survive for years. "Heart attacks," acute myocardial infarctions, might not always be fatal. This was a revolutionary observation.

How could a patient survive the complete shutoff of blood supply from one of the two large coronary arteries? Surely this catastrophic event would cause such extensive heart muscle damage that escaping death was impossible. According to Herrick, the answer came from of the work of the pathologists of the late nineteenth century.

The heart and its arteries were of intense interest at the time. The basic pattern of the structure of blood vessels was known for years. Both the arteries and the veins start out as large visible tubes and then become smaller and smaller, as branches spread out from the main highway of blood to become "arterioles" and "venules," and then eventually "capillaries," the smallest of the blood vessels that actually unload the oxygen to the cells. The blood supply of the heart was crucial, to be sure, and something was obstructing blood flow in many patients. Were the coronary arteries simply fixed tubes that began and ended, like a highway closed from road construction at one end? Did they branch into smaller tubes and spread their life-giving blood throughout the muscle?

Theories abounded, and some were given more credibility than others. One of the great German pathologists of the nineteenth century, Julius Friedrich Cohnheim MD (1839-1884), was convinced that the heart's arteries were "end-arteries," that is, they began as large arteries, then became smaller and smaller until they formed capillaries, but that was the end of the line for the blood flow. Because Cohnheim worked in the laboratory of the renowned Rudolf Virchow MD (1821-1902) in Berlin, he had great credibility in the medical world. When he said that the coronary arteries were "end-arteries," most doctors simply accepted this belief. This helped explain why a sudden occlusion of one of the heart's main two arteries would cause an abrupt end to a life. Blood flow to the muscle simply ceased, without any other options. But Herrick thought otherwise. There had to be a reason that not every patient with a severe coronary artery blockage died quickly. Millennia of human evolution must have developed a way to deal with a shutoff of blood supply through an artery.

Herrick took the spark of his ideas from the surgical exploits of John Hunter many years prior. Planning on operating on aneurysms of arteries in the back of the knee, Hunter had believed that the arteries of the body could create new pathways for blood if the main thoroughfare became diseased or was surgically removed. Hunter's patients were English coach drivers. The drivers developed these aneurysms because of the chronic trauma to their legs as they drove the wealthy around the streets of London, wearing heavy leather boots that went above the knees. The aneurysms caused permanent disability and often burst, leading to sudden death from bleeding. If Hunter had been around in the twentieth century, he could have used a metaphor of modern life to explain his idea. All of us have been caught in a traffic jam due to an accident or roadwork, and we know what happens—cars flood onto the side roads to get around the holdup. Many city dwellers pride themselves in knowing how to negotiate this common affliction of modern life.

Hunter felt that the leg's arteries must have emergency highways, tubes of arteries that were normally very small, but when a blockage occurred in a big artery, the pressure behind the blockage would stretch the smaller ones open. Blood would then divert into the smaller arteries and pass around the detour. These newly opened arteries could be lifesaving. Hunter called his theoretical new arteries "collaterals," a Latin word meaning "side by side." Hunter knew that he could isolate and remove the aneurysm from a patient in about five minutes. Then the collaterals would open up and supply enough blood to allow the lower leg to live. When he contemplated doing his first patient, most of his colleagues thought this was only his enormous ego bragging. But the surgery was a success, and the patient was even able to go back to work.

Over a century later, in 1912, Herrick spoke to a group of his colleagues in Chicago and reviewed the previous work and knowledge of the effects of coronary artery disease. He acknowledged that a complete obstruction of a large coronary artery was "almost always suddenly fatal." In an understatement, he said, "It must be admitted, also, that the reputation of the descending branch of the left coronary as the artery of sudden death is not undeserved." This was the first description of the classic work of the Widowmaker.

Herrick pointed out that the effects of blocked coronary arteries were very variable when the pathologists were able to get their hands on the heart. An obstruction could result in sudden massive necrosis, death of tissue that was obvious on sight, but it could also result in scar formation, a process that took months or even years to occur. Sometimes the heart muscle formed not just a scar, but also an aneurysm of the wall of the left ventricle, similar to the leg aneurysm that Hunter repaired in the 1770s. Herrick noted that the pathologic findings were "patchy," with a significant variability even when the obstruction of the main artery was identical from case to case.

However, Herrick's talk was not the great success he had anticipated, and it would be a while before his contributions were recognized as valuable.[8] By 1919, Herrick had collected many more cases to bolster

---

8   John Hunter would have admired Herrick's observations. Herrick suspected that "the hope for the damaged myocardium lies in the direction of securing a supply of blood through friendly neighboring vessels so as to restore so far as possible its functional integrity." The collaterals were crucial to surviving a heart attack, and modern research would prove that Herrick was correct.

his beliefs and his publication in *The Journal of the American Medical Association* in that year finally achieved the recognition he thought his work deserved. James Herrick's insights served as a "stepping stone" to understanding the nature of a heart attack. His work gave hope that coronary artery atherosclerosis was not a death sentence in all people and that perhaps in the future new treatments would allow patients to live longer lives and even prevent heart attacks altogether.

But there was another finding that still continued to confuse the doctors of the time, including Herrick. This was the significance of the pathologists sometimes finding a "coronary thrombosis," a blood clot, inside of the coronary arteries of people who had died from a heart attack. There was atherosclerosis, to be sure, but why had a blood clot formed? Was it important or was it just a bystander of the more chronic process of atherosclerosis? More importantly, what did cause atherosclerosis anyway? What was that gritty sometimes calcified debris inside of the arteries made up of? Accepting that people can live with the problem for years, why then do so many have acute heart attacks and die quickly, or just die almost instantaneously, like John Hunter did?

By the 1920s, the four diseases of atherosclerosis of the heart arteries were pretty clear though largely untreatable: angina pectoris, myocardial infarctions or heart attacks, sudden death in those with angina and history of heart attack, and most alarming those who died suddenly with no history at all of heart disease (the problem only found at an autopsy). In an era where diagnostic tools were limited, the patient's description of the pain was usually the best path to a diagnosis, and for some time, this would be the focus.

A KEY SIGN

Samuel Levine MD (1891-1966), a cardiologist from Harvard, also saw patients with coronary artery atherosclerosis, and he noted unique physical movements by his patients with angina. When asked to describe and point to the area of pain of angina, patients held a clenched fist over the middle of the chest to emphasize the sense of "squeezing" caused by the disease. Levine wrote about the clenched fist as a sign of angina, still called "Levine's Sign."[9]

As one of the great cardiologists of the first half of the last century, Levine made other contributions as well. In his textbook *Clinical Heart Disease* published in 1936, he was one of the first to use the term "coronary thrombosis" to describe a heart attack. Levine went on to train generations of medical students, residents, and cardiology fellows at Harvard, many of whom went on to great careers as clinicians and researchers.

Another early observer was also a major contributor to the field of medical education. It is crucial to instruct medical students in the practice of history taking and to learn how to sort out which patient's chest pain might be due to heart disease. For those visual learners, illustrations are key. Fortunately for many medical students, including me, a great artist would provide just what was needed.

THE MICHELANGELO OF MEDICINE:
DR. NETTER AND HIS DRAWINGS

The drawings in the large green bound volumes were seductive and seemed surreal. All medical students of my era were familiar with the work of Frank Netter[10] MD (1906-1991). The Netter drawings

---

9   In a study done in the 1990s of 138 patients who had a diagnosis of coronary artery disease established after admission to a coronary care unit, eighty percent used one of the typical hand movements to describe their chest pain. Levine's Sign has stuck in the minds of all good clinicians to this day.

10   Frank Netter was an unusual combination of skills and training. Passionate about art and drawing at a young age, Netter earned a medical degree and became a surgery intern at Bellevue Hospital in New York City. Though he never practiced medicine himself, in 1936, he produced an advertising piece about the use of digitalis for heart disease for a Swiss manufacturer, CIBA. The drawings became a hit with the physicians who were the advertising targets. His medical experience then allowed him to produce brilliant drawings of the human anatomy and his *CIBA Collection of Medical Illustrations* is an, eight-volume work. In his honor, the medical school of Quinnipiac University in Connecticut is named the Frank H. Netter School of Medicine.

were never part of the "official" curriculum in medical school, but if you wanted to get an idealized picture of the circulation or the lungs, looking through a Netter volume was always spectacular. As I turned the pages in the Netter volume on the heart and the circulation, I saw exquisite depictions of patients with heart failure, short of breath, with swollen legs from edema due to their bad hearts. But there was a drawing of a middle-aged man clutching his chest that stood out for me then and over the next forty-five years.

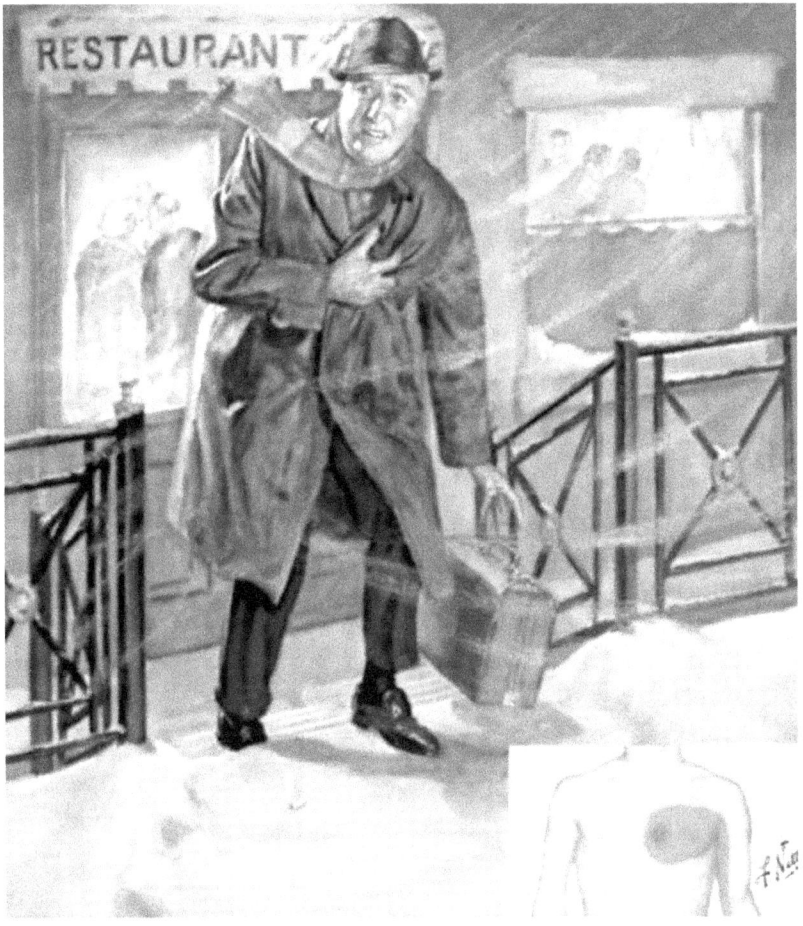

Figure 3. Typical symptoms of angina pectoris in a man. Frank Netter drawing. (Copyright Netterimages.com)

In this one drawing, Dr. Netter managed to capture some of the risk factors and provocateurs of angina, as well as the most common humans thought to suffer from this malady: middle-aged men.[11] Netter's angina was associated with being overweight, the symptoms often occurring after eating a big meal. In addition, the symptom frequently comes on with exertion and is more likely to occur in winter weather, when the blood vessels' walls constrict in response to the cold. The pain is most often felt in the left chest, with "radiation" into the left arm.

Knowledge of the symptom of angina has changed over the years, and we now recognize that the chest pain can occur at rest as well as with exertion. But to a medical student in the 1970s, Netter's drawing was memorable, serving as a key starting point to make a diagnosis of angina due to coronary artery disease. I still see that man on the restaurant steps in my mind when I interview people with chest pain. Netter captured so many of Heberden's observations in one drawing almost two centuries later, that if I were asked to teach a medical student about coronary artery disease, angina, and the heart attack, I could not do better than to have them read Heberden's description and look at Netter's drawing.

The collective work of these early observers documented in oral lectures, texts, and illustrations signaled the dawning of a new era, one in which scientists and doctors would begin to move from diagnosis alone to treatment of the symptoms and causes of heart attacks. One of the first of these new and exciting tools researchers discovered to track down the illusive Widowmaker would come from a startling source.

---

11 History would prove that belief false—women were also suffering from this malady, just usually at an older age than the men.

CHAPTER 3

THE EXPLOSION OF CHEMISTRY: AMYL NITRITE AND NITROGLYCERIN

You think I have disdain, but I have nothing but envy.
The perfection of muscles pumping in unison, blood flowing
seamlessly from one chamber to the next.
Yet that is only part of the picture. The unseen has its role,
too, the chemistry of motion.

It is in this hidden arena that the scientists find something that will give me pause. A way to stop the haywire, just long enough ...

A POWERFUL LITTLE PILL—SPRING 1976

He was such a dignified man, tall and thin, always dressed in a suit and tie outside of the operating room, in the later years of his surgical career, but still performing surgeries and involved with running the Department of Surgery at the Hospital of the University of Pennsylvania. I was honored to be assisting him that morning in completing a straightforward surgery, a repair of a hernia in a man's groin.

Jonathan E. Rhoads MD (1907-2002) was a legend at Penn. An internationally renowned surgeon and scholar, he was the chairman of the department for many years and helped train generations of residents who went on to outstanding careers in surgery. But by the spring of 1976, he had slowed down his operating schedule. He was no longer the boss but still a steady presence in the hospital.

Dr. Rhoads watched me closely but was silent. I had accrued enough experience after ten months to know what to do next, and the procedure was going well, very routine. After concentrating on my suturing for a few minutes, I glanced up to look at Dr. Rhoads, hoping for an acknowledgment that my work was satisfactory. His skin was pale to begin with, but now he was ashen, even if only the upper half of his face was visible above the surgical mask. I didn't know what to think, but I was immediately worried, and my heart rate picked up. The man just didn't look right.

For a brief moment, our eyes crossed, and he quickly glanced down. "Arnold, you can finish up now. I'll be outside if you need me." He left the room. I looked at the anesthesiologist, who was also stunned. Regaining my focus, I was able to close all of the tissue layers and the skin and finish the surgery.

Leaving the operating room, I saw Dr. Rhoads sitting on a stool. Some color was back in his face, and he asked me if I had any problems finishing the case. I hadn't and went to write the post-op orders for the patient.

My day was so busy that I forgot about Dr. Rhoads, what was wrong with him, and how he had recovered so quickly. But I would soon come to find out...

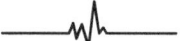

SHATTERING A PRISON OF BELIEF: ORGANIC CHEMISTRY AND SCIENTIFIC DRUGS

As frustrating as it was for the doctors of the nineteenth century to identify the cause of the disease of patients with angina and heart attacks, even more demoralizing was the lack of any medication to even temporarily relieve the frightening chest pain. Any drugs that might help people came from chance observations about the possible benefit of a "natural" compound on a disease process. There seemed to be no other way to discover new medications.

The long-standing "roadblock" to the development of new drugs that needed to be overturned was the idea of "Vitalism." This was a simple idea that espoused that all "vital" compounds derived their power from a mysterious "vital force of nature," hence the term Vitalism. For centuries, Vitalism held sway, but in 1823, a German chemist, Freidrich Wöhler MD (1800-1882), mixed together two "inorganic" compounds from jars and produced urea, a known "vital" molecule excreted into the urine by the kidney. The mystery of Vitalism was over and allowed a new breed of chemists to experiment with the compounds and molecules of life—organic chemists.

A new idea evolved, destroying a centuries-old one, and organic chemistry was the new science, one that opened the path to new medications to treat so many human diseases and in particular the disease of the Widowmaker. By the middle of the nineteenth century, a foundation was laid for the first time in history for further research into medications, a bedrock of scientific principles that would guide the decisions that doctors would make about the treatment of patients. New organic compounds could be rigorously tested and their effects documented using more and more tools for measurement.[12] One product in particular would prove quite effective though startling in its origin.

THE MEDICAL EXPLOSIVE: NITROGLYCERIN

Ascanio Sobrero PhD (1812-1888) was one of many medical doctors of his time who saw his future in organic chemistry, not medical practice. He moved from his native Italy to Paris and worked with Theophile-

---

12 Two of these new compounds would revolutionize the treatment of atherosclerosis of the coronary arteries. It would take decades until these brand-new drugs broke through to become standard treatment for angina.

Jules Pelouze PhD (1807-1867), a well-known chemist. Pelouze was exploring the chemistry of glycerol, a common substance found in the triglycerides, a fat component of the cell walls of animals and plants.

When Sobrero experimented with glycerol in 1847, the project took a strange turn. He combined glycerol with nitric acid and sulfuric acid, and something very striking resulted: a brand-new explosive. He named it "pyroglycerin" and was terrified of his own work. His new molecule would explode, sometimes without warning. The least amount of physical stimulation, such as an insect landing on it, might set it off. To make matters worse, tasting the stuff, or even handling it, caused an intense headache. He had firsthand knowledge of the organic chemical's effect. An explosion scarred his own face, and he was so frightened by the substance that he kept his discovery secret for a year.

In spite of his fear of his invention, Sobrero did recognize its industrial potential,[13] as did other chemists of the time. As an easy to produce substance, they considered its potential use as a great explosive for the mining industry. But how to use this material without it exploding accidentally? A young student in Pelouze's lab thought he might have the answer.

Alfred Nobel (1833-1896) was born in Stockholm, Sweden, to a family involved in engineering and technology in Czarist Russia.[14] He became an influential scientist and took great interest in Sobrero's discovery. In the late 1850s, young Alfred ended up in Paris and met Dr. Sobrero and his explosive, quickly realizing this organic compound might be a great product for his family business. Returning to Russia in 1862, Nobel and his family began experimenting with different compounds to try to "stabilize" the pyroglycerin, now renamed "nitroglycerin." Nobel stumbled on an additive that calmed

---

13 Years later, Sobrero expressed some regrets about discovering pyroglycerin. He wrote, "When I think of all of the victims killed during explosions, which in all probability will continue to occur in the future, I am almost ashamed to admit that I am its discoverer."

14 Surprisingly, considering his later accomplishments, Nobel only spent one year in a "school" outside of his home.

down the explosive. Nobel called it "kieselguhr," diatomaceous earth, and when mixed with pyroglycerin, it created a much more stable explosive. Nobel's new invention, dynamite, was patented in 1867 and revolutionized the world of industrial explosives.

But fortunately for the world of medicine and victims of the Widowmaker, dynamite alone was not the end of the story for Sobrero's powerful compound. Its chemical formula, $C_3H_5(ONO_2)_3$ indicates that each molecule contains three carbon atoms, five hydrogens, nine oxygens, and three nitrogens. It is the chemistry of nitroglycerin that makes it so powerful. Some thought this awesome power must have been directly related to the headache it caused. If that was true, what was happening in the human body to cause that nasty effect? As it turns out, when activated, the gas of nitroglycerin takes up more than 1,200 times the volume of the original compound and liberates heat to about nine thousand degrees Fahrenheit. The pressure wave generated is twenty thousand times greater than the pressure of the atmosphere at sea level, a wave moving at more than seventeen thousand miles an hour. No wonder Dr. Sobrero was terrified of his invention. Imagine the power that such a molecule could have on the blood vessels of humans, even in tiny amounts. Perhaps nitroglycerin could do more than just cause a headache. A brave medical doctor thought he would explore the idea.

The adventurer was the German Constantine Hering MD (1800-1880), who was a strong believer in a new and controversial school of medicine and pharmacy: homeopathy. Hering was a devotee of Samuel Hahnemann MD (1755-1843), who was also German, and began his career as a traditional medical doctor before becoming frustrated at the inability to predict the effectiveness of drugs. Ultimately, Hahnemann reached the conclusion that "Nothing remains but for us to experiment on the human body." Instead of waiting to try medications on the ill, Hahnemann settled on the idea that first drugs needed to be tried on healthy people, and Hering was sure that nitroglycerin would be an interesting compound to "prove."[15]

Hering began his experiments with his newly renamed compound "glonoine," an acronym combining glycerol trinitrate (G), glycerol (l), oxygen (O) and nitrogen (N), with oxide (ine) at the end. Since one of the basics of homeopathy was that very small, sometimes infinitesimal doses of medication would be effective, Hering was not concerned that the dilute nitroglycerin he was using would explode. He prepared the drug in the usual manner for homeopathic physicians, as sugar pellets infused with an alcoholic solution of glonoine, placed on the tongue. Almost all of Hering's subjects developed an intense headache immediately after ingestion of even the smallest amount of glonoine. In his initial report of his studies in 1851, Hering noted that in addition to the headache, the medication sped up the heart rate.

Herring moved to the United States and continued his homeopathic studies in Philadelphia but did not work any further with glonoine. But on the other side of the Atlantic, interest in glonoine resurfaced. In the 1850s, Alfred G. Field MD, an English physician, procured some from a homeopath and tried using it on himself and a few animals. Field found the drug very useful in one particular patient, a sixty-eight-year-old woman who was having many episodes of "intense pain in the epigastrium (*the upper abdomen*), extending up to the top of the chest, and then down the inside of the arm." This woman was suffering from angina pectoris and told Field that the spells began suddenly, lasted about thirty minutes, and appeared to have no effect on her after they disappeared. The glonoine, she reported, when used shortly after the episodes began, quickly aborted the pain. Dr. Field had no idea why the glonoine worked, but it was doing a wonderful job for his patient, much better than any other therapy at the time.

As striking as Field's report was, there was no great rush to use glonoine in patients with chest pain. Most physicians at the time felt

---

[15] The process of "proving" was Hahnemann's controversial and ultimately flawed theory that argued that a drug that produced specific effects in the normal "provers" would be effective in treating a disease with symptoms similar to the reaction from the drug. So a medicine that caused a headache in normals should help people with headaches.

that the disease of angina pectoris was rare and saw very few people with problems similar to Field's woman. Still, the findings of doctors like Field, and those of the researchers before him, were instrumental in discovering a treatment that would eventually resurface as a highly useful drug to counteract the symptoms of the Widowmaker.

As the glonoine story went dormant and remained on the back burner for a few more years, another finding from the expanding world of organic chemistry struck the fancy of a few Scottish and English doctors trying to understand the action of potential drugs on the circulation. They were convinced that chemistry was the means to effective results with new medications, and with this belief, a new path to the treatment of angina might be opening.

A BRAND-NEW MEMBER OF THE NITRITE FAMILY

Frederick Guthrie PhD (1833-1886) was a chemist and physicist at the University of Edinburgh in Scotland. Looking for new organic compounds to study, he procured an unstudied chemical named "amyl nitrite" from a French chemistry professor, Antoine Balard (1802-1876). In 1844, Balard mixed an alcohol with nitrous oxide and produced a compound known as an "ester"—a new combination of carbon, oxygen, and nitrogen atoms. He was another organic chemist just trying out different concoctions of atoms and molecules in his laboratory. He named his new molecule "amyl nitrite."

Much like Sobrero, Guthrie was shocked by the effects of Balard's invention. He described the effects of inhaling just a small amount of the amyl nitrite: "One of the most prominent of its properties is the singular effect of its vapor upon the action of the heart." In less than one minute, the arteries of the neck would throb, the heart rate increased, and the face flushed. The effects were similar but even more rapid in onset than those Hering saw with glonoine.

Other medical faculty in Scotland and England began to investigate the effects of amyl nitrite. They were unsure of how the compound worked and had no idea how it might help patients with diseases, but they were going to look into that potential. What they needed was a clinician, a person who knew patients and their problems, to use the data from experiments with amyl nitrite and try the substance in people. Thomas Lauder Brunton MD (1844-1916), a Scotsman, became that person.

Brunton was learning his craft as a doctor when he first encountered patients with angina pectoris and began to explore treatments. It is not possible to determine how many of his patients had chest pain from atherosclerosis. Whatever the cause, Dr. Brunton was dissatisfied that there was no effective recourse for this chronic, often disabling, and ultimately fatal condition. Oddly enough, there was one treatment for chest pain that intrigued Brunton, because sometimes it did work for a time: therapeutic bleeding. When Brunton bled patients with chest pain, many did receive temporary relief of their symptoms.[16]

More significant than the short relief this provided his patients, Brunton could do something that no one was able to do before: he could make measurements of the physiologic effects of the bleeding, that is what was actually happening to the circulation. He had a new tool called the sphygmograph. With this device, Brunton could measure the blood pressure before and after he gave medication, as well as the heart rate. For the first time, a doctor could correlate an effect with objective measurements rather than only documenting what the patient felt. This was a major advance in medicine.

Using his portable sphygmograph, Brunton noted that when the pain of angina occurred, the patient's "pulse becomes smaller and the arterial tension rises." He observed that when the patients were bled, the blood pressure fell, although slowly, and that at times this effect was enough to relieve the chest pain. But Brunton was much

---

[16] Future research would explain why the bleeding did help some of his patients. By decreasing the amount of blood in the body, the pressure on the walls of the heart chambers decreased. Work in the mid-twentieth century showed that the "wall tension," like the pressure inside an expanding toy balloon, is a major driver of the heart muscle's need for oxygen. Less blood volume in the heart from bleeding then could occasionally relieve angina pain.

more interested in the effects of amyl nitrite. When his patients having chest pain inhaled the preparation, the pulse also became slower and "fuller," and the blood pressure returned to a lower level. Based on data, not on speculation, Brunton concluded that angina pectoris was due to "contracted arterioles," the small blood vessels of the arterial side of the circulation. The fact that he was not right about his conclusions doesn't diminish the importance of the intellectual process Brunton pursued. He was one of those laying the groundwork for the future of the new field of pharmacology.

Amyl nitrite worked and was the first drug ever found to relieve angina, the chest pain of atherosclerosis; however, the path forward in understanding was difficult, independent of the clear-cut response of many of the patients with angina. An American, Horatio C. Wood Jr. MD (1841-1920), did extensive work with amyl nitrite and came away from his work more confused about its true effects than when he started. Furthering Wood's frustration was the lack of understanding of what truly caused angina pectoris. In 1876, he summarized the "state of the art" about this form of heart disease: "The truth is we have no positive knowledge of the real nature of the disease alluded to. How futile then to attempt to explain the physiologic effect of a medicine by its effect upon it... Surely this reading the unknown by the unknown resembles the youthful gambols of a kitten in pursuit of its tail, a circle of useless labor."

But the willingness to confront the data at face value, without vested interest, was a crucial path on the road to scientific medicine. Ideas need to be tested, reviewed by peers, discussed, and re-tested. More fundamental work would lie ahead. By the time of his death in 1916, Brunton was well recognized for the major contribution he had made to the treatment of patients through his work with amyl nitrite. One of his obituaries commented, "His famous discovery, therefore, has been called a lucky shot, but such hits are only made by persons who have profoundly studied the conditions."

THE EXPLOSIVE COMES TO MEDICINE

Another Englishman brought to patients with angina the second drug that changed their lives for the better, a medication that has stood the test of time. William Murrell MD (1853-1912) was educated as a medical doctor at University College London. After graduation, he looked to study drugs that had effects on the nervous system and the hearts of experimental animals. He came upon the scattered publications about the use and physiology of the compound invented by Sobrero decades earlier: nitroglycerin.

Early on, Murrell knew he was dealing with something very powerful. In 1879, he recounted his personal encounter with the drug. While seeing a patient, he accidentally used his tongue to moisten the stopper on a bottle of liquid nitroglycerin. Almost immediately, he developed a violent headache and an alarming increase in his heart rate. Murrell wrote that the tachycardia "seemed to shake my whole body. I regretted that I had not taken a more opportune moment of trying my experiments, and was afraid the patient would notice my distress, and think that I was either ill or intoxicated."

Murrell also knew of Brunton's experiments with amyl nitrite and the similar effects of the nitroglycerin on headaches and tachycardia. But the amyl nitrite effect dissipated within a few minutes. Using his own sphygmograph, Murrell was able to see that the blood pressure and heart rate effects of the nitroglycerin lasted up to one hour. But the key questions remained: Would the drug really help patients? Would it relieve or prevent the chest pain altogether, and would a patient of Murrell's respond in the same way that Alfred Field's woman had two decades earlier?

Murrell decided to put these questions to the test. His experimental subject was a sixty-four-year-old male with angina whom he instructed to take doses of one percent nitroglycerin solution dropped into half an ounce of water three times a day. The compliant patient's report the next week was astounding. The man reported three observations after using the nitroglycerin: the spontaneous chest pain episodes were many fewer, the duration of suffering was markedly less, and finally, taking an additional dose after the chest pain began aborted the episode in only a minute or two. Amazingly, Dr. Murrell had confirmed that there was an effective treatment for the increasingly most common form of heart disease, angina pectoris. Two drugs, amyl nitrite and nitroglycerin, had almost identical effects on human circulation: a lowering of blood pressure and an increase in heart rate.

For the first time in the history of the treatment of heart disease, a compelling treatment was directly correlated to the physiology of the effects of a medication.[17] The use of nitroglycerin rapidly expanded in Europe and then into the United States. More and more patients with angina could expect relief from seeing their physician. By the mid-1880s, Parke Davis & Company of Detroit, Michigan, was producing five different forms of nitroglycerin. Today the tablet dissolved under the tongue is still widely used, and an intravenous form was developed many years later to treat the acute pain of a myocardial infarction. Today, a "close relative" of nitroglycerin, called isosorbide dinitrate, is a tablet taken once or twice a day that controls angina in many patients.

By the end of the nineteenth century, there was hope that coronary artery disease could be controlled with medication, drugs that had definite although incompletely explained measurable effects on the circulation that somehow relieved the chest pain. The first attempts at scientific drug development created the new discipline of pharmacology and held the promise of not just better medications but also an understanding of the normal function of the heart and how the heart responds to the injury of a heart attack.[18]

---

17 History would later confirm that the initial explanations of the cause of angina, and the physiology and pharmacology of the drug, were only first estimates of the truth.

18 Almost one hundred years later, three scientists from the United States, Robert Furchgott PhD (1916-2009), Ferid Murad PhD (1936-), and Louis Ignarro PhD (1941-), through years of meticulous work and collaboration, finally proved that nitroglycerin actives a molecule called nitric oxide, which causes rapid dilation of blood vessels throughout the body, and in nitroglyerin's case especially the large veins in addition to the coronary arteries. Furchgott, Murad, and Ignarro won the Nobel Prize for their discovery in 1998.

At the end of his life, Alfred Nobel again made his mark on the world, a long-lasting contribution far different from his invention of dynamite. Understandably unhappy to see the future of his legacy, Nobel rewrote his will in November 1895, indicating he wished that ninety-four percent of his fortune, over thirty-one million Swedish kroner, be set aside to establish the Nobel Prizes. The first Nobel Prizes were awarded in 1901 in Chemistry, Literature, Peace, Physics, and Physiology or Medicine. These honors continue to be the penultimate acknowledgements of achievement in the academic and scientific world.

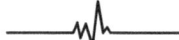

AN EXPLANATION IN THE MIDDLE OF THE NIGHT— SPRING 1976

. . . It was just another night on call for me just a few days later. I was paged to pick up an outside call. It was Dr. Rhoads, wanting to talk to me at two a.m.

"Arnold, I just got off a plane from a meeting I was attending and would like to meet you to make rounds on my patients. I'll be there in about thirty minutes, and I'll page you again when I arrive."

Rounds in the middle of the night? Well, it was Dr. Rhoads. In addition to the twenty-five different things I needed to do before the next day in only a few hours, I now needed to wake up sleeping post-op patients so they could tell their attending surgeon that they were doing fine.

Rounds took about thirty minutes, and I was already racing ahead prioritizing all of the other jobs ahead of me. But Dr. Rhoades asked, "Arnold, would you like to have a cup of coffee with me down in the canteen?"

Wow, I thought—a personal audience with Dr. Rhoads, in the beautiful setting of the vending machine room in the bowels of a one-hundred-year-old hospital, with the chance to imbibe a fresh cup of bitter coffee made by a machine. This was a thrill, but the timing was not one I would have chosen.

Dr. Rhoads did inquire about how the internship was going, where I was from, and what my future plans were. I didn't disclose that I was thinking about changing careers from surgery to cardiology. After about twenty minutes, Dr. Rhoads stood up and half turned away from me, exposing the pocket in his starched white shirt under his suit.

Then I saw it—a small smoky-colored glass bottle of pills. I recognized them immediately from my internal medicine and cardiology training as a medical student. Dr. Rhoads was having angina and taking nitroglycerin. Now it became clear that an attack of angina had forced him out of the operating room a few days earlier. How often Dr. Rhoads needed the drug was unknown to me, but the nitroglycerin was allowing him to go on with his life, relieving the smothering pain and anxiety of coronary artery disease. He lived to age ninety-five.

Little did I know at the time that Alfred Nobel had such a hand in the development of this amazing substance. Nor was I aware that closer to Nobel's lifetime, a Nobel Prize would be given to a Dutch doctor and scientist who created a device that, as we will see, would be the single most powerful advance in the diagnosis of all forms of heart disease.

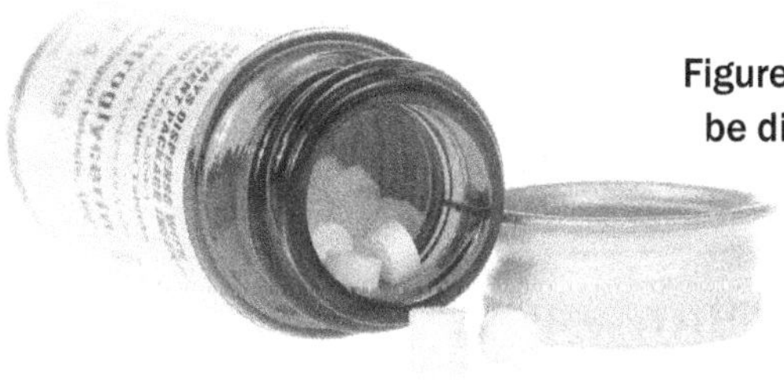

Figure 4. Nitroglycerin tablets to be dissolved under the tongue. First used in 1880. (Copyright Shutterstock)

CHAPTER 4

THE DAYS OF THE DUTCHMAN: ENGINEERING THE ELECTROCARDIOGRAM MACHINE

From outside they cannot catch me, the body providing a barrier to their even knowing what I am up to. Often it is only after I strike a lethal blow that they are able to pry inside and unearth the handiwork I have left behind.

But what if the doctors can find the message the heart is sending? Like the flashing of a lighthouse on the rocks it would signal where the danger lay.
If only they could see it.

TECHNOLOGY TO THE RESCUE—LATE SPRING 1974

Something wasn't right about this man, and you didn't need to be a doctor or a nurse to see it. As I walked into the room to introduce myself, I took a quick look at his face. He was sitting bolt upright and was breathing heavily. Obviously, he was in distress. I asked him his name and why he was in the hospital. He couldn't complete a sentence without stopping to gasp for air. I tried again. Was he having pain? Was he having trouble breathing? All I heard was a grunt.

Seeing this man was just another "pre-op H and P" (medical history and physical examination prior to surgery) for a medical student on the general surgery service. Normally, it would be time to practice your history and physical examination skills, write it up, and then show it to the intern or resident, who would "sign off" on it. The paperwork said "inguinal hernia repair" and "male, age 66." This job should have been quick and easy.

I checked his blood pressure—normal. I felt for a pulse, at each wrist, then the carotid arteries in the neck next. I wasn't sure I could feel the heartbeats consistently. When in doubt, you take the stethoscope and listen to the heart. I listened through the black rubber tubes attached to the stethoscope's diaphragm, the piece of plastic that amplifies the sound and carries it to your ears. I heard a rapid beat, all over the place; there was no regular pattern. I was sure it was well over one hundred beats a minute (normal is sixty to one hundred). His face looked dusky, and some foamy liquid was coming out of his mouth. Now my heart rate went up and cold sweat formed on my back against the green surgical top under my short white coat.

As I leaned over his back and put the stethoscope on his chest, it was clear he was gasping for air every second. I heard loud crackles and grunts, in and out with each rapid and shallow breath, and a gurgling sound. What was going on here? I looked around for a nurse to help the patient—and me. But we were down at the end of the hall, far from the nursing station. I was alone with a very sick man.

I calmed myself for a minute with some self-talk: *Go back to the basics, go through your routine, what you have learned and already done before. You couldn't get a good history, you've taken the blood pressure, listened to the heart and lungs, and checked the pulse. My God -this man's in acute congestive heart failure!* His heart continued to beat incredibly fast.

An overly rapid heartbeat for sure, but what was it telling me?

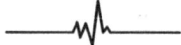

THE FIRST TECHNOLOGY:
THE DOOR TO THE HEART OPENS

1889—Basel, Switzerland

The young Dutch doctor, a serious medical scientist, must have thought that he was at the circus. Attending his first international conference, Willem Einthoven MD[19] (1860-1927) didn't understand what he was seeing. An Englishman named A.D. Waller[20] MD (1856-1932) came on stage and had a stunt to perform. His bulldog Jimmy was the star of the show. With the canine's one leg sitting in a bucket of saltwater and the other three legs wired up to a contraption known as Lippman's capillary electrometer, Waller entertained the audience of doctors with a photographic recording of Jimmy's heartbeat.

As a medical doctor, Waller was aware that his performance was not groundbreaking science, for scientists had known for over a century that animal tissue, especially nerve and heart cells, carried electricity. Luigi Galvani MD (1739-1798) at the medical school in Bologna, Italy, showed that he could make a frog's leg contract by passing a small electric current through it. Waller had done his act with Jimmy many times throughout Europe and regarded the cardiac electrical currents that he recorded as a simple curiosity. But for the Dutch doctor in the audience, the performance sparked a new reaction in him. Something about the spectacle he was witnessing made Einthoven recognize his new life's work.

This epiphany was surprising given Einthoven's opinion of himself as a "true scientist"—devoted to empiricism, not opinions or flashy

---

19   Willem Einthoven was born into a medical family. Willem's father Jacob was a doctor, as well as Jacob's father. He lived his early life in the Dutch East Indies, returning to Holland for his formal education.

20   A.D. (Augustus Desiré) Waller was just four years older than Willem. Born into a scientific family in Paris, he moved to London to work and perform research at St. Mary's Hospital. Waller knew that nerve and heart cells carried electricity, and he was out to prove that day in Basal that once again he could record the signal of the heart's beating from the surface of the body of a dog.

displays. At age twenty-nine, he had published interesting work in ophthalmology and orthopedics, and believed that mathematics and physics would pave the future for medical research. Einthoven was already the chairman of the Physiology Department at Leiden, Holland, in 1886, just one year after graduating from medical school. He wanted to be at the forefront of the scientific revolution of his day.

Nonetheless, for Einthoven, Waller's sensationalized performance had given him a grand idea. He knew as a medical doctor that the only tools the doctor had to try to figure out a problem with the human heart were checking the patient's pulse or listening to the heart with a stethoscope. Ultimately, a definite diagnosis was only made when the patient died and an autopsy was performed. But what if there was a way to record an electrical signal from the heart while the patient was alive, a message that could be analyzed and compared to the patient's symptoms? What if the recording of this signal could be sent to other physicians to examine and analyze, an objective measure of the heart's electrical activity? That would be a spectacular achievement. Then and there, Einthoven began to pursue the innovative idea of an "electrocardiogram."

In European medical schools, driven by the German influence on scientific medical research, students were expected early on to involve themselves in an area of research. Unlike in the modern era, where the clinical skills of patient care are the major emphasis in medical school education, research drove a career in Einthoven's time. After all, there really wasn't too much doctors could do for patients. There was scant scientific basis for much of what was tried. Anecdotes, such as "this seemed to work," were often the basis for treatment. Driven by a fluke accident to his wrist that made him question currently accepted ideas of orthopedics, Willem began his entry into medical research. He presented his study of elbow and shoulder motion at the Dutch Royal Academy of Sciences, directly contradicting the beliefs of the time. Knowing how little professors regard the intellect and original thoughts of medical students, this was no small accomplishment. This was a harbinger of more to come from the Dutchman, who was a man on the move.

The nineteenth century was a cauldron of scientific inquiry into the relationship between electricity and chemistry. There was an explosion of interest in the behavior of atoms and electricity, even in an era when the understanding of the electric charges of subatomic particles, the electron and the proton, was a mystery. Einthoven's attendance at the conference with Waller and his performing dog[21] would not only bring the work of both of these men together but that of an earlier scientist fascinated by "electro-chemistry."

Gabriel Lippman PhD (1845-1921) was aware of the work of William Henry (1774-1836), who had proved that when a mercury electrode was placed in a bath of sulfuric acid, the liquid *moved* when a voltage was applied to the electrode. Further, he showed that liquid mercury in an acid bath also moved when a current was applied through a nail or a wire. What was happening here? Magic? Electricity caused a liquid and mercury to move?

Lippman wanted to accurately measure and document these unexplained movements in response to electricity and created a "capillary electrometer" as his tool. Lippman built a glass tube 1.0 meter long that tapered to only 7 mm in diameter and was hung vertically. The glass tube was filled with mercury, and at the very end of the tube was a capillary point, a tiny .005 mm in diameter. Attaching a microscope to the side of the glass tube, Lippman could observe the capillary point clearly. He then connected platinum electrodes to the mercury at two points and ran a current through the electrodes. The mercury moved, and Lippman recorded the movement with his tiny microscope. Now there was a way to measure this strange movement of the interaction between electricity and atoms. Maybe in the future these movements could explain the movement of the heart muscle.

---

21 A member of the House of Commons felt that Waller was being cruel to Jimmy and challenged Waller on the floor of that chamber of the British Parliament. In response to the questioning of how Jimmy felt during his shows, Waller said, "If my honourable friend had ever paddled in the sea, he will appreciate fully the sensation obtained thereby from this pleasurable experience."

Lippman's capillary electrometer intrigued others, especially Waller, who wanted to use the tool to prove his theory that electrical "potentials" could be found in the muscles of animals and man, both the muscles of the skeleton and the heart. Waller thought, if he could focus a light beam on the end of the column of mercury in the electrometer, he could produce an image and record it on a photographic plate. He would hook up an animal or a person's limbs to wires and send them to the mercury column in the electrometer. If the mercury moved, then electricity had flowed from the animal or human to cause that motion.

The eccentric Waller[22] thought to use an invention of the 1860s, toy trains, to demonstrate his discovery. He attached the photographic plates to slowly moving toy train wagons and placed the plates behind his electrometer and the beam of light, thus making a moving record of the electrical movement changes. Using this clever technique in animals first, his theory was correct.

Waller continued his research, now on the human heart. Reminiscing about the summer of 1887 years later, he wrote, " . . . it occurred to me that it ought to be possible to use the limbs as electrodes and thus lead off from the heart, i.e. from the intact and normal organ. Obviously man was the most convenient animal to use so I dipped my right hand and left foot into a couple of basins of salt solution, which were connected with the two poles of the electrometer and at once had the pleasure of seeing the mercury column pulsate with the pulsation of the heart . . . " He had recorded his own heartbeat. He published the first recordings of the electrical current of the heart in humans in the *Journal of Physiology* in 1887—the electrogram, using Lippman's tool, photographic plates, and toy trains.

---

22 By all accounts, Waller was not the typical medical university professor of the nineteenth century. He did not wear a morning coat and a silk hat. He was described as a "short stocky man, very light on his feet. His grey beard and double-breasted blue jacket make him look exactly like a skipper in the Merchant Navy. Like Sir Winston (Churchill), he seemed to be habitually smoking cigars, and was invariably followed by his bulldog, Jimmy, who also had a Churchillian quality . . . " It has often been said that some people strongly resemble their pets.

A.D. Waller died in 1922, and his legacy of work is impressive for his insights and ingenuity in inventing a way to record the heart's electricity, yet he had failed to unearth its even more impactful use. Waller did not recognize the chance for viewing this "signal" from within the living human organism to understand both the normal function of the heart and also what changed in disease. He did not see the potential application of his invention in diagnosing and further understanding heart disease.

Willem Einthoven did see that potential. He first wanted to improve Lippman's electrometer and then learn the mathematics and physics of mercury. He found Lippman's device was too sensitive to the effects of the mechanical environment of the electrometer, leading to inconsistent measurements. Working feverishly in his laboratory, he had spent his initial years trying to develop complex mathematical corrections for the Lippman electrometer readings. His own variant of the device was slow to respond to the changes in electrical current, but the recordings were still much better than the "waves" produced by Waller. Five discrete cardiac electrical deflections were found—named P, Q, R, S and T.[23] These names have lasted the test of time.

Frustrated and unnerved at times,[24] Einthoven did not give up and pursued the invention of an even better instrument. For the next five years, he worked diligently on a new and innovative device: the string galvanometer. The working part of the new machine was a single thin wire of silver-plated quartz placed between two electromagnets. When an electric current was applied the wire moved, creating a shadow. Just as Waller had done with the movement of mercury, Einthoven recorded the movement of the shadow and magnified it many times over. But the thin quartz wire had remarkable qualities; its tension, sensitivity and response time could be adjusted easily.

By 1901, Einthoven's machine was poised to change medical history, but the next challenge was how to put it to use. The genius of

---

23   Why Einthoven did not use A, B, C, D, and E remains a mystery of medical history.
24   In a letter to his brother Johan in 1896, he described himself as "a very ordinary little professor who is not equal to the task he set himself."

the memorable innovator is how to apply a tool, and Einthoven was not just a physicist and mathematician—he was a medical doctor. Einthoven's goal all along was to use his new "electrocardiogram" machine to study humans. He quickly came to understand the timing of the normal rhythm of the heart and saw that the atria and the ventricles of the heart had separate electrical signals. The signal from the ventricles was a much stronger signal, and that made sense—their muscle mass was much greater than the atria. Einthoven identified most of the common abnormalities on the EKG signals that still form the basic learning requirements of medical students to this day. These changes included slowing of the heart rhythm and "dropped" beats known as "heart block." He saw irregularly timed heart beats from the upper heart chambers, the atria, an erratic pulse that clinicians had long identified but didn't understand. Now these "arrhythmias" of the atria and the ventricles, atrial fibrillation, atrial flutter, and ventricular abnormal beats, could all be documented with the electrocardiogram.

By 1906, Einthoven was recording "telecardiograms" from patients. He had his laboratory containing the immobile galvanometer[25] connected by telephone lines to the hospital in Leiden. He worked with the clinicians caring for the patients (not always a smooth relationship). Some of his colleagues became jealous that so many of the patients were requesting a telecardiogram. But Einthoven continued to innovate. Once he knew he could record a consistent signal with the electrocardiogram leads attached in a particular way, he began to experiment with combinations of lead attachments. The electrocardiogram could view the heart from many different points of view, similar to a photographer looking at one subject from the front, the back, and the side. Einthoven found that the signals differed depending on the way in which he attached the leads and that these varied signals would give even more insight into the heart and its physiology.

How was this of use to the clinician? A doctor now could determine if the atria were enlarged if there was a larger and longer signal from

---

25   The first string galvanometer was massive, weighing about six hundred pounds.

the P wave, the first portion of the electrocardiogram. A century ago, one of the most common forms of heart disease was rheumatic fever. Rheumatic fever often damages and blocks the mitral valve on the left side of the heart—and the left atrium becomes enlarged. Now a doctor could see this on the EKG, an electrical signal of a disease in a living person. Another disease, high blood pressure or hypertension, caused the heart muscle, especially the left ventricle, to enlarge and thicken, another important signal the cardiologist could see on the EKG tracing. The study of diseases of the heart had entered a new world, a world not yet able to alter the course of a heart problem. A new specialty had emerged: cardiology.

By 1905, other investigators began using the electrocardiogram. Einthoven contracted with Edelman and Sons in Munich, Germany, and then the Cambridge Scientific Instrument Company, Ltd. in London, England, to manufacture the electrocardiogram. The EKG quickly became a standard of medical practice[26] and attracted much attention both in Europe and the United States. In 1908, a young English physician, Thomas Lewis MD, wrote to Einthoven, asking him for a copy of his groundbreaking publication of 1906, *Le Telecardiogram*. Lewis' inquiry began a long-term collaboration, a synthesis of the right people at the right time, Einthoven the mathematician and physicist and Lewis the clinician. It was Lewis who was able to show the wider medical world that this wonderful tool was far more than the electrical curiosity of A.D. Waller.

Though the long-term impact of Einthoven's work was slow to arrive, fame did come to him within a few years. In 1924, he was awarded the Nobel Prize in Medicine. In a letter congratulating Einthoven, his colleague H.A. Lorenz MD (1853-1928) wrote that the Prize's "recognition of ingenuity and perseverance is the more striking, because you have always worked in perfect simplicity and modesty." That year, Einthoven toured the United States, giving

---

26 We in the profession still use a variant of the string galvanometer; it is just much smaller and portable than Einthoven's six hundred–pound, two-room behemoth.

lectures in New York City, Minneapolis, Boston, Ann Arbor, and Cleveland. He saw new work using his tool, for the first time to confirm the diagnosis of that most dreaded of heart diseases, the myocardial infarction, the heart attack. Here was the crucial link between all of Einthoven's work and the pursuit of the Widowmaker.

Willem Einthoven continued his work until he died in 1927. In his eulogy, Wenckebach commented on the string galvanometer with this flowery language of his time: "This wonderful instrument was born out of Einthoven's head, fully developed like Pallas Athene from that of Zeus." Perhaps there was some exaggeration in comparing a machine to a legend of mythology, but considering the EKG's impact on medicine, perhaps not.

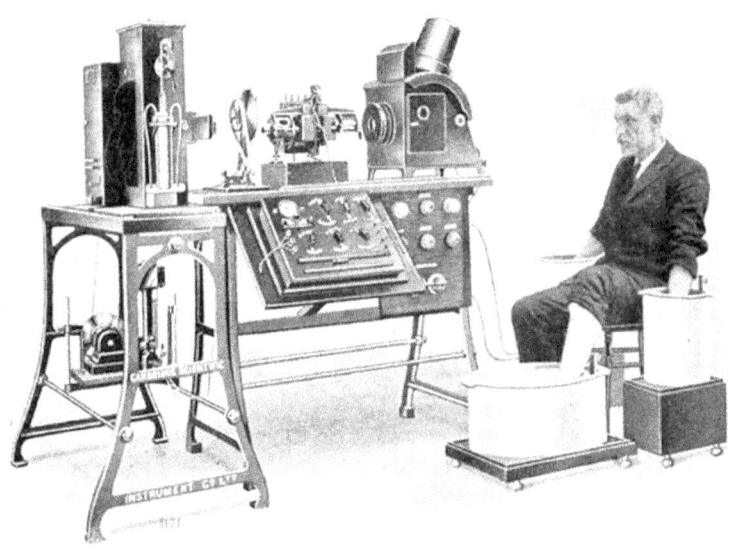

Figure 5. Einthoven's very early EKG machine, with the patient's left foot in a bucket of saltwater (around 1910). Copyright Alamy

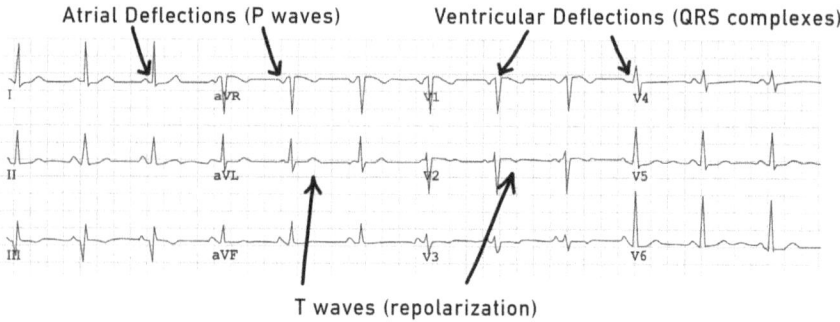

Figure 6. Normal 12-lead electrocardiogram demonstrating electrical activity of the atria, the ventricles, and "repolarization" of the ventricles.

THE TRUE PROMISE OF EINTHOVEN'S INVENTION

As great as Einthoven's accomplishment was, it was only the beginning. By 1909, others were using his machine to unlock the secrets of the most important and common form of heart disease, coronary artery disease, the cause of angina pectoris and acute myocardial infarction. Doctors recognized angina pectoris as a cardiac disease for many years, but not all types of chest pain are caused by blocked coronary arteries. The pain could be from the lungs, or the aorta, or just the muscles or bones of the chest wall. How could a doctor be sure of the cause? But that same year, Simmons and Nicholai in Germany reported a change from the normal electrical signal of the EKG in a patient with angina. Nine years later, Bousfeld, an Englishman, also showed that the electrocardiogram changed from normal when a patient had chest pain from angina. The signs were becoming clearer and easier to read.

By 1909, Edelman and Sons were exporting their EKG machines to the United States. In New York, Harold Pardee MD (1887-1973) acquired a device for the New York Hospital. In 1920, Pardee wrote an article describing a patient he had taken care of in 1917. A thirty-eight-year-old man began to have chest symptoms, and Pardee's account of this man's history is remarkable for its similarity to the story told by so many suffering from coronary artery disease:

> "Otherwise he had been in the best of health until August, 1916, when he had a slight attack of 'indigestion,' with epigastric (*abdominal*) distress and eructations (*belching*) of gas. At this time his physician told him that he had heart trouble, although he had never had reason to suspect this himself. About December, 1916, he began to notice that his 'wind' was not so good as it had been, and during February, 1917, this trouble became distinctly worse and he also noticed occasional slight aching precordial (*chest*) pain.
>
> "On March 4, 1917, suddenly, while he was in bed, asleep, he felt a sharp stabbing pain beneath the sternum (*breast bone*). This radiated about the left chest and down the left arm and was very severe. He felt very weak and prostrated and thought he was going to die. His heart was beating very heavily, he said, and very slowly. He was not short of breath and did not lose consciousness (*pass out*). After twenty or thirty minutes he vomited, and this was repeated several times during the course of the day. The pain continued severe, although less so after the vomiting."

Throughout his hospitalization, the episodes of chest pain in Pardee's patient continued, and he was able to "hook" the man up to the cumbersome EKG machine when he was having symptoms. During these episodes, he saw remarkable changes in the EKG, specifically elevation of the signal between the end of the QRS, the large signal from the ventricles, and the T wave, the signal indicating "repolarization" and the end of a single contraction of the heart. This change was ST segment elevation, now a classic sign of severe myocardial lack of blood supply. The T wave also changed—it became very large and came to a distinct large "point" at its peak—very different from the T wave appearance seen when the man was not having the symptoms.

Though there was not much that Pardee could do for the man, what the doctor recorded would stand the test of time. The patient went on to pass away from another "heart attack" within two years, but Pardee showed that Einthoven's machine, the EKG, could be used to obtain a definite signal from the heart that something was wrong—the heart muscle was not getting enough blood. To this day, the precise understanding of why the EKG signal changes in exactly the way Pardee saw almost one hundred years ago is still not certain. The changes that Pardee saw in his patient are seen thousands of times a year across the globe in patients suffering from coronary artery disease, either an attack of angina pectoris or an acute myocardial infarction.

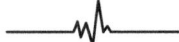

AN URGENT ANSWER AND SOLUTIONS

... I knew that the answers I needed for the gasping man in front of me would come from hooking him up to an electrocardiogram, an EKG. I ran back to the nursing station and found the old beat-up device. I rolled it as fast as I could back down the hall to the patient's room, plugged it in, and turned it on. Then I found the four electrode leads for the limbs, both arms and legs. Now I needed the "goop," the tube of gel that allows the heart's electrical signal to be transmitted to the EKG machine.

As the patient continued to struggle for air, I knew this process was far from over, and I would have to hurry. I squirted just a spot of gel on the limbs and then attached the rectangular gold-plated electrodes, sliding the color-coded wire from the EKG machine through the drilled-out metal on top of the electrodes. White for the right arm, black for the left, then red and green for the legs. The memory trick went through my head: "The way to remember the correct leg leads during the Cold War? 'The reds are on the left.'"

With the four limb leads done, next came the six chest leads, and there was still no nurse to help me. I undid the tie on the back of the man's thin blue-striped gown and slipped it over the shoulders. Then I squirted the "goop" on the chest, just a little, not too much (the sound said it all). One squirt went to the right of the breastbone in the middle, then five more spots on the left, in a downward arc from the upper chest to just to the left of the nipple. I tried to find spots without much obstructive chest hair. Then I needed the six suction cups that were those chest leads. I squeezed the first cup and placed it on top of the first spot of gel on the right side of the chest—lead V1. I made sure the cup attachment read "V1." Then came the next five, and I needed to get the right ones in the right spots, V2 to V6, but some slipped off and had to be re-applied. Finally, the EKG machine and I were ready to go.

I flipped the lead switch on the machine. Lead I: I ran a tracing through the machine, the EKG's stylus burning the heart's signal on the paper. This took about ten seconds. I tore off the tracing and made sure I saved it. Next I turned the dial to Lead II. The same process started, and I did it for all twelve leads in a standard EKG. I had gotten pretty fast at doing this during my internal medicine rotation. I was done in about two minutes.

Now what? The man looked like he might stop breathing soon. I studied the tracings. I saw no P waves, the first small signal that comes from the two atria, the upper chambers of the heart. I did see the QRS signals that come from the two ventricles, the two lower chambers. The signals were spaced very close to together on the paper and had no organized time pattern. This told me what I needed to know, and I knew this man's problem: atrial fibrillation. And indeed, his heart was beating very fast. In addition, my patient had pulmonary edema—"lung water"—due to his rapid heartbeat.

I had made a diagnosis: congestive heart failure due to rapid atrial fibrillation. Congrats to the young medical student, but there was still a sick man in front of me struggling to breathe. I paged the surgery resident, my immediate supervisor, who fortunately was not operating at that moment. He could sense panic in my voice and came right over. He looked at the man and then the EKG. He agreed with me. The man was in rapid atrial fibrillation. He also pointed out that a portion of the EKG signal, the ST segment, was down below the baseline signal. This was a sign of a lack of blood supply to the coronary arteries due to the rapid heart rate and probably partially blocked-up coronary arteries.

Now the resident knew what to do. He ordered oxygen and intravenous medication, first morphine sulfate. Yes, morphine, and it calmed him down, opened up the veins, and dropped the pressure inside the heart. This happened very quickly, within minutes. *Remarkable!* I thought. Then he injected a syringe of a diuretic known as furosemide (trade name Lasix) to force the kidneys to pump out large amounts of urine quickly. He and I placed a catheter in his bladder to catch that urine so we were sure that the diuretic was working. Finally, we gave the man intravenous digoxin, a medicine used for two hundred years to treat atrial fibrillation. The digoxin slowed the heart rate down.

In about ten minutes, the man was feeling better and was quickly transferred to the Cardiac Care Unit, owing his life to the information we were able to obtain from the EKG. It was this machine that gave us the answer, as it has in countless cases over the last century, without an incision or an autopsy. The invention of the Dutchman Willem Einthoven changed medicine forever and has saved an inestimable number of lives, including that of my patient in 1974.

Einthoven's work opened the door to the future. However, the cause of the heart attack still eluded researchers. While Einthoven was still laboring in his laboratory, another researcher had been trying to solve the mystery of atherosclerosis.

CHAPTER 5

THE RUSSIAN AND HIS RABBITS: CHOLESTEROL AND ATHEROSCLEROSIS

I have begun to hear murmurs of how I am predestined to strike, my occurrence embedded from conception in your DNA.

This gives me peace. For then I am simply the blameless executioner, acting on a message which has long ago dictated how much hindrance to lay down and how much to let flow, whether your artery can remain supple or become a tightening noose.

RESEARCH IN ANIMALS—EARLY SPRING 1971

The professor walked me to the back of his lab and opened the door to a room with about twenty very large cages. The noise was deafening from screeching and the rattling of metal bars. I stared at orangutans, up close and personal, each one weighing over one hundred pounds and four to five feet tall, swinging back and forth in their prisons and screaming every few seconds. They were frightening gymnasts.

I was starting medical school that fall at Penn when an opportunity presented itself. The flame of my interest in the heart and its diseases was still there and now gaining some new oxygen, so I thought I was ready to do some authentic research in animals. Answering a post for student jobs, I walked over to the laboratory of David Kritchevsky MD (1920-2006) located in the Wistar Institute, a historic research facility on the University of Pennsylvania campus. For the senior member of his research team, he was very informal and engaging. In his not-so-clean white coat, he began to show me around.

Standing inside the orangutan room, Dr. Kritchevsky simply waited for my reaction. Finally, I said, "So I guess these are the animals you study?"

He smirked a little and said, "Good guess." After a few more awkward minutes, I asked him to describe what I would be doing. He said, "Well, the students take a large syringe full of different kinds of fat and proteins and inject the orangutans. Then we sacrifice them a few months later and see what their arteries look like."

"Inject the orangutans?" I murmured, then more clearly asked, "Do you put them to sleep first?" He shook his head. I tried again. "Wow, that sounds like it's pretty hard to do."

Kritchevsky replied, "Yeah, it's a real sport. We all take a look to see who gets injected first, the orangutan or the med student."

That summer, I chose instead to work in the pulmonary lab at Penn, making breathing measurements from patients with lung disease. They didn't move very much. I eventually did animal research in heart disease but never in orangutans. Yet over the years I developed great respect for those who could do animal research as a career. Without this work, the cause of atherosclerosis and the heart attack would still be unknown. Still, I suspect if that summer's project involved rabbits, I might have been up to the task.

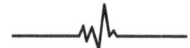

UNLOCKING THE DOOR: WHAT CAUSES ATHEROSCLEROSIS?

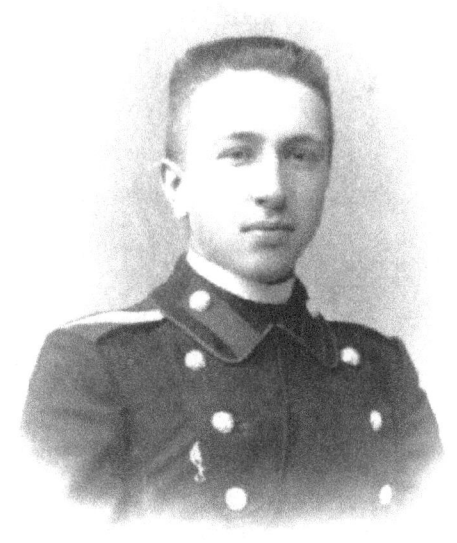

Figure 7. Photograph of Nikolai Anichkov as a young man (Courtesy of the Journal of Lipid Research, Hindawi Publishing, 2004)

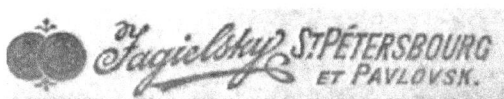

If he walked into an imaginary bar of great scientists in the 1940s, no one would know his name. Nikolai Nikolaevich Anichkov MD (1885-1964) was a man whose achievements remind us that the luster of fame in science and discovery is often in retrospect and even then clouded by that of others. For example, in the United States, all children were taught that Christopher Columbus (1451-1506) discovered America in 1492; only years later did some of us realize that the Viking sailor Leif Eriksen (c. 970—c.1020) came to the New World centuries before Columbus. So too it would be with Anichkov and his wonderful discoveries.

At the dawn of the twentieth century, the focus of medical research was on infectious diseases like syphilis and tuberculosis, and immunization and the first drugs to treat these terrors were making inroads. But to many doctors, especially the pathologists examining the hearts and blood vessels of people dying from "arteriosclerosis," this increasingly common disease was a mystery.

Doctors were stymied by arteriosclerosis. Sir William Osler MD (1849-1919) was the foremost American clinician of his time. In 1892, Osler published a 1,050-page textbook, *The Principles and Practice of Medicine*, and yet he could only include two paragraphs to describe the treatment of the dreaded disease causing the chest pain of angina pectoris, the heart attack, and sudden death. Osler's advice consisted of the following: "In the early stages, before any local symptoms are manifest, the patient should be enjoined to live a quiet, well-regulated life, avoiding excesses in food and drink. It is usually best to explain frankly the condition of affairs, and so to gain intelligent cooperation." Essentially, he told his patients to not do very much and to get their affairs in order before they would suffer a heart attack or die suddenly.

While scientists could see it, they couldn't explain it. Under the microscope, arteriosclerosis was just a jumble of fat molecules, white blood cells, smooth muscle cells from the middle layer of the arteries, platelets, blood clot, red blood cells, and cells that just defied description. But what was the cause for all of this chaos and destruction of blood vessels, especially in the heart? There were many choices. Careful research was needed to answer the question and answer it in a way that embedded skepticism and the willingness to allow others to confirm the results of the "first movers." Nikolai Anichkov wanted to be included in that group.

Anichkov was born in St. Petersburg to an upper-class family and enrolled in the Imperial Military Medical Academy in St. Petersburg in 1903. Formally named in 1798, the Academy was the incubator for researchers such as Ivan Pavlov PhD (1849-1936). As is evidenced by Pavlov's breakthrough work on conditioned reflexes, which won him the Nobel Prize, this was not a "third-rate" institution. Anichkov was in the right milieu for a budding researcher.

But Anichkov's work first required an understanding of the pathology of arteriosclerosis uncovered by those who came before him. Rudolph Virchow MD (1821-1902), "The Pope of Medicine," had thought arteriosclerosis was caused by the "metabolism" of the artery, but he had no clue as to what the metabolic problem was. Somehow, he thought, the artery itself was producing the "hard gruel" blocking the flow of blood in the arterial tubes: "plaque." Carl von Rokitansky MD (1804-1878), a pathologist from Vienna, Austria, reasoned that blood clots were the primary culprit that led to the final pathology. A clue to the cause of the artery problem did emerge in 1901. Adolf Windaus PhD (1876-1959), a chemist from Germany, found out that the plaques contained a particular fatty molecule in much greater amounts than normal arteries, first named cholesterine.[27]

Arteriosclerosis was a topic attracting many researchers looking to make their reputation and answer the plaguing questions. For example, was the cholesterine the real cause of the disease or just an innocent bystander? In 1904, the German pathologist Felix Marchand MD (1848-1928) added the term *"atherosclerosis"* to the medical world, plaque made up of gruel containing a particular molecule, cholesterol. It was known that cholesterol was common in the body and made up a good percentage of the contents of the membranes of most of the cells of the body, especially the brain and nervous system. But what was it doing inside of arteries?

The Russians in St. Petersburg knew of Windaus' discovery of the cholesterol in the plaques and were eager to expand on the knowledge. Alexander Ignatowski MD (1875-1955), a young professor at the Imperial Academy, was doing experimental work with rabbits, feeding them different foods. Since atherosclerosis looked like fat, and cholesterol, a form of fat, was a known component of various foods, maybe the problem was from the diet. Indeed, Ignatowski found that when rabbits were fed meat and eggs, they quickly developed fatty deposits in the liver and atherosclerosis of the aorta, the major blood vessel that originates from the top of the heart. The atherosclerosis was also destroying the coronary arteries of the heart. But what specifically was in the meat and eggs that did this?

---

27 We now call this molecule cholesterol.

Anichkov wanted to carry the work much further. It wasn't good enough to say that atherosclerosis was just caused by food. After he received his medical degree in 1909, Anichkov stayed on as a faculty member at the Academy. A medical student, Semen Chatalov MD (1884-1951), volunteered to help Anichkov conduct more rabbit experiments on atherosclerosis and confirm their suspicion that cholesterol alone was the culprit. This molecule in the food first entered the body through the intestine and then the liver somehow engulfed it. The Russian's belief was that these same molecules must have gotten out of the liver and were carried into the blood vessels, where they took up residence in the walls of the arteries. The result was atherosclerosis.

The outcomes were slow to present themselves. The Russians fed the rabbits three different dietary supplements—protein, egg white, and egg yolk—and waited to see which rabbits had the plaque form. It would be weeks and months before they would get their answer. Would Anichkov's patience be rewarded? Staring and squinting through his microscope, Anichkov saw no plaque in the aortas of the rabbits fed protein and egg white. But in the egg yolk–fed animals, he found plaques that were "doubly refractile." Then using polarized light through the scopes, he also saw "double cross figures." Only one molecule was to appear under the microscope as "doubly refractile" and contained "double cross figures" —cholesterol. The egg yolk had to be the culprit.

Anichkov and Chatalov set about disseminating their findings. In December 1911, they presented their work at the Russian Society of Pathologists. Their paper "Response of the liver to different sorts of food fat" is one of the classics of research into the cause of heart disease. Anichkov was a careful scientist. He pointed out the strengths of his work as well as the unanswered questions but was uncertain what future research should focus on. He and Chatalov published a summary of their work, as well as the research of others, in 1913. Among their first comments was "The very fact that we start with a diversity of viewpoints and observations strengthens our conclusions and gives them scientific validity." Even with success, they were maintaining healthy skepticism, looking for independent verification of their results and conclusions.

Anichkov and Chatalov were not satisfied with their egg yolk results alone, nor to confine their findings to animals alone. Next they did experiments with purified cholesterol. They reported convincingly that "after only 4 to 8 weeks of feeding cholesterine (dissolved in oil) we produced in the experimental animals a rich infiltration of the entire liver parenchyma with the same liquid spherical crystals that one of us (Chatalov) has seen in the livers of rabbits fed egg yolk." Anichkov quickly recognized that his discovery might be directly related to human disease: "As noted in the literature, the human body does not seem to be indifferent to cholesterine. In many pathological changes of both localized and generalized nature, one finds cholesterine and its compounds deposited in the tissues in great quantities. *Many authors have even associated fluctuations in blood cholesterol content with the origin of some pathological processes."* [28] This was a remarkable insight at the time, and the future would prove that disregarding this belief would be a lost opportunity to save lives.

Soon Anichkov became a sought-after young researcher and was offered traveling fellowships by others, enabling him to further climb the academic ladder. In 1913, he moved to Austria and then took a position with Karl Aschoff MD (1866-1942) in his laboratory in Freiburg, Germany. Aschoff was fascinated by Anichkov's rabbits and their atherosclerosis. Under his own microscope, Aschoff noticed certain strange-looking white blood cells working as "scavengers," gobbling up diseased cells in order to protect the overall organism. These cells, now called phagocytes or macrophages, are an important part of the body's immune response to many diseases, like bacterial and viral infections. They respond vigorously to anything that shouldn't be there, like atherosclerosis, not just pathogens. The immune system of these rabbits was not taking atherosclerosis lying down!

---

28   Italics mine.

Anichkov also found the scavenger cells. He saw that some of the phagocytes were filled with a substance that looked like foam.[29] He was an eyewitness to the microscopic "war" that takes place inside the artery when something that doesn't belong there penetrates into the artery wall, especially cholesterol. Yet it would be many years before medical science would realize that it was the breakdown of this repair process, the erosion of the carefully built "wall" over the cholesterol plaque built by the immune system cells, that leads to an acute myocardial infarction—the heart attack.

But the outside world of politics and World War I caught up with Anichkov and all of the other non-Germans working in the Kaiser's research laboratories. He was arrested and sent to a prisoner of war camp. Through Aschoff's influence, he escaped to neutral Sweden and then traveled home to St. Petersburg. Nikolai was assigned to the Russian military medical corp. He was a physician-in-charge in an evacuation train from the front lines until Russia left the war in 1917. To continue to work at a prestigious post after the Revolution must have required something else. Did he become a Bolshevik and join the Communist party? His political beliefs remain a mystery, but he did what he needed to do to continue his career as a Soviet doctor.

By 1920, Anichkov returned to his research roots and became a Professor of Pathologic Physiology at the Academy. He vigorously pursued his work on atherosclerosis, wrote papers, and spoke at international meetings in Asia and Europe. But his work was ignored by many in the Western world. As the age of Joseph Stalin's (1878-1953) Russia took root, the outside world grew disinterested and skeptical of the work of Soviet scientists. Anichkov's work on atherosclerosis was in the winter of a long hibernation.

Despite the lack of interest from outsiders, Anichkov's ideas about atherosclerosis progressed over the years, and he continued to work out the kinks. He realized that there was a major problem with his theory—how come other animals, specifically dogs and rats, common

---

29 Today these cells are indeed called "foam cells."

research models, did not develop the same aortic plaques as the rabbits when fed the cholesterol-high diets? The gap in Anchikov's theory was the same as it has always been in "translational research" —how does a finding in a laboratory, in a small animal like a rabbit, relate to a disease in human beings? This was why he continually pushed for much more work in the lab and people. Anchikov thought the difference between humans and some animals must be in the blood or the liver. There was something in the blood or the liver of the dogs and rats that broke down the cholesterol before it had a chance to form the plaques.[30]

In addition, Anichkov realized that although atherosclerosis of the aorta was a serious problem in human disease, it paled in comparison to what this disease did to the small arteries of the heart, the coronary arteries. Disease of these arteries was causing people young and old to die, often suddenly.

But given that almost all of Anichkov's work was published in Russian, it is not surprising that it was not until the late 1940s that there was any recognition of Anchikov's groundbreaking work outside of the Soviet Union. When searching for references, how many Westerners would take the time to try to decipher the title of an article written in the Cyrillic alphabet, particularly in the age when Soviet Russia was largely cut off from the outside world? How could other researchers communicate or collaborate with people like Anichkov? While the hurdles were formidable, other researchers finally began to examine his work.

Even though Anichkov's work was re-discovered and valued by the 1950s, there was still great skepticism that diet alone was the cause of atherosclerosis, angina, and myocardial infarction, and it is no wonder. It is difficult to imagine that the people of the world would have accepted the need to alter their diet during the years of the extreme economic disaster of the post-World War I era of the 1920s in Europe, followed by the worldwide Great Depression of

---

30 The future would prove him correct, and the complex metabolism of cholesterol would be discovered by others.

the 1930s, and the six years of World War II through 1945. Similarly asking people to stop smoking cigarettes in those decades would have been fruitless. For millions at the time, living constantly within sight of their cigarettes and lighter is similar to our current obsession with our cell phones.

Anichkov's work, however, was undeterred. His lab continued to study the effect of atherosclerosis on the heart. Just like James Herrick found, his autopsies told him that the severity of blockage in one of the coronary arteries did not necessarily mean that the heart muscle supplied by this artery was damaged by a myocardial infarction. In fact, sometimes a heart attack occurred in another part of the heart, where the artery supplying that part of the muscle was not as badly blocked. Anichkov's work confirmed the importance of the collaterals first suggested by John Hunter when he repaired aneurysms of the legs and given much further credence by James Herrick's study of patients with coronary artery disease.

In addition to opening up collateral blood vessels or "detour routes" around blockages in the major arteries, Anichkov discovered that the heart was clever in other ways. The arteries with the blockages became larger and allowed more blood to pass around the fatty plaque buildup. Even when a blood clot or thrombus was found inside the arteries, slits where blood could still get by were found in some of the hearts. These insights help lead to the understanding that coronary artery atherosclerosis was a long-term and complicated process. The idea that atherosclerosis was simply a "rusty pipe" process was much too simplistic. Thousands of years of evolution weren't going to pass without the human body learning how to deal with its imperfections.

PROGRESSION OF ATHEROSCLEROSIS

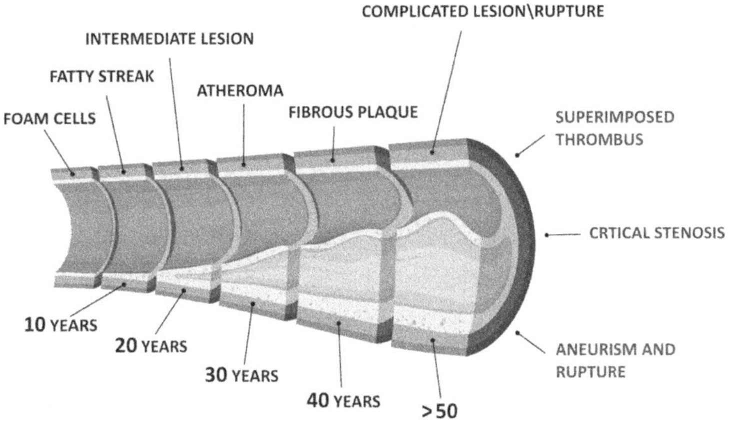

Figure 8. Long timeline of worsening of atherosclerosis
(Copyright Shutterstock)

In 1958, William Dock MD published an editorial in *The Annals of Internal Medicine* entitled "Research in arteriosclerosis: the first fifty years." By that time, the effect of cholesterol in the diet on atherosclerosis was beginning to be accepted. Dock wrote, "Thus the early work of Anchikov bears comparison with that of Harvey on the circulation and of Lavoisier on the respiratory exchange of oxygen and carbon dioxide." Those of us who have studied science and medicine recognize the names of William Harvey MD, the discoverer of the circulatory system, and the Frenchman Antoine Lavoisier (1743-1794), who identified oxygen as the key element to life of all kinds. To be mentioned with those two is quite remarkable for a man who lived through the Russian Revolution, two World Wars, and the Soviet Union of Stalin. He must have been one tough Russian; however, his Russian origin likely deprived him of a Nobel Prize.

By the time of his death, Anchikov's work had achieved the recognition of the scientific world that it deserved. Anichkov's belief about the underlying cause of atherosclerosis and heart attack was finally accepted. Cholesterol was not just an innocent bystander. In March 1964, Anchikov's article "Compensatory Adjustments in the Structure of Coronary Arteries of the Heart with Stenotic Atherosclerosis" was published in *Circulation*, the official publication of the American Heart Association. His work was finally in the Western literature. By the time the door of knowledge was opening in the West, it had been creaking softly out of earshot for almost forty years. Nikolai Anichkov died in December 1964, ironically, of a myocardial infarction, a heart attack. He was seventy-nine years old.

While Anichkov's achievement remained buried in obscure Soviet research archives, the rest of the world struggled with the enormous problem of at least making a diagnosis of disease of the coronary arteries. There had to be a better way other than waiting for an autopsy.

CHAPTER 6

DIVINING THE SIGNALS: THE CREATION OF THE STRESS TEST

*Climbing the stairs, raking leaves, lifting a heavy suitcase—
a pattern is before them and yet they do not see. Why does it take so
long for the doctors to harness their understanding of the moments
I so frequently strike?*

*A new wave of researchers, however, is in hot pursuit, and their
ability to apprehend my design will soon be put to the test.*

THE DOCTOR'S STRESS TEST

The sweat began to pour off of his head, face, and chest, percolating up in larger and larger beads. He stared straight ahead, mentally whipping his leg muscles to continue with the uphill climb and increased speed of the mechanical treadmill. His face, ruddy several minutes earlier, was ashen.

Standing right next to him, I swung my gaze from the man to the electrocardiogram signal. I'd seen the signal change almost two minutes prior and now was convinced that it was time to stop the test. He had only been exercising for five minutes.

"That's enough, Dr. Stein. We need to stop," I barked to him as well as the technician.

"Why, Arnold? I'm doing fine," the older man said. Doctors make the worst patients.

"Well, we'll talk about that. Let's get you to sit down now."

He stumbled over to the chair, with the sweat continuing to drench his chest and the electrodes pasted to his body. He was breathing heavily but still believed this was just his normal response to exercising.

"What's wrong? Do you see anything?" he asked.

"Let's have you rest for another minute or two," I said in my practiced calm voice.

Dr. Hyman Stein was my mentor in the early days of my private practice, and we had grown quite close. He was in his mid-sixties and very vigorous, and I had never had any reason to believe he had any health issues. Then one day he had paged me and said he wanted me to perform a stress test on him. I asked why. He said that he wanted to begin an intense exercise program and that, although he felt great, his wife had insisted that he have the test first, "just to be safe." I remember having asked him if he had any cardiac symptoms, like chest pressure or shortness of breath, either at rest or with exertion, but he had laughed off my questions, claiming "Of course not. Don't you think I would have called you if I was having any problems?"

"Okay, we can do it, but as you know it's not really indicated unless someone has symptoms or an abnormal electrocardiogram."

"Let's just see if you can schedule it," he had replied.

I could not refuse the man, and now staring at his pale face, I was glad for that fact . . .

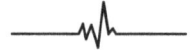

THE BLOOMING OF THE ELECTROCARDIOGRAM: MORE THAN A CURIOSITY

The medical world was astonished by Einthoven's electrocardiogram and rushed to put it to its best use. Taking the EKG of patients with all types of possible cardiac symptoms, like chest pain, shortness of breath, palpitations, dizziness, and passing out would offer great opportunities for correct diagnosis and possible treatment.

But the looming question of greatest importance centered on the diagnosis of angina and the myocardial infarction. Were there EKG abnormalities that could identify that "mischief" of Heberben, coronary artery disease? If that were true, the first step toward scientific diagnosis of the work of the Widowmaker would be a reality. But similar to the ancient Greek Oracles of Delphi trying to predict the future by examining the entrails of birds, the progress was difficult. It was so clear that the EKG could identify with great accuracy abnormalities of the heart's rhythm, but rhythm problems are usually markers of the underlying disease, not the disease itself.

With so much unknown, the science was ready to reap many new discoveries and foster careers. The EKG and its signals would drive many into the new field of cardiology to try to make their mark in research and unlock its potential. In 1918, nine years after Einthoven's machine became commercially available, a British doctor, Guy Bousfield MD, was planning to photograph an EKG in a patient with disease of the aortic valve. He was very surprised by what he accidentally discovered.

While setting up his recordings, Bousfield's patient began to have chest pain. With little hesitation, Bousfield asked his associate to go to the pharmacy to bring the patient amyl nitrite to relieve the chest pain, but as the patient was already "hooked up" to the EKG machine, Bousfield decided to record the heart signals while waiting for the medication to arrive. Bousfield was stunned by what he saw. First, there was a delay in the time it took for the ventricles to contract, known now as a "bundle branch block," a common finding in patients with aortic valve disease. But those changes were present all of the time in a patient without chest pain; in Bousfield's patient, however, the electrical delay disappeared when the patient's chest pain resolved! So clearly his damaged aortic valve was not causing the EKG changes he saw. What in the world was going on?

In addition, the Englishman saw something brand new: the T wave, the end of the ECG complex, which normally pointed upright on the tracing, was deeply *upside down*—it was "inverted." Even more surprising was that this change was only temporary, with the T wave appearance returning to normal when the patient felt better. Bousfield thought that the changes had something to do with pressure inside of the heart and an effect on the heart muscle surrounding the aortic valve.[31] His brief article was a "case report" on one patient only. It is doubtful that too many doctors noted it, even those already using the EKG machine. But his report was a start.

Around the world, others were discovering the value of this new device. Across the Atlantic Ocean in New York, Harold Pardee MD (1886-1973) acquired an EKG machine for the New York Hospital. Pardee received his MD degree from Columbia, served in the United States Army Medical Corp in World War I, and in England had the opportunity to work with Sir Thomas Lewis, Einthoven's collaborator.

In 1917, Pardee discovered a brand new finding that would prove quite valuable while taking care of a thirty-eight-year-old man with classic symptoms of coronary artery disease—"indigestion," chest pain, and radiating pain down the left arm. In the hospital, the man continued to have chest pain, but Pardee was able to attach him to the cumbersome EKG machine when he was having symptoms. He saw changes on the tracings even more profound than those noted by Bousfield a few years earlier: a striking elevation of the normally "flat" electrical baseline signal between the end of the QRS, the large

---

31 The idea that these changes were due to the work of the Widowmaker, atherosclerosis of the coronary arteries, was not yet a consideration.

signal from the ventricles, and the T wave, the signal indicating "repolarization" and the end of a single contraction of the heart. This change is called "ST segment elevation," now seen as the most important EKG abnormality of a severe acute myocardial infarction.

The machine was able to record another new abnormality: the T wave became large and came to a distinct "point" at its peak, so sharp that you wouldn't want to sit on it, very different from the T wave appearance seen when the man was not having the symptoms. The changes that Pardee observed are now called "Pardee's sign," for the elevation of the ST segment on the EKG, and "Pardee's T waves," for the abnormalities of the T waves. Pardee was sure that his patient had coronary artery disease. The EKG findings clinched the diagnosis, later confirmed when the man died and underwent an autopsy.

Prior to the invention of the EKG and x-rays there were innumerable "signs" in medicine, often with names attached honoring the doctor who first noted the "sign," always a physical examination finding, like Heberden's nodes of arthritis. But now a sign was named for something discovered by using technology, an electrical signal from the heart itself, an accurate depiction of the reality that the heart muscle was not getting enough blood. For the first time in the history of coronary artery disease, doctors could say with certainty that blocked arteries were the cause of a person's chest pain, a diagnosis made before one was made on the autopsy table.

While great strides were being made in diagnosis, the problems of treatment and how to expand the use of the machine were still daunting. Pardee could only advise the man to take nitroglycerin as needed, and he died from a myocardial infarction less than two years later, an early victim of the Widowmaker's epidemic.[32] Pardee had a "prepared mind" to make his discovery and was in the right spot at the right time with his patient. But how could this apply to general

---

32 The changes that Pardee saw in his patient are now seen thousands of times a year in patients suffering from coronary artery disease, due to an attack of angina pectoris, or an acute myocardial infarction.

practice? Sure, you could hospitalize people with chest pain, wait until they had an episode, and then run an EKG, but that didn't seem too practical. There had to be a better way to use Einthoven's creation.

STRESSING THE PUMP: THE ELECTROCARDIOGRAM SHOWS ITS POWER

Francis C. Wood MD (1900-1990) of the University of Pennsylvania in Philadelphia had another idea. Wood quickly rose through the academic ranks at Penn, and his research focus was how to diagnose angina pectoris. Wood and his colleague Charles Wolferth MD (1887-1965) wanted to be just like auto mechanics. If you take your car to a shop because the engine isn't running right, the mechanic doesn't just turn on the ignition and test the engine at idle; he increases the RPMs, knowing that "stressing" the engine is much more likely to find the problem. So Wood and Wolferth applied this principle to the heart. The two knew that angina often came on with the stress of exertion. Wood and Wolferth believed that physical exercise could induce chest pain in people with angina and that an EKG during exercise might demonstrate new types of abnormalities, answering the question, "What caused their symptoms?"[33]

The Penn professors collected a series of thirty patients who they were certain had coronary artery disease based on their symptoms; six of the patients developed angina spontaneously, and twenty-four required physical work to induce the chest pain. Understanding the potential danger of their work, Wood and Wolferth noted in their publication of 1931 that the exercise "was stopped by the first suggestion of pain." They were going to record an EKG before, during, and after the chest pain episode and also record the blood pressure every few minutes. In addition, Wood and Wolferth had a

---

[33] It is unlikely that Wood and Wolferth, given the limited options of the time, gave much thought to ethical questions required of today's researchers: Was it safe to induce chest pain in patients with a potentially life-threatening disease? Could the exercise actually induce a heart attack?

"control" group of one hundred patients, fifty who had no known heart problem at all and fifty who had another form of heart disease, disease of the heart valves. They assumed that the controls would show no changes in their EKGs with exercise.

Wood and Wolferth tried different forms of exercise, including stooping many times, doing sit-ups, walking around the room with arms swinging, walking up flights of stairs, and stepping up on a chair and back down again. The patients assumed to have coronary artery disease would often develop chest pain, and their EKGs became abnormal, with changes identical to the changes seen by Bousfield and Pardee, as well as some new changes that had not been seen before. The abnormal changes were seen with exercise but not at the beginning of the test. After a few minutes of rest, the EKG returned to normal.

But there were problems with the results. Only fifteen of the thirty (fifty percent) developed abnormal EKG changes when they had chest pain while exercising. This meant that the "sensitivity" of the EKG, the ability to detect an abnormality associated with coronary artery disease when that patient did in fact have the disease, was only fifty percent. In the other fifty percent of patients, all thought for sure to have coronary artery disease by Wood and Wolferth before the test, their doctors would still be in the dark about a diagnosis. They would likely still believe their assessment that the patient's symptoms were due to atherosclerosis even though the stress test EKG did not become abnormal.

However, one other observation from their data was significant. Five of the thirty people died, not during their stress test, but within a few months. All five had developed abnormal EKGs with exercise. A modern cardiologist would say then that an abnormal stress test had a high "positive predictive value" of mortality. Wood and Wolferth missed the abnormal test as a valuable prognostic tool.

The research duo wanted more information about the effects on the heart when a coronary artery was artificially occluded. So Wood and Wolferth went back to the animal laboratory and performed some of the first studies on the effects of lack of blood supply to the heart in living animals. Studying dogs and cats, they found that putting a clamp around a coronary artery and cutting off the blood supply completely but temporarily caused dramatic visible changes to the heart within fifteen seconds! Words failed them. They wrote, "The cardiac contraction changes character in a manner that defies description." They could see the muscle of the left ventricle change color, to the gray-dusky of "cyanosis" due to lack of oxygen. The heart would "dilate," increase in size, and then the heart would quiver—it would "fibrillate." But when they released the clamp, the heart recovered.

What they showed was that in the animal lab, completely occluding a coronary artery caused consistent EKG changes that could be reversed by releasing the occlusion or giving medication. The animal "model" was just that—important to explore but very different from the disease caused by slowly progressive coronary artery atherosclerosis. The disease in people was much more complex than creating an artificial problem with the heart's blood supply in healthy animals.

Wood and Wolferth had shown that physical exercise could indeed change the EKG signal in addition to often inducing angina. Even armed with their surprising new animal data and the discovery of new EKG abnormalities with exercise, they were still not satisfied with the statistical "sensitivity" of their exercise tests. In their very small study of thirty, only half of the people who had typical symptoms of angina had EKG changes that confirmed their "clinical" diagnosis of coronary artery disease. A fifty percent sensitivity is similar to guessing heads or tails when you flip a coin, odds not nearly good enough to predict disease. This kind of result is now called "hypothesis generating," interesting but raising more questions than answers.

The two Penn professors knew that much more study was needed before stress testing could be recommended for widespread use. Wood and Wolferth's concerns, however, did not put an end to the quest to use the EKG to diagnose coronary artery disease. Arthur M. Master MD (1895-1973) would push the research forward to confirm a diagnosis of this often-fatal disease.

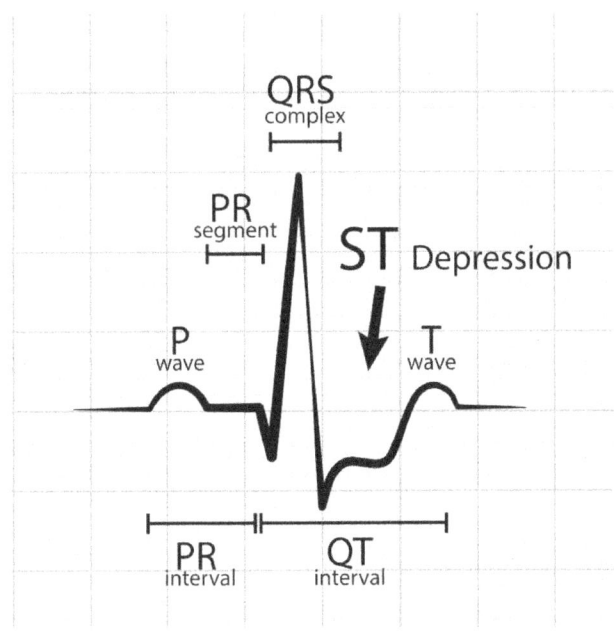

Figure 9. Typical "ST segment depression" of the EKG signal below the baseline electrical signal seen with exercise-induced lack of blood flow through the coronary arteries due to atherosclerosis—myocardial ischemia (Copyright Shutterstock)

Master, born in New York City and in 1921 receiving his MD degree from Cornell University, was interested in heart disease and was in the right place. As a medical student, he introduced himself to none other than the discoverer of his own EKG sign: Harold Pardee. Pardee suggested that Master meet with his colleague Bernard Oppenheimer MD (1876-1958), a leading cardiologist at The Mt. Sinai Hospital. Soon Master was traveling from Cornell to Mt. Sinai, spending two afternoons a week working in Oppenheimer's EKG lab.

In the 1920s, performing an EKG was a major endeavor. Later in life, Master wrote about those days, describing how a technician needed to push a large cart with the EKG equipment, including three-inch wide gauze bandages soaking in brine-filled jars to apply to the patient's arms and legs, the salt solution causing a major mess to the bedsheets that the nurses needed to change after the test. The machine was plugged into the wall electrical outlet and the signal sent electronically back to the laboratory, with Master using a speaker and a headset to communicate with the lab as the test was proceeding.

Knowing the right people was one of Masters' strengths. Soon he followed in Pardee's footsteps, completing advanced cardiology training in England with Einthoven's friend Sir Thomas Lewis. When he returned home to New York City, Master established his own private practice with an emphasis on cardiac disease and became an excellent and sought-after clinician. Fascinated by the electrical and mechanical function of the heart, he continued to work with Oppenheimer at Mt. Sinai. Together they pursued the work that Einthoven had started but did not live long enough to complete. The "EKG project" link had now gone from Einthoven in Holland, to Lewis in England, and to Pardee, Oppenheimer, and Master in America.

Analyzing what was known about stress tests in the late 1930s, Masters learned two important things: first, there was crystal-clear data proving that exercise could cause angina; secondly, the patient's chest pain correlated with the increase in heart rate and blood pressure caused by exertion. As impressive as these facts were, he still thought the science needed to take a step back.

Master knew that there just wasn't enough knowledge about the physiology of the normal heart subjected to exercise to make an accurate diagnosis. He wanted much more information than just the EKG findings. How many steps could a "normal" person, one without heart disease, do in a fixed amount of time? If patients with coronary disease could do less, how much less? Did the heart's capacity vary by age, weight, and sex? Was the information from the EKG alone really sufficient to make a diagnosis, or were other variables like blood pressure and heart rate also helpful? Did the EKG change in normals as well as those thought to have coronary artery disease? So much was unknown. Only when these questions were answered could a doctor really compare the performance of their patient during exercise to the normal standard and feel confident in a diagnosis of heart disease or not.

First, Master and Oppenheimer set out to "standardize" the capability of the normal heart. They wanted their patients to perform the exact same exercise protocol each time they were studied; they weren't going to swing their arms one time, and another time jump up and down. A simple wooden device would be the answer: two nine-inch-high steps. Master and Oppenheimer invented, not a new country line dance, but what came to be called the "Master Two-Step Test." The patients would just walk up the two steps and then down the two steps, over and over again, at first for ninety seconds and later for 180 seconds.

The electrocardiogram was not used in the initial studies but, rather, took a "backseat" to other information. The patients, 1,500 total from ages four to seventy-four, just exercised, and the heart rate and blood pressure were measured at rest, during, and after the test.[34] They organized the data into detailed tables of the normal work capacity of the heart, with variables including age, sex, and weight. Not surprisingly, cardiac "efficiency" decreased with age, and with weight gain, and could be improved by weight loss. By the mid-1930s, Master was ready to use his Two-Step Test on patients.

Master was convinced that his test was reliable and reproducible and could be used by any doctor willing to invest in a small wooden Two-Step platform for office use. With the information from the test, a doctor could determine whether or not heart disease was causing

---

34 Their study is an example of the meticulous science and work that is necessary to create a "breakthrough" discovery in medicine. It's hard to believe how these two fit this often-tedious work into their schedules, and they must have really charmed the parents of four-year-olds to participate in the studies.

significant impairment of the heart's function. The Master Two-Step Test could help answer the common question of patients receiving a cardiac diagnosis: "How much work can I do?" Master also noted, "At the other end of the clinical spectrum, it could help sort out patients with true cardiac disease from malingerers." But the bigger question was whether Wood and Wolferth were correct when they claimed that the exercise test EKG was not accurate enough to establish a definite diagnosis of coronary artery disease or even to determine that some patients with chest pain did not have atherosclerosis as the cause of their symptoms.

The avid researcher set out to answer those questions. He figured out a way to attach electrocardiogram leads securely to a patient hopping up and down on his wooden steps. Designing electrode leads that would not fall off during exercise and would also remain stable when the patient started to sweat was no minor feat. But with this engineering problem solved, Master could turn his attention to his major interest: patients with coronary artery disease, those with angina, and those who had had a myocardial infarction in the past. He was determined to see if his test could establish both a more definite diagnosis and prognosis for his patients.

Most significantly, Master knew an important fact: too much exercise done too quickly could cause changes in the EKG signal even in a normal heart. So he needed to "stress" his patients' hearts, gradually and in stages, first using ninety seconds of stepping and then later only 180 seconds. As the patient's workload increased, he saw the kind of EKG changes seen by Wood and Wolferth, and then, as predicted, he saw the tracing return to normal with rest after the exercise. The Cardiology "Oracles" were getting better at EKG interpretation.

By 1942, Master and his colleagues had enough patient studies, 201, to publish their results. He had five groups of patients: 1) normals without obvious heart disease, 2) those with angina and a normal EKG, 3) those with angina and an abnormal EKG at rest, 4) patients with a history of a coronary occlusion and a normal EKG, and 5) those with a history of a coronary occlusion and an abnormal EKG. Much to his relief, none of Master's normals developed abnormal EKG changes after exercise. This was a very important finding, as it meant that the test had a low "false positive" rate, that is becoming abnormal in people without disease, a misleading finding.

In patients with definite coronary artery disease, as best as could be determined at the time based on clinical judgment and the resting EKG, in the 136 cases who exercised for ninety seconds, fifty-nine were abnormal, forty-three percent. In the seventy-eight able to exercise a second time for 180 seconds, thirty-nine were abnormal, fifty percent. These were the "true positives," patients felt to have the disease because of their symptoms, and now also an abnormal EKG during the test. The highest sensitivity of the test for the four "disease" groups was in those with angina and abnormal resting electrocardiogram, sixty-seven percent.

From the perspective of 1942, these were remarkable results. In an era where a diagnosis of coronary artery disease had no objective basis other than clinical judgment, a resting EKG (often normal even in patients with significant disease) and an autopsy, the standardized Master Two-Step Test could both establish the diagnosis and also "rule it out," meaning being able to tell patients that their heart was fine and not the cause of their chest pain.

More importantly than even the EKG findings of the test, Arthur Master's work reaffirmed a fundamental principle of cardiac function: there was a link between exercise and the demand of the heart muscle for an increased blood supply and that about fifty percent of the time, patients with chest pain from coronary artery atherosclerosis developed an abnormal EKG reflecting "ischemia," an impaired blood supply. An abnormal test was proof that the disease described by Heberden and Herrick could be detected using objective data, not just the patient's descriptions of the symptoms.

As the Two-Step Test quickly was used more and more, the "law of large numbers" came into play. Casinos depend on just this kind of mathematics. If you think you have a "system" to "beat the house" playing Blackjack you may have great success playing one hundred hands, but if you play one thousand hands, your results for sure won't be as good. The game is just set up that way, unless you can count cards from multiple decks and risk getting tossed out of the casino. All medical tests, including a blood sample, an x-ray, or a stress test, will first surface in the medical literature when the researchers report their great initial results (otherwise few editors would publish the data). But there was a major bias problem in Master's test patients, all of whom had a very high chance of atherosclerosis before they were stressed. Their diagnosis was actually in little doubt as far their doctors were concerned.

The likelihood of an abnormal stress test in these first patients with chest pain should have been very high, but the growing number of investigators were going to study a much more varied group of patients, those with chest pain not typical for angina, and normal EKGs at rest. These people had a much lower incidence of true coronary artery disease. Their results were not going to be as good as Master's initial report, which even at best was only fifty percent accurate.

The greatness of Master's work was that it provided the foundation for further progress. A test with a much higher "sensitivity," the statistical term that indicates the percentage of time a test will reveal the presence of a disease, was needed. He succeeded in establishing that all of the aspects of exercise—the EKG, the amount of work performed, the patient's symptoms with exercise, and the blood pressure and heart rate response—provided information that held out hope for a challenging but exciting future for research into the diagnosis of the work of the Widowmaker.

MACHINES FOR EXERCISE

It would fall on the next generation of cardiologists to lift the diagnostic fog. Robert A. Bruce MD (1916-2004) was a New Englander who after his training was lured to the Pacific Northwest. In 1950, he became the first chairman of the cardiology division at the University of Washington in Seattle. Dr. Bruce had concerns with the Master's test. He felt it was cumbersome to use, and although it gave some insight into the physiology of the heart, it could not assess how the lungs functioned. He thought he had a better idea. He and his colleagues built a motorized device that could increase its speed and angle of walking in a predetermined way.

Bruce called his device a "treadmill."

Using his skills as a mechanical and electrical engineer, Bruce and his colleague Paul Yu first used their new equipment to assess the lung capacity of workers exposed to a lung toxin, beryllium. In 1949, they reported using a "staged" exercise test of three-minute increments, starting the treadmill off slowly and on a flat level and then increasing the speed and incline gradually. Patients exercised until they were fatigued, usually in less than ten minutes. Comparing these results to the results in normal people, they were able to determine which patients were severely disabled from beryllium-induced lung disease.

Bruce and his colleagues then looked to see if they could improve on Master's results in patients with chest pain. Early on, Bruce found one of the major reasons for the inaccuracy of the Master's protocol: the changes on the electrocardiogram with exercise were just too sensitive. The slightest shift in the EKG signal was viewed as abnormal, but many times, the alleged abnormality was just the random shift of the electrical signal from the heart to the machine while the patient was exercising.

What Bruce observed is a potential problem with all forms of medical testing. For example, early on in the use of CT scanning of the head, small scars on the brain were interpreted as signs of multiple sclerosis, the serious degenerative disease of the brain and spinal cord. But ultimately doctors learned that these changes were just "normal variants." Not everyone's head CT scan looks identical;

neither does their EKG at rest or with exercise, whether they have coronary artery disease or not.

By the late 1960s, Bruce was confident of his findings using new EKG change criteria for determining if coronary artery disease was present or not. In 1969, he compared the results of a study done by A.J. Brody in 1959 on patients without known heart disease, using the Master's criteria for an abnormal test, comparing the results using his new criteria for abnormal. In the Brody study of 756 men, 280 of the patients (thirty-seven percent) had very slight changes in the EKG or a cardiac arrhythmia with exercise that Master said was abnormal. Yet in four years of follow-up, only thirty-one (eleven percent) developed symptoms of coronary artery disease. Those who had a normal test by Master's criteria had more accurate results; only 4.2 percent of those people developed coronary artery disease. Overall, the results of the Brody study were distressing; thirty-five percent of the patients were misclassified as either having or not having coronary artery disease. These results were not even better than flipping a coin.

Bruce then evaluated similar patients, some with chest pain and others without cardiac symptoms, using his own criteria for abnormal. He looked at their EKGs for the ST segment depression, that dipping of the electrical signal below the baseline signal when the heart is at rest. He knew that the ST segment needed to be quite deeply depressed before one could conclude that the change was truly abnormal. Using the Bruce criteria, only twenty-three (three percent) of his 756 patients were abnormal, much lower than using Master's criteria. More importantly only 2.7 percent of the patients were misclassified.

Here was a hint of the problems that occur in "screening" a population containing patients without symptoms of heart disease. The likelihood of an abnormal test truly representing a disease depended upon the incidence of the disease in the group being studied. Men in their sixties with chest pain on exertion are going to have a much greater chance of having an abnormal stress test than a woman in her twenties with chest pain not consistent with angina.

Bruce and his Washington colleagues began to collect large amounts of data on thousands of patients, particularly those who were without symptoms of coronary artery disease, to see if stress testing in this group was a great value or not. The Seattle Heart Watch study began in 1971 and ended ten years later, following up over four thousand patients. Bruce was also the first to use computers to more accurately interpret the changes in the EKG with exercise, markedly decreasing the subjectivity involved in looking at small changes in the electrical signal.

What they found was that stress testing was only useful in people who had risk factors of coronary artery disease and not in those without. The implications of these results were significant, indicating that widespread screening of asymptomatic people was not helpful in predicting who would develop coronary artery disease, even in the midst of an epidemic of the disease. To diagnose lack of blood supply to the heart due to coronary artery atherosclerosis, you needed to "stress" the heart in gradual stages and stress the heart's demand for blood and oxygen by increasing the heart rate and the blood pressure. For sure in order to test the heart, you did need to take the pump out for a spin on the mechanical highway of the treadmill.

By the 1970s, stress testing was used widely to sort out whose symptoms were due to coronary artery disease or not. On the treadmill, some people would become short of breath, with no chest pain, or even more alarming have no outward symptoms at all as the EKG changed to expose the lethal potential of their disease. Data acquired from thousands of people indicated that simply being able to walk for more than five minutes using Dr. Bruce's protocol carried a good prognosis over the next several years. But more work and science were mandatory to crank up the accuracy statistics of the stress test. The desire for new images of the heart and its blood supply would take front and center to improve the diagnosis of the work of the Widowmaker before it was too late. The diagnostic fog was lifting, but the morning was still misty.

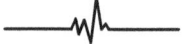

A LIFE-SAVING WALK

. . . His breathing slowed and the sweat stopped pouring out as he rested on the table under the nuclear camera imaging his heart's blood supply. I took a deep breath and began.

"Dr. Stein, you had very significant changes in the electrocardiogram just now. The ST segments dropped four millimeters from the baseline. I'm pretty sure you have coronary artery disease." I let that sink in before continuing. "You told me you hadn't had any symptoms, but are you sure?"

Dragging the words out of his mouth, he said, "Well, maybe a few times I have had some chest pressure when I exercise, but it went away quickly when I rested."

I pressed him further. "Did you feel that today, that chest pressure?"

"Well, just a little, but it was there and now it's gone."

I sighed. "I don't need to tell you what this means. I think we need to look into this further. You need a cardiac catheterization."

My friend had his cardiac catheterization two days later. The doctor in his sixties, and in apparent wonderful health, had severe blockages of all three of his largest coronary arteries. In another two days, he underwent successful coronary artery bypass surgery and was back at work full time in eight weeks.

The stress test saved his life, and he was another fortunate human who escaped the grasp of the Widowmaker. The work of eighty-five years, from Willem Einthoven's invention of the electrocardiogram in 1905, and the groundbreaking work of medical scientists Francis Wood and Charles Wolferth, Arthur Master and Bernard Oppenheimer, and Robert Bruce and his colleagues allowed me to rescue my mentor. As diviners of the heart signal, they were the true Oracles of Cardiology, able to diagnose the present and foresee the future.

As the first Oracles did their work in the 1930s, they were unaware that a breakthrough that would change the face of cardiology forever had already occurred, work that would remain obscured for years by the arrogance of his mentors and the horrors of the Second World War.

CHAPTER 7

DESTROYING THE FIRST SHIBBOLETH: THE PREMIER HEART CATHETERIZATION

*The correct path to find me often lies hidden
inside the beating heart.
But how to get at it?*

*For if the heart is cold, so too is the trail. And without the right skill,
it only takes the slightest of touches
to do my job for me.*

A VIRGIN'S FIRST RIGHT HEART CATHETERIZATION—SUMMER 1979

"Looks good. The third time *was* the charm," said Dr. Stan Lewis when the procedure was over. He was just a year ahead of me in cardiology fellowship training. When you're in training, the best teachers are often those who have barely twelve more months of experience than you do.

I had just successfully inserted a piece of plastic into a woman's heart to obtain detailed information that would help save her life.

Less than a decade earlier, this procedure was unimaginable. How it came to be is even more so. Long-held iconic beliefs—shibboleths—are difficult to conquer ...

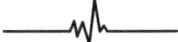

HOW TO DO YOUR OWN HEART CATHETERIZATION
A PRIMER BY WERNER FORSSMANN MD

> The Laws of Arthur C. Clarke (1917-2008),
> noted science fiction writer:

FIRST LAW: When a distinguished, but elderly scientist states that something is possible, he is almost certainly right. When he states that something is impossible, he is very probably wrong.

SECOND LAW: The only way of discovering the limits of the possible is to venture a little way past them into the impossible.

THIRD LAW: Any sufficiently advanced technology is indistinguishable from magic.

Despite being an unlikely candidate for medical greatness, Werner Forssmann MD (1904-1979) was about to perform an impossible magic trick. Born to a middle-class, supportive family, Forssmann loved his uncle Walter, a country doctor, who had stepped in as a role model after the boy's father was killed in World War I. As graduation from medical school approached in 1921, Forssmann decided he wanted to pursue residency training in internal medicine but was turned down everywhere he applied. Through a family connection, he was able to gain a spot in a surgery training program at the Auguste Viktoria House, a hospital not in the pantheon of great German medical training institutions.

Forssmann was obsessed with the human heart, the lack of knowledge about its true function, and the challenges to treating it. He wondered about the heart's physiology after someone suffered a heart attack or had a heart valve problem but was also aware of how difficult it would be to research it. Specifically, Forssmann knew the prohibition in Latin, handed down from generations of surgeons to all young trainees: *"Noli me tangere,"* meaning "Don't cling to me," written in the Gospel of John as the words of Jesus when Mary Magdalene recognized Him after the resurrection. The medical variant of this phrase was, "Don't touch the heart," because your patient will die almost immediately if you do. Therefore, trying to repair a damaged heart, such as in the case of trauma to the chest, was a futile effort. Performing surgery on a beating heart meant death would come quickly either from uncontrollable bleeding or a sudden irreversible "quivering" of the heart muscle, ventricular fibrillation. *Noli me tangere* was a sacred teaching never to be violated.

But young Dr. Forssmann wasn't so sure about that. He knew that French physiologists in the nineteenth century had placed tubes inside the hearts of horses and as a result gained important knowledge about blood pressure and how the heart worked. He wondered how the animals' hearts tolerated those experiments, and, he reasoned, horses being mammals just like humans, couldn't humans be studied as well?

Forssmann sought to find out. He read the works of Claude Bernard MD (1813-1878), the veterinarian Auguste Chauveau (1827-1914) and Etienee-Jules Marey (1830-1904), who were all able to measure the pressure inside the right side of the animal hearts. He was "haunted day and night" by an image he had seen in a textbook of Marey's experiment with a horse, where a man was holding a tube that he had inserted into the jugular vein of the neck of the horse. The tube was pushed into the right side of the heart, the right ventricle, allowing Marey to record a pressure curve on a graph depicting what was occurring in the ventricle. Forssmann was intrigued with this signal from within, the same principle Einthoven used with his electrocardiogram, but now, to his wild amazement, the pressure signal provided "in real time" information obtained from a *living* animal. So much for "*noli me tangere*," at least where horses were concerned.

Emboldened with this data, Forssmann devised a plan to record this internal pressure signal in living people. Step-by-step, he considered his options. He did not want to put a tube in a human being's jugular vein because no one would agree to a neck incision that would leave a large scar. Instead, he thought, he could use a vein around the elbow, one easy to find and dissect out. But what kind of tube could he use to insert into the vein? There were catheters that urologists used to place inside the bladder through the urethra, the small short tube in women and the longer one in men through the penis. One of them might work. Finally, and most importantly, where could he find a patient for this first-one-of-its-kind experiment?

By the summer of 1929, Forssmann felt he had worked out the details as best he could and was ready to try out his idea. Working up his courage, he presented his proposal to his boss, Dr. Richard Schneider. Schneider listened politely and then categorically said no. The risks were far too great to let him do his experiment on a research volunteer. Forssmann then asked if he could do the experiment on himself. Schnieder could not believe what he was hearing. What would he tell the young man's mother if her son died in his hospital trying to put a catheter in his own heart? Schneider left no doubt about his decision.

Undeterred, Forssmann somehow convinced a nurse, Greta Ditzen, that she should be his subject for this experiment. On the chosen day, she was available to help him and there were no afternoon cases scheduled, leaving an empty private surgical theater. Ditzen arranged all of the necessary equipment and sat down on an operating table, holding out her left arm. Forssmann asked her to lie down, explaining that sometimes the local anesthetic he planned to inject under her skin could make people dizzy. She agreed, and

Forssmann strapped her legs and hands tightly to the table, putting the operating instruments behind her head so she couldn't see him.

And then Forssmann began to work not on her, but on himself!

The young surgeon took the needle and inserted it into the bottle of anesthetic, drawing out one cc of the clear liquid. Then he watched as the needle disappeared under the skin of his left arm just above the elbow. He pushed the plunger down slowly, injecting the medicine. The expected numbness set in quickly. Forssmann then took the surgical blade he had carefully laid out on the cart and cut into his skin, immune to the sight of his own blood coming out of the wound. Next he located the large vein he was looking for, expertly sliced it open, and pushed the urethral catheter into his vein, advancing it about one foot. He took a look at his work and was pleased; the procedure thus far had only taken a few minutes.

Forssmann packed the surgical site with gauze and with his right hand released Nurse Ditzen from her restraints. He said proudly, "There we are, it's ready now. Please call the x-ray nurse." She spun around and looked aghast when she saw Dr. Werner with a urethral catheter hanging out of his left arm! Ditzen did her best to recover her professional composure and called to alert the x-ray nurse. The new co-conspirators ran quickly down the hall to the x-ray department and demanded that she perform a chest x-ray immediately.

After pushing the catheter in further to actually reach the heart, Werner ordered the stunned x-ray nurse to do her job; the image she produced would reverberate through medical history. Here was a photo of a catheter inside of the right side of a human heart, and *unbelievably*, the heart's owner was not lying dead on the cold hospital floor. He got up and was walking, talking, and thrilled by the experience! Forssmann had performed the first human cardiac catheterization, on himself, and the news spread like a tsunami throughout the small hospital.

Next came a meeting with Dr. Schneider where he accused Forssmann of betraying his trust, but fortunately the senior doctor also realized the importance of what his young trainee had just accomplished, congratulated him, and insisted that he immediately write up a report of his experiment for publication. He warned Forssmann, however, not to discuss the experiment with anyone outside of the hospital until his report was published, lest they try to steal his idea. Schneider helped Werner write his paper, and two weeks later, they shipped the text plus the x-ray images to the editors of *Klinische Wochenshrift*, the most prestigious German medical publication of its time. The article entitled "Probing the Right Side of the Heart" was accepted and scheduled to appear in the journal on November 5, 1929.

After a brief and tumultuous hiatus at a much larger Berlin hospital,[35] Forsmann returned to August Viktoria House and was allowed by Schneider to perform additional studies and have much freer rein. Still passionate about his research, he made his first attempts to use his heart probe to inject x-ray contrast dye into the circulation. He captured the images of the heart and the large surrounding blood vessels, images never recorded before using x-ray. He also catheterized his own heart *nine* more times. Perhaps author Oscar Levant was referring to people like Forssmann and himself when he wrote, "There is a fine line between genius and insanity. I have erased that line."

Forssmann's experiments led to several more publications on "angiocardiography," a brand-new imaging technique of the heart and blood vessels using x-ray contrast dye, and Forssmann may have continued on this path if it had not been for the ire his work had produced. In his autobiography *Experiments on Myself: Memoirs of a Surgeon in Germany*, Werner Forssmann sums up his failure to advance his research at that time:

---

35   An account of Forsmann's conflicted time with the Chief of Surgery at Charite Hospital in Berlin, Ferdinand Sauerbruch MD, is a key example of how research and medical advancement can be stalled by conflicting interests and personalities.

"For a doctor in the twenties and thirties the heart was not just an organ like any other. Subconsciously he still clung to the ancient mystical idea of the heart as the center of life. As late as the 1890s, Theodor Billroth MD (1829-1894),[36] having pioneered stomach surgery, announced that surgery could now go no further. He thought it would be criminal to touch the heart. So I had committed the cardinal sin; I had broken into the sanctuary and wantonly destroyed a taboo. So it seemed to many of my contemporaries, and they hated me for it."

Even though he was shunned by the German medical community, not everyone ignored Forssmann's work. Andre Cournand MD (1895-1988) was a French immigrant who became a lung specialist at Columbia-Presbyterian Hospital in New York City, where he met another young pulmonologist, Dickinson W. Richards MD (1895-1973). They both believed that understanding the "pulmonary circulation," the manner in which blood flows from the veins into the right side of the heart and then the lungs, would give a clue about the effects of lung diseases, especially tuberculosis. Almost nothing was known about this neglected portion of the circulation.

Cournard and Richards thought that if an obscure German surgery trainee was able to put a ureteral catheter into the right side of the heart, then certainly trained pulmonologists could do it. They improved on the methodology, using pressure monitor catheters developed by engineers instead of urinary catheters, and in 1941, they published their first article on the pulmonary circulation based on information obtained from a catheter.

The two Columbia lung specialists opened the door again for new research, not only into lung diseases, but also heart diseases. Patients with poor heart function were often severely short of breath, and now

---

36 Billroth was a world-renowned German surgeon of the nineteenth century.

the new procedure, cardiac catheterization, gathered a wealth of new information about both the physiology of the lungs and the heart and how medication could affect the way the heart performed. Surgery became available for diseases of the heart valves and congenital heart disease. While laudable, surgery to repair the Widowmaker's work was still unimaginable.

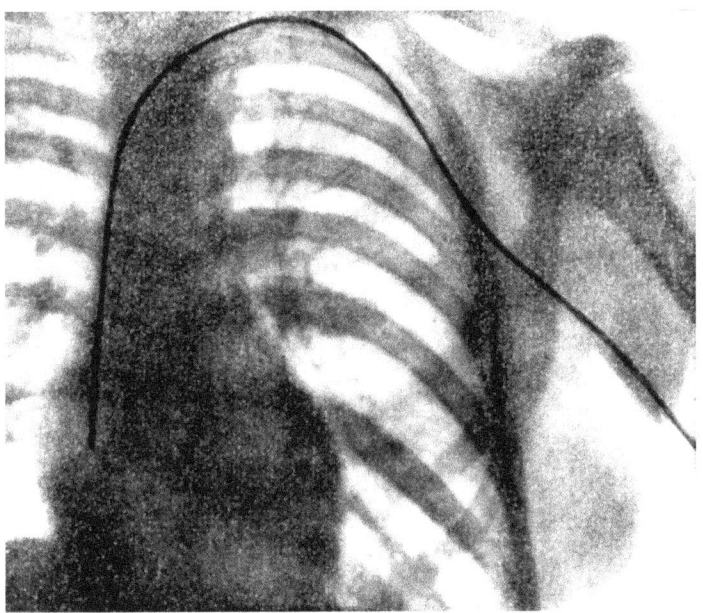

Figure 10. World-shaking chest x-ray demonstrating urethral catheter inserted into the right side of the heart by Werner Forssmann MD, October 1929. (Copyright Alamy)

FAME FROM OUT OF NOWHERE

Werner Forssmann was unaware of the scientific developments stemming from his self-experiment in 1929. Despite his passion for cardiac research, he had resigned himself to living a good but quiet life in obscurity. Then, one day in 1950, a pediatrician friend of Werner's told him that he was sending young patients with congenital heart disease to a clinic in Basel, Switzerland. He told Forssmann that this clinic was using heart catheters to diagnose and treat these children.

In fact, one of the doctors in Basel had referred to Werner as "the father of the whole thing." His friend insisted that Forssmann travel to Basel to see what they were doing there.

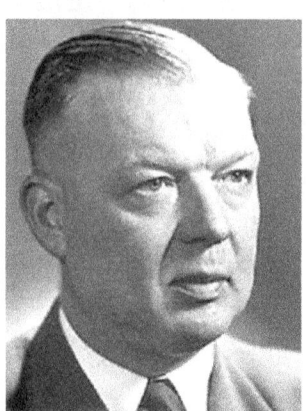

Figure 11. Werner Forssmann MD (1904-1979), Nobel Prize winner 1956 (Courtesy of cardiacathletes.com)

Forssmann did travel to Switzerland, and his fame gradually increased. In February 1951, Professor Dr. John McMichael (1904-1993), the "Father" of English cardiac catheterization, invited Forssmann to London to participate in the production of a documentary film about cardiac catheterization. Five years later, he was even more surprised to learn that the world's most prestigious scientific organization was aware of Forssmann's landmark work. On October 12, 1956, he received a telephone call from the Nobel Prize committee in Sweden announcing that he, along with Andre Cournand and Dickinson Richards, would receive the Nobel Prize for Medicine.

After his trip to Sweden, Forssmann returned to practicing medicine and surgery and spending time with family. He published his autobiography in 1974 and died of complications of congestive heart failure in 1979.

The essence of research in any field is to thoughtfully explore new ideas but to use some logical previously known basis for the new concept. Many ideas will still turn out to be wrong. Forssmann's work was thoughtful and based on previous animal experiments. His ideas were not wrong, led to more and more groundbreaking work, and eventually treatment for the work of the Widowmaker. Cardiology without cardiac catheterization is not cardiology.

OPENING MORE DOORS: PROBES OF THE LEFT SIDE OF THE HEART

In the late 1940s, there were still uncharted areas of the heart and its circulation. The three Nobel Prize winners of 1956 had explored the right side of the heart, but the left side of the heart remained a mystery. This left side, the heart's "business end," holds the chamber that pumps the blood to the rest of the body. The left ventricle, the largest and thickest heart chamber, was, in particular, poorly understood. The tiny tubes that run along its surface and provide its blood and oxygen, the coronary arteries, could not be seen or studied in a living person. Despite the enormous progress in cardiac medicine, knowledge about the coronary arteries that cause angina pectoris and myocardial infarction had not changed much since the eighteenth century.

In 1950, Drs. Henry Zimmerman, Roy W. Scott, and Norman Becker of Case Western Reserve University in Cleveland ventured into this unmapped area. They placed a catheter not inside of a vein, but an artery in the arm. They pushed the tube against the force of blood coming into the artery from the heart, through the artery of the upper arm, into the chest, and then into the heart, into the *left* ventricle. This had never been done before. And the patient survived!

The procedure was even more daring than it seems. To get the tube into the left ventricle, Zimmerman and his colleagues also needed perfect timing to advance the catheter past the leaflets of the aortic valve at the top of the ventricle. These leaflets open and close with each heartbeat. Pushing a stiff catheter against closed leaflets could severely damage them. Great hand-eye coordination, in addition to timing, was needed. They had just a second to safely pass the catheter past the valves as they opened. Imagine trying to capture that perfect photograph of your dog or one of your children—the "crucial moment" is so brief!

The three investigators thought carefully about what type of patients to enroll in their upcoming study. In the late 1940s, before the widespread use of penicillin, there were still unfortunate patients suffering from advanced syphilis, the destructive venereal disease affecting many organs of the body. The aorta and its valve were often victims of the long-term onslaught of syphilis. The damage from syphilis to the wall of the aorta made it increase in size and the damage to the valves made them leak when they were supposed to close up tightly after the left ventricle ejected blood into the aorta with each heartbeat. Unfortunate as this condition was, it was the perfect situation to try to push a plastic tube from the aorta into the heart's left ventricle, because in these patients the aortic valve leaflets were always partially open enough to allow a small catheter to slide by them.

The Cleveland team was successful; ten of the eleven patients they studied survived the procedure easily. Zimmerman and his colleagues proved that the left heart was now no longer "off-limits." Another destroyed shibboleth entered the history books. More and more cardiologists joined the chase in their newly constructed cardiac catheterization "laboratories" to gather exciting new information about how the left ventricle functioned, both normally and in patients with diseases of the heart muscle, heart valves, and most importantly, the coronary arteries plagued by atherosclerosis.

What Werner Forssmann began was not finished, however. Cardiac catheterization still had one more crucial unexplored area of the heart's anatomy to try to image: those pesky small coronary arteries running along the surface of the heart. These were the tubes that were actually getting blocked up with plaque and causing the epidemic of death from heart attacks. Images of where those blockages were located in the coronary arteries, and how severe they were, would be crucial information for possible treatment and prognosis.

There were very strong convictions in the 1950s that still relegated the heart's own arteries to unchartered territory. These little "tubes" of blood vessels are less than an eighth of an inch wide, half the size of a drinking straw. No engineer could design a catheter smaller than that, and if you tried to put one of those firm plastic tubes into the entry point, the orifice of a coronary artery, you would probably tear the artery, a disaster that would likely instantly cut off the blood flow and create a heart attack. Even if a catheter could "engage" the opening, if you then injected contrast dye to take a picture, the dye itself would replace the blood and deprive the heart of oxygen in a flash. The heart would likely fibrillate and then stop beating altogether.

But in 1958, an accident in the cardiac catheterization laboratory at the Cleveland Clinic spurred the imagination of a courageous doctor who seized the opportunity that luck had presented to him. F. Mason Sones Jr. MD would prove that the prohibitions against imaging of the coronary arteries with contrast dye were ideas that also needed to be discarded, like many other concepts of the past.

Discovery and then more discovery is not a smooth path; it proceeds in fits and stops, and unpredictably. It can follow many false paths, but persistence and the willingness to fail and try again is its history. In his Nobel lecture in December 1956, Forssmann summed up very well his own contribution, an observation that applies to most human exploration of the unknown: "Thus we guard ourselves against the mistake which runs all through the history of medicine: that of concentrating dogmatically upon first one, then another facet of research, instead of standing back to view this whole as a growing entity."

The research would expand dramatically after the rest of the medical world discovered Werner Forssmann's first self-experiment. But it would still take decades until treatment and prevention of the work of the Widowmaker would yield fruit. Forssmann was almost certainly not aware that answers were coming from small town America, new tools, bold surgery, and medications he knew nothing about.

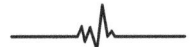

THE CATHETER TO HELP SAVE A LIFE

. . . The woman before me had come into the hospital with severe chest pain and shortness of breath due to another heart attack. Her chest x-ray showed lungs full of water, pulmonary edema, and the electrocardiogram and blood tests confirmed the myocardial infarction. The damage was done, but would we be able to help her survive?

We needed a key piece of information: what was the pressure inside of her heart? When a heart attack damages the left ventricle, pressure builds up inside of it, pushes a pressure wave back into the left atrium, and then into the lungs, causing a leak of fluid. What was the number of that pressure? The range of normal was well known, and that number would guide her treatment. Too high meant she needed more diuretics to increase her urine output and drop the pressure inside of the heart; too low and she needed more intravenous fluid to increase the pressure. We also wanted to know how much blood her heart was pumping each minute, the "cardiac output." Maybe she needed medication to increase that number.

By the mid-1970s, there was a bedside procedure that answers these questions: placing a catheter to measure the pressure inside of the right side of this patient's heart, not the left side, where the most important datum lies. This was my job, and I had never done one. I needed a guide; that was Dr. Lewis' job.

The access point to the heart for the catheter was the large vein in the upper chest, the subclavian vein. Once I put the thin pressure monitor embedded in the catheter inside of that vein, I would push it forward and it would "float" through the circulation into the right side of the heart, finally into a position where it could measure the pressure of the left side of the heart.

But how was that even possible? The blood vessels leaving the right side of the heart and entering the lung to obtain oxygen get smaller and smaller and then just end. The oxygen transfer to get blood to the other side of the body, by pumping it out of the left side of the heart, happens between the tiniest of blood vessels. How could a plastic tube, a catheter, measure a pressure in such a small area, and what would it mean anyway?

This was the audacious goal, the idea that by pushing a catheter from the right side of the heart into the small blood vessels of the lung, I could measure pressure inside of the left side, not the right side of the heart. The whole concept was counterintuitive. But it turns out that the pressure reading from those tiny lung blood vessels is almost exactly the same as the pressure reading in the left side of the heart!

Stan and I gathered the necessary equipment and went to work. I put the patient in the proper position to maximize the chance that the needle would hit the subclavian vein under the collarbone. After numbing the skin well, I took a deep breath and pushed a large needle into the skin, hoping to strike the vein. This was a "blind stick." I couldn't see the vein but knew where it was supposed to be. I pulled back on the syringe attached to the needle, looking for that flashback of dark blood that would signal I was in the right spot. I still hadn't exhaled.

I knew I would only get a few tries, and my first puncture was a "swing and a miss." Strike one. I glanced at Stan, who didn't say anything but his eyes above his mask said, "What do you want from me? Try again." I finally needed to empty my lungs, took another deep breath, and tried again. Strike two—no blood flashback. The unwritten rule was that the younger person got only three tries; then the senior person would take over. I shifted the position of the woman's collarbone just a bit, thinking that a subtle change in the angle of inserting the needle might work. One last quick thrust of the needle and another breath held on my part. I drew the syringe back slowly, and there it was, a beautiful dark blood from the vein, quickly filling the syringe as I pulled back. My breathing normalized.

The rest of the procedure went easily. As the catheter passed from the vein into the chambers of the right heart, I could see the pressure tracings that I had memorized change so nicely, telling me that the catheter was headed in the right direction. The catheter pressure "waveform" told me when it entered the pulmonary artery. I advanced the catheter just a few more centimeters, watched the waveform closely, and then slowly inflated the balloon on the end of the catheter, using less than one cc of air. It was time to hold my breath again.

As soon I inflated the balloon, the waveform changed again— the catheter was "wedged" into a very small pulmonary artery, transmitting back the actual pressure inside of the left side of this patient's heart. And the pressure was too high. Now the CCU team could measure the pressure any time they wanted by inflating the balloon as I had done earlier. They knew she needed more diuretic medicine to "whip" her kidneys to eliminate the fluid. We measured her heart's output of blood, and it was just slightly low but acceptable.

Stan and I saw her for a few days more, and her breathing improved. The lung water dissipated, allowing her to be removed from the ventilator, and she went on to an uneventful recovery. She had survived her heart attack.

I knew about the value of catheterization of the right heart; now I saw its utility directly. I also knew that the catheter I used was invented by two cardiologists from California: Drs. Swan and Ganz. But Werner Forssmann? I had never heard of the man. Soon I would learn about another dynamic group of people who would do more than anyone else to label the work of the Widowmaker for the epidemic it had become.

CHAPTER 8

TRACKING AN EPIDEMIC: THE FRAMINGHAM HEART STUDY

If you want to know one of the keys to my success, it is isolation. Each case, each doctor, alone stabbing at a solution that is often guesswork. There is no power in these numbers, no army of information to assault me.

It is this lack of cohesion that I count on.

NO SURPRISE

Mr. D was a self-proclaimed "guy's guy," a rough and tumble person who liked to party, travel, ski, and hit the beach. He had a solid job and felt pretty invincible. He had only come to see a cardiologist because his family doctor was worried about him, since Mr. D had suffered a heart attack and now two weeks later was recovering.

I was glad he came to see me. In my office, his blood pressure was 180/110, quite elevated, and his recent lab tests showed that he had a very high cholesterol. He loved to smoke and considered exercise a colossal waste of time. To make matters worse, he had uncontrolled diabetes, a problem he had ignored for several years. Mr. D was just short of fifty years old. For many, the first fifty years is a free pass to do pretty much anything we want, except use illegal drugs and drink too much alcohol, without experiencing serious consequences. After that, we often receive a loud and clear message that we need to change our ways. Mr. D had received his message. Would he listen? I had my doubts.

I was not surprised to learn about his recent heart attack. A research study conducted decades earlier in a small town outside of Boston had given me the necessary clues.

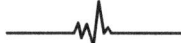

CAN SCIENCE DEAL WITH EPIDEMICS?

In 1948, forty-four percent of all deaths in the US were due to cardiovascular disease, a twenty percent increase in just eight years. By 1950, predictive models estimated thirty-three percent of American men would develop cardiovascular disease before the age of sixty. Its prevalence would be twice that of cancer. Some of the best minds had been studying the disease for centuries but still could not figure out what was causing so much death and disability. It was time to look at the problem from an entirely new perspective.

Surprisingly, this would require looking back almost a hundred years: the science of epidemiology was about to be discovered in a water pump.

London, England, 1854

Just like the previous outbreaks, the latest deadly cholera flare-up was unexpected. John Snow MD (1813-1858), a London gynecologist, had lived through these epidemics before. When another one hit Soho, a suburb of London, in August of 1854, Snow was determined to prove his theory that there was evil in the water supply. He searched through the hospital and public records of the people who died from cholera. His meticulous sleuthing paid off. The surprising data were clear—he found five hundred fatal cases of cholera reported within 250 yards of a community gathering spot where Cambridge Street joins Broad Street. At the center of that spot? The community water pump. Snow didn't know the exact culprit, but he was sure that something in the water was killing people. He was ahead of his time with his suspicion; the idea that waterborne microscopic organisms caused disease was yet to be discovered. By forcing the pump's closure and stopping the epidemic, Snow had simultaneously saved the day[37] and created the field of epidemiology.

Fast forward to the middle of the twentieth century when medicine had changed dramatically in two important ways. First, the post–World War II scientific and technical advances such as the development of antibiotics and a new understanding of gene function and protein structure combined to drastically improve the practice of medicine. But while progress had also been made in the field of cardiology, unfortunately, heart disease was still like a plague, slower in its attack rate but just as deadly.

In 1945, however, heart disease and stroke began making headlines. The wartime President of the United States, Franklin D. Roosevelt, had a long history of very high blood pressure, congestive heart failure, and hypertension, a disease for which his personal physician could only prescribe a sedative. Roosevelt's personal physician, Admiral Ross McIntyre MD, an ear, nose, and throat specialist, declared that the President's blood pressure was "no more than normal for a man of his age." The President died from a cerebral hemorrhage, a form of stroke, in April 1945. Roosevelt's death spurred great concern about disease of the heart and blood vessels, and the health of the United States entered into politics. This is when another dramatic change occurred in medicine: the introduction of social medicine, using science to determine the causes and treatment of the most common disease of an entire population, not just one unique patient.

---

37   Modern science has now taught us that a microorganism known appropriately as *Vibrio cholerae* causes cholera.

The experts knew that the onslaught of heart disease could not wait any longer to be addressed. If a national health system was politically untenable,[38] could research, divorced from politics, lead the way to a better understanding of heart disease? A determined woman would pave the way for the science of epidemiology to find the answers.

A ZEALOT ARISES

"You can solve any problem if you have money, people, and equipment," she would say. Born in Watertown, Wisconsin, Mary Woodard Lasker (1900-1994) led a middle-class American childhood, but disease stalked her family. Mary suffered from chronic ear infections, and both of her parents had hypertension. Her mother and father died from strokes when Mary was in her thirties.

In 1938, Mary found her calling for medical advocacy. She first became the secretary of the Birth Control Federation[39] and then in 1940 married Albert Davis Lasker (1880-1952), a man equally committed to using basic research to change the future of medicine. Together they established the Albert and Mary Lasker Foundation in 1942 and began awarding prestigious prizes for basic and clinical research, as well as medical journalism. Fortunately for those pursuing the Widowmaker, Mary's focus was clear: "I am opposed to heart attacks and cancer and strokes the way I am opposed to sin."

In 1944, the Congress of the United States passed the Public Health Act, which expanded the role of the Public Health Service and Congress to provide grant money for any field related to public

---

38 Harry Truman, Roosevelt's successor, advocated for a national health system, but it was labeled as a "communist act."
39 Later to become The Planned Parenthood Federation.

health.[40] Before his untimely death, President Roosevelt wrote, "In establishing a national program of war and postwar prevention, we will be making as sound an investment as any government can make; the dividends are payable in human life and health." Seeing an opening, Mary Lasker leveraged this new government interest in public health. She recruited many other women to converge on Washington and Capitol Hill, badgering the powerful to expand funding for the crucial areas of research: heart disease and cancer. In a typical male chauvinistic saying of the times, her group of lobbyists was referred to as "Mary and her little lambs."

But the constant pressure worked. In 1948, Congress passed the National Heart Act, a bill that allowed the National Institutes of Health to establish a specific branch devoted to the study of heart disease.[41] Mary Lasker left a great legacy and advanced the study of heart disease in immeasurable ways.[42]

THE HEART PROBLEM TAKES CENTER STAGE

By the late 1940s, the political milieu shifted due to the convergence of three societal changes: a new enthusiasm for far-reaching medical

---

40   The origins of the state's role in public health were modest. In 1798, a Marine Hospital Service was established to care for merchant marine sailors. Its purpose was to investigate possible transmission of infectious diseases from sailors returning from abroad to the general population and to use quarantine procedures if necessary. The name of the agency was converted to the United States Public Health Service. In 1889, President Grover Cleveland signed a bill creating the Service into a military branch under the direction of a "Supervising Surgeon," later known as the "Surgeon General."
41   Funding for the National Institutes of Health grew rapidly, and a clinical center, renamed the Warren Grant Magnuson Clinical Center in 1980, was built in Bethesda, Maryland. Further funding for heart disease research came in 1972 when the National Heart, Blood Vessel, Lung and Blood Act was passed, expanding the role of the National Institute of Health (NIH) in cardiovascular research. At last count, research from the NIH has yielded eighty Nobel Prizes, and more are certain in the future. As of 2019, the NIH had a budget of $39 billion, covers three hundred acres of land, has seventy-five buildings, and over twenty thousand employees, including six thousand scientists.
42   Mary Lasker died in 1994 at age ninety-three and left $10 million to the Lasker Foundation, an organization that still thrives. The Foundation supports young scientists with early career grants and offers a series of lectures and internships. The Lasker Prize is America's equivalent of a Nobel Prize in Science.

research, the acceptance of using taxpayer money to pay for it, and the further refinement of the science of epidemiology. Out of this arose the idea that it was time to conduct a major research study to uncover the causes of the cardiovascular disease epidemic.

Enter Joseph Walter Mountin MD (1891-1952), a revolutionary thinker in epidemiology whose interest in the field was sparked early and often. Joseph was exposed to the horrors of untreatable infectious disease as a toddler when he and his brother both contracted diphtheria. Joseph survived, but his brother did not. Mountin went on to receive his MD degree from Marquette University in Milwaukee in 1914. During World War II, malaria epidemics were widespread in American forces training in the southern states and then fighting in tropical islands in the Pacific Ocean. Mountin worked to implement preventive measures, directing the Malaria Control in War Areas division of the Public Health Service.

Mountin believed that the same tactics used to study and control infections could be used to discover the causes and prevention of heart disease. He was convinced that atherosclerosis was *not just due to aging* but that there were other factors at play. When the National Health Act established a $500,000 grant for a long-term epidemiology study of heart disease in 1947, Mountin saw his opportunity. He delegated the project development of this idea to a young physician named Gilcin Meadors MD (1915-1988). Meadors began his work to "study the expression of coronary artery disease in a 'normal' or unselected population and to determine the factors predisposing to the development of the disease through clinical and laboratory exam and long-term follow-up." It was a tall, complex order.

One of the biggest hurdles was finding a place to conduct the trial. Suggestions poured in. The strongest one came from a prestigious source: Harvard Medical School. Paul Dudley White MD (1886-1973), the pre-eminent cardiologist of his time, and his colleague David Rutstein MD (1909-1986), Harvard's Chair of the Department of Public Health, believed they knew the perfect spot.

A "TYPICAL" AMERICAN TOWN: THE 1940S IN FRAMINGHAM, MASSACHUSETTS

Just twenty miles west of Boston lies Framingham, Massachusetts, a town that held great promise for more reasons than one. In the 1940s, it was a very stable town of twenty-eight thousand people, overwhelmingly Caucasians of European origin, boasting successful industries and commercial businesses, including a General Motors automobile plant. More importantly to White and Rutstein, the town had two good hospitals and was geographically close to the cardiologists at Harvard. White and Rutstein realized the study's academic research potential, and they wanted to be involved. They argued that Framingham's population accurately represented American society at the time. Convinced, Meadors turned his attention to the real work of smoothly navigating the local political waters of this small town.

How could he best enroll the local residents and doctors of Framingham in the project? Meadors had one big advantage: the town had participated in a six-year epidemiology study of tuberculosis between 1917 and 1923. He wondered, "Twenty years later, would the doctors of the town view the study as interfering with their patient interactions or would they see it as a chance to participate in something grand?" Meadors met with the people of Framingham and talked to the Massachusetts Medical Society. He assured the doctors that the examination every two years would not jeopardize their doctor-patient relationships nor their incomes. Meadors was pleasantly surprised that Framingham's lone cardiologist agreed to help and that the younger physicians in town expressed great interest in the project. He had the buy-in he needed to proceed.

Next, Meadors and his colleagues debated research methodology. Should the study emphasize *preventing* heart disease or just be an *observational* study, i.e. letting the natural history of cardiac disease evolve over time while the participants received their usual medical care from their own doctors? Meadors realized that epidemiology, at its core, is a natural history acquisition process, not one that offers treatment, prevention, or even a fundamental physiologic and biochemical understanding of the causes of disease. John Snow in the 1850s did not understand what really caused cholera, but he figured out where it was coming from and then how to stop and prevent it. Meadors decided The Heart Epidemiology Study, later known as the Framingham Heart Study (FHS), would have the same goals about heart disease.

Meadors also knew that he had to be very clear about exactly what areas of heart disease he would study. Of course the first would target atherosclerosis of the coronary arteries and its two manifestations—chest pain i.e. angina pectoris, and heart attack, a myocardial infarction. But there was a second focus—hypertension. He wanted to uncover the relationship of high blood pressure to stroke, heart attacks, and congestive heart disease.

After meetings with an advisory committee of specialists from many areas of medicine, the Framingham investigators came away with hypotheses and data that needed to be gathered over the next twenty years. It was a long, ambitious list that included factors that might have a relationship with heart disease: increasing age, male sex, hypertension, high blood cholesterol levels, tobacco smoking, habitual use of alcohol, high body weight, a high level of hemoglobin in the blood, diabetes mellitus, and finally, gout, a disease of the joints due to high blood levels of uric acid. They also decided to gather information on two factors that might lower the risk of heart disease, including increased levels of physical exercise and high levels of thyroid hormone in the blood.

The study's goal was to enroll six thousand local residents, and on October 11, 1948, the researchers enrolled their first study volunteer. From 1948 to early 1950, nearly all the volunteers were twenty to seventy years of age. Each underwent an initial examination including a history, physical exam, an electrocardiogram, and electrokymogram (a now obsolete method of recording the heart's movements), and blood tests for cholesterol and thyroid hormone levels. A few years later, enrollment was limited to people between ages thirty and fifty-nine, estimating that the study could attract sixty percent of the estimated ten thousand people in this age bracket living in Framingham. The investigators came very close, and remarkably, especially for the times, fifty-five percent were women. This was in sharp contrast to other studies of the last several decades which enrolled very few women and often excluded them altogether.

The FHS study population had other strengths from a research point of view. Only eighty-two people in the original group had a history of coronary artery disease. Thus the prevalence rate, defined as the rate of a particular disease present at a specific point in time, was very low at 1.6 percent. This was just the type of group that the investigators wanted to best study the true incidence of cardiac disease, the rate at which people would develop heart disease over time. The purpose of the FHS was to track the development of new heart disease over time, not follow the course of people who already had the disease.

The hard work continued, with consistent examinations of the study participants over the years and keen oversight. To meet the study requirements, doctors saw the patients promptly, a new phenomenon in the doctor-patient relationship. The patient reaction was quite positive, and in over thirty years of the study, the "dropout" rate of participants was an astonishingly low three percent! In 1949, a new director was appointed, Thomas Dawber MD (1913-2005). The Harvard Medical School graduate had devoted his entire career to public health efforts. Enthusiastic about the study, Dawber felt strongly that medicine needed major changes. Caring for patients when they were already ill was not enough; disease needed to be prevented, and, in particular, heart disease.

In 1957, nine years after its inception, the study presented its first breakthrough finding: hypertension, defined as 160 millimeters of mercury (mm Hg) systolic over 95 mm Hg, was associated with a four-fold increase in the incidence of coronary artery atherosclerosis. A few years later, the study reported that stroke was strongly associated with hypertension. For the first time, medical science identified a definite target for treatment with medication that could thwart the epidemic of coronary artery disease and stroke: high blood pressure.

Over the next decade more data accumulated, all supporting most of the initial hypotheses of the trial. It was clear that there were seven key factors that contributed to the risk of heart disease—increasing age, total cholesterol level, body weight, an abnormal change on the electrocardiogram, blood hemoglobin level, extent of cigarette smoking, and hypertension, especially the systolic pressure, the upper number of the blood pressure. This multiplicity of factors, all adding up to markedly increased risk, led Dawber and his successor in 1966, William Kannel MD (1923-2011), to coin the term "risk factors" for heart disease. The Framingham investigators had taken a new stand in the world of medicine—"epidemiologic activism."

THE MAJOR FINDINGS

The Framingham findings led to more mathematical and statistical analysis and ultimately surprising realizations. Although each risk factor was important, it was also true that the common risk factors often clustered together in one person, that is someone with high blood pressure was often obese, had high cholesterol, and diabetes as well. Although the risk of atherosclerosis was significantly increased by each factor, if someone had multiple risk factors, their total overall risk was far greater than the risk posed by each single risk factor simply added together. The ramifications of this discovery, that the sum of risk was greater than the parts, cannot be understated. For the first time, physicians could produce a mathematical "score" of risk. The Framingham Risk Score model pointed the way for doctors to identify high risk patients and treat them to lower blood pressure and blood cholesterol levels, control diabetes, and stress the need for weight control and regular physical exercise.[43]

And the lessons kept coming. William Kannel summarized key conclusions of the FHS in a publication and lecture in 1990. He pointed out that twenty percent of American men would suffer a heart attack before age sixty. Women had a much lower incidence when they were young, but they, too, were frequent victims, with a lag period of about twenty years compared to their male counterparts. After menopause, the risk in women increased three-fold. Even more disturbing, thirty-three percent of heart attacks went unrecognized, identified only later on the basis of an abnormal electrocardiogram. The prognosis of these people was just as poor as those in whom a heart attack was identified by typical symptoms, electrocardiogram findings, and laboratory tests. Both high blood pressure and heart attack were truly "silent killers."

The Framingham risk factors continued to pile up. Kannel reported that blood cholesterol in the high end of the "normal" range at the time posed a five times increased risk. He went on to stress the devastating effects of high blood pressure and shattered the myth that the elderly and women were immune from its complications. For many years, doctors believed that it was the lower number of blood pressure, the diastolic pressure, that posed the most risk, but the study found that elevation of the upper number, the systolic pressure, was a more ominous finding. Glucose intolerance and diabetes; cigarette smoking (the number smoked each day rather than the years smoked); and poor lifestyle choices like obesity, high fat and cholesterol diets, and a sedentary lifestyle, all led to increased risk. On the positive side, Kannel reported that even a modest degree of physical exercise decreased the long-term risk.

The ever-present electrocardiogram, the ancient machine of

---

43 These ideas seem commonplace now, but the evidence supporting these recommendations came directly from the Framingham Heart Study. While some cardiologists believe the Framingham Risk Score should include family history in its assessment and that one needs to consider that its conclusions arose from an almost exclusively Caucasian population, it is still in use thirty years later and remains a major achievement in the public health assessment of the risk of atherosclerotic heart disease.

Willem Einthoven, was still important and remained the simple and most effective way to detect changes that were harbingers of risk, like the silent heart attack and left ventricular hypertrophy, the abnormal thickness of the left ventricle caused by chronic, poorly controlled high blood pressure. Doctors now had the evidence to act on these findings and use medication to lower blood pressure and prevent problems before they occurred.

Finally, there was the influence of genetics. It wasn't a simple relationship, as it is for some genetic diseases like sickle cell anemia, but atherosclerosis, just like cancer, ran in families. In those families, one often found a high incidence of the other major bad actors such as hypertension, diabetes, and increased cholesterol levels.

One of the most important conclusions of Kannel's report was that "normal" levels of cholesterol, blood pressure, or blood sugar in 1990 were misleading. Normal values come from sampling many people without symptoms of a disease, but from the 1940s to the 1980s, these so-called normal values were obtained in a population with an epidemic of atherosclerosis. How useful were these values? Hadn't President Roosevelt's doctor declared that his patient's blood pressure was "no more than normal for a man his age"? Normal levels needed to be replaced by a different metric—"optimal."

Despite reporting his alarming statistics, Dr. Kannel ended his Bishop Lecture at the American Heart Association meeting on a very positive note. He pointed out that overall mortality rates had decreased in the United States over several years prior to 1990, and that life expectancy had significantly lengthened. Some good changes were occurring.[44]

The FHS also began investigating the importance of an increasingly common cardiac arrhythmia in an aging population, atrial fibrillation, and its role as a major risk factor for a stroke. The Framingham data,

---

44 Over the next almost thirty years, the Framingham Heart Study, now under the auspices of Boston University and headed up by Daniel Levy MD, has continued to investigate the causes of congestive heart failure, often a long-term consequence of coronary artery disease, hypertension, and myocardial infarction.

as well as many other studies, have confirmed the strong relationship between atrial fibrillation and stroke, leading to thousands of people being treated with chronic anticoagulants, "blood thinners," to reduce the dreaded complication of a stroke.

In my 2018 interview with Paul Sorlie PhD, the head epidemiologist for the FHS for forty-eight years, he emphasized that the study has always tried to explore new technologies and look at cardiovascular problems that were not part of the original trial. In recent years, the study has worked to try to unravel the complex genetics of atherosclerosis, using the most modern techniques available. The study is also exploring the differences in cardiovascular disease in different ethnic and racial groups. The volume of data the study compiled and the thousands of blood samples collected will continue to serve as a unique resource for future inquiries into the causes and then lead to new treatments for cardiovascular disease. The Framingham Heart Study celebrated its seventieth anniversary in October 2018. Hopefully, it has many more decades of work ahead of it.

The Framingham Heart Study was a turning point in the use of epidemiology in medicine. Although its original purpose was just the acquisition of data, in an era when causes of cardiovascular diseases were obscure, Kannel summarized well the results of the study and pointed the way to the future: "Appraisal of this 'natural history' suggested that awaiting symptoms was a form of brinkmanship that could no longer be condoned. Further," he said, "a coronary attack, it would appear, should be regarded as a medical failure rather than the first indication for treatment."

Armed with the Framingham data, doctors and scientists had a research and therapy path to follow, led by the basic scientists, the pharmacologists, the drug industry, and the practicing cardiologists. The treatment battle was engaged, and many were becoming aware that the heart disease needed to be thwarted early on. This would require further understanding of one of the key signs of the Widowmaker's impending arrival of atherosclerosis. This understanding would come from an unusual machine and its quirky inventor.

CHAPTER 9

SPINNING INTO CONTROL: LIPOPROTEINS AND CHOLESTEROL

In a foxhunt you may arrive at a moment when one of the dogs catches the scent and barrels down a trail. But what if the pack does not follow?

So too it is with science. I am grateful for those rare moments in time when the hint of a way to track me down is lost on all but the lone pursuer.

MILKY BLOOD

The whirring and spinning of the machine were ingrained in my mind by the time I was an internal medicine resident. I had just drawn blood from the arm veins of two patients into tubes with the red top rubber stoppers and walked samples down the hall to the small laboratory room on the patient floor. I put the tubes in the holes in the device, making sure they were roughly equal by weight so the machine wouldn't wobble and eject the blood tubes out onto the floor. I flipped the start lever. The smooth sound told me that the tubes were balanced.

I waited just a minute or two, flipped the lever down, and let the centrifuge machine slow and then stop its rapid rotation. I removed the tubes and took a look at the blood inside to make sure that there were two layers—the dense red blood cells pushed by acceleration and gravity to the bottom of the tube, and the clear layer at the top, the serum, with its electrolytes, sugar, and other molecules of interest for us to measure.

In the days before laboratory technicians drew blood samples almost every hour, the techs came only once a day. If I needed a blood test after that, it was my job as a resident to do the deed. I always asked the patients if they had eaten recently because I didn't want blood that had an artificially high sugar level in it. Even in people without diabetes it takes time for insulin to secrete out of the pancreas in response to a meal and do its work to force the sugar into the cells. If the patient had eaten within an hour or two before the resident vampire did his job, the serum layer didn't have a clear yellow color. It looked like milk. Sometimes there was another layer at the top of the tube, frothy foam like the whipped cream on top of a cup of hot cocoa. I was pretty sure I didn't want that stuff floating around in my bloodstream for too long.

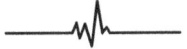

FOOD JOURNEYS: UNRAVELING THE COMPLEXITY OF CHOLESTEROL AND FAT

The notion that atherosclerosis had a great deal to do with the human diet was swirling around in the minds of medical scientists ever since the mid-nineteenth century when Rudolph Virchow used his microscope to demonstrate the yellow hard substance inside of arteries; it just looked like fat. The observation of the milky and fatty appearance of blood after a meal was also nothing new. If somehow fat and the diet were related to human disease, first doctors needed to understand how fat got into the body after we ate a piece of meat, a slab of butter, or drank milk. Even more remote was a possible link to the arteries of the human heart.

But the makeup of the milky fluid confused the early organic chemists. Was it only fat? Were there protein molecules also present? A German named Nerking, working with horses, was the first to be convinced that the lipids in blood were not just fat, but instead, were fat molecules bound to protein. And what was the role of cholesterol, the molecule found in the bile and gallstones? Cholesterol is a major component in the human diet; was it absorbed with the fat or not? How did it end up in bile and gallstones?

First would come an inkling of some order amidst the confusion before a more solid finding would be unearthed. In 1924, Simon Henry Gage and Pierre Augustine Fish of Cornell University in Ithaca, New York, using a specialized microscope and contrast dye, identified particles of about one micron in diameter (one millionth of a meter) in blood after eating; they named these particles "chylomicrons." The particles were only present for a few hours after eating and then disappeared. But how these molecules were broken down and what happened to the metabolites continued to puzzle these scientists. The answer came decades later from an unpredictable source. In the 1940s, John Gofman MD PhD (1918-2007) fell in love with a machine, a very special centrifuge, a device that spins incredibly fast and separates all kinds of mixtures into distinct layers based on the weight of each molecule. The "spinner" took him on a convoluted path to unravel the mystery of atherosclerosis and the human diet.

The young John Gofman, who loved both science and medicine, would find himself in the right place at the right time. He began medical school in his hometown of Cleveland, Ohio, at Case Western University, but after just a year he changed his career goal and moved to Berkeley, California, to study physics, mentored by two future

Nobel Prize winners, Ernest O. Lawrence PhD (1901-1958) and Glenn T. Seaborg PhD (1912-1999).[45] Dr. Seaborg's work was to try to synthesize and identify new elements of the periodic table. His tool was the fastest ultracentrifuge in the world at that time. The spinning device generates intense centrifugal force. If you place a liquid mixture in tubes into the slots in the machine, it will push heavier, denser particles to the bottom while the lighter ones float to the top, much like a washing machine on spin cycle draws out the moisture of wet clothes. Gofman devoted himself to learning how to use this device.

After a war assignment isolating plutonium, Gofman returned to medicine with a unique skillset and a new focus in mind. Driven by the death of his father from heart disease, Gofman wanted to use the ultracentrifuge to study the lipids of the blood and try to figure out what they might have to do with the atherosclerosis that took his father. He joined the Division of Medical Physics at UC Berkeley. His goal was to establish a brand-new type of laboratory to study a unique set of molecules: the lipoproteins.

Gofman and his team, especially Frank Lindgren PhD (1924-2007), went to work quickly. They had a powerful "spinner;" their ultracentrifuge had a speed of just less than sixty thousand revolutions per minute. To put into perspective the force their machine created, consider that 1 g is the force exerted at the earth's surface. Astronauts subjected to the pressure of launch into space through the earth's atmosphere experience maximum g forces of less than ten. *Gofman's device could generate a gravitational and acceleration force of 240,000 to 300,000 gs!* Using this force to spin down blood samples, especially "post-prandial" samples (after eating), his team could identify specific layers of molecules. Using a sophisticated method of imaging, they could measure the particular way each layer changed light, indicating

---

45 Lawrence won the Nobel Prize in Physics in 1939 for his invention of the cyclotron, and Seaborg in Chemistry in 1951 for his synthesis and discovery of ten new elements.

the relative densities of each molecular layer. And they had another trick; they discovered that adding table salt (sodium chloride) to the blood samples added density to the serum as a whole and increased the density differences between the molecules. The salt enabled the researchers to better see the foam (the lower density molecules) that floated to the top of the centrifuge tube.

In his first major paper published in 1949, Gofman reported that the floating molecules, which he called lipoproteins, were combinations of fat, cholesterol, and protein, comprising only 2.5 to 6.0 percent of the total proteins in the serum. He was able to differentiate three different classes of lipoproteins, based on their Svedberg units—the Sf.[46] These units measure the size of a particle based on how fast it migrates to the bottom of a centrifuge tube. It is a measure of time and is defined as 10-13 seconds. Svedberg told Gofman that his idea of centrifuging lipoproteins to separate them into discrete molecules wouldn't work. Gofman believed differently. Using the Svedberg units, the team was able to find lipoproteins of four distinct sizes—those with Sf of 100-200 units, Sf of 30-70, Sf of 10-20, and the lightest ones, the "foam" at the top of the tubes, of 3-8 Sf. Gofman named them High Density Lipoprotein (HDL), Low Density Lipoprotein (LDL), Very Low Density Lipoprotein (VLDL), and chylomicrons.

In addition to the amazing discovery of what we know now as HDL and LDL, Gofman was convinced that the explanation for atherosclerosis, by then suspected as the major factor causing heart attacks, came from one of these. Cholesterol is not a free-floating molecule in the human body; it is bound to proteins when ingested. When it travels through the gut and into the lymphatics, it combines with other proteins in different ways. Gofman suspected the LDL molecule caused the buildup of plaque and went to work investigating his hunch. He and his group began studying rabbits,

---

46 Named after the original ultracentrifuge researcher, the Swede Theodor Svedberg (1884-1971). S for Svedberg, f for flotation.

just like Anichkov had done many years before. Gofman found that when he fed rabbits high cholesterol diets, sure enough, the levels of the LDL molecules increased dramatically, and the animals developed much more severe atherosclerosis very quickly.

Armed with these data, Gofman turned to humans and thought carefully about who he wanted to study. While patients who had had heart attacks, or those who had angina pectoris were logical subjects for inquiry, his interest also stretched to other problems associated with an increased risk of atherosclerotic heart disease and possibly high levels of total cholesterol. These included patients with diabetes mellitus, hypertension, hypothyroidism (low levels of thyroid hormone), and nephrosis, a form of kidney disease known to be accompanied by high lipid levels.

Over several years, Gofman collected blood samples from over 1,500 patients with these disorders, plus a good number of "normals." In 230 males who had suffered a myocardial infarction, *ninety-one percent had higher than expected LDL levels*, often significantly higher than what was felt to be the normal range at the time. In his paper in 1950, Gofman commented that these patients may have had even higher levels of LDL before their heart attack, as many of them were on restricted fat diets when he studied them. Gofman also found elevated levels of LDL in the patients with angina, diabetes, hypertension, hypothyroidism, and nephrosis, again compared to normal standards of that era. Most remarkably his data revealed that the *total* cholesterol level in the blood had no consistent relationship with the level of the LDL. If cholesterol build up caused atherosclerosis, as Anichkov had insisted, that was true because the body's metabolism combined cholesterol with a specific protein to form LDL.

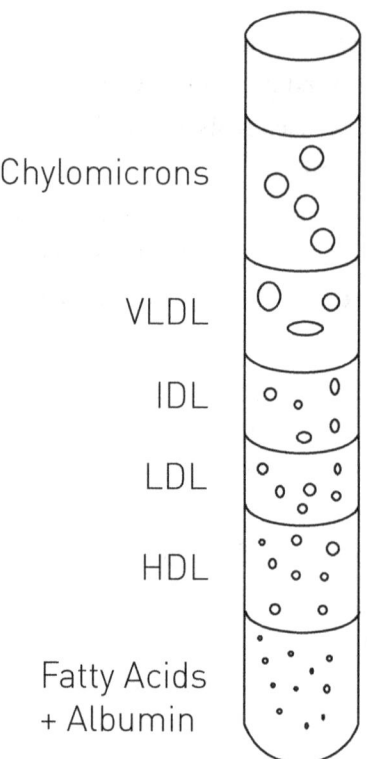

Figure 12. Separation of blood lipoproteins by ultracentrifugation; layering of molecules based on molecular weight and density of each lipoprotein molecule. (Courtesy of Meredith Dawson Designs, LLC)

Gofman reached other startling conclusions. The good news was the LDL level was not affected by ingesting just one fatty meal. Instead, LDL levels reflected someone's dietary choices in the long run, not for just a week or so. Gofman noted that consistent dietary changes could lower LDL levels. A healthier *pattern* of eating could work. He also found that the LDL levels in women rose significantly over the age of sixty; future research confirmed that women after menopause have higher LDL levels and an increasing incidence of coronary artery disease and heart attacks.

John Gofman continued his work on lipoproteins and published his amazing findings. In 1950, his discoveries appeared in *Circulation*, the official journal of the American Heart Association. In describing the difference between the LDL levels of the normal and those who had suffered a heart attack, Gofman wrote, "This difference is unequivocal evidence that the presence of these molecules is in some way associated with the presence of atherosclerosis." In 1959, he published a prescient book entitled *Dietary Prevention and Treatment of Heart Disease*. Along with two colleagues, Alex Nichols PhD and E. Virginia Dobbin, a dietician, Gofman outlined for a general audience a concise description of the long-term process of "hardening of the arteries" and also the possible role of blood clots superimposed on top of the atherosclerosis in causing heart attacks. The book emphasized again that the major culprit causing atherosclerosis was the specific lipoprotein LDL.

Gofman emphasized that most of these damaging lipoproteins came from animal fat and perhaps replacing that form of fat with liquid vegetable oils would reduce the levels of LDL in the blood. But to change the LDL levels over time, dietary changes needed to become consistent. Skipping hamburgers for a few days wasn't enough. He also noted that the fat in fish did not seem to raise the levels of the damaging lipoproteins. Clearly John Gofman would not have been pleased by the nutritional contents of the K-rations so many of his contemporaries had consumed just a decade or two earlier.

Gofman's focus then shifted to dietary prevention. He wrote, " . . . a great deal of education is required so that people will understand that the real time to do something about a problem like heart disease is *not* after that heart disease has become obvious but *long before.*" He had grand ambitions to educate people and wrote one of the first of innumerable "self-help" books to be published in the last sixty years. It contained pages of suggestions for low fat, low carbohydrate meals and snacks, recipes developed by his wife and "taste-tested" by his son. Gofman realistically understood how hard it would be to convince many people to change their dietary patterns in the early 1960s. Meat and fat-laden dairy products filled most plates in the Western world. He predicted that some of those who read his book and tried his recipes would rather take their chances of having a heart attack than give up their dining pleasures.

In the early 1960s, Gofman abruptly left his research into heart disease. William Virgil Brown MD, editor of the *Journal of Clinical Lipidology*, reported that Gofman became angry when the National Institute of Health rejected his proposal to include LDL measurements using ultracentrifuge techniques in a trial of the treatment of coronary artery disease. The NIH felt that measuring total cholesterol alone would provide enough information, flying directly in the face of his discovery of LDL's crucial role in atherosclerosis.

In retrospect, it was not Gofman's technical laboratory prowess that made his work so impressive, but rather it was the interpretation of his research. By looking at clinical and laboratory data, he unraveled a major part of the food's path from the mouth to the coronary arteries. His rigorous data analysis led to the understanding that atherosclerosis was caused not by cholesterol alone but by a specific form of a cholesterol-protein molecule, only detected by a blood test. Gofman also subscribed to W. Edward Denning's notion that "In God we trust, all others bring data."

All of Gofman's conclusions have stood the test of scientific scrutiny and time. It is not possible to prevent heart attacks without understanding the role of the LDL particle. His research paved the way for the advances in treatment of the last seventy years. In particular, Gofman's Sf 10-20 molecule inspired two young scientists at the National Institute of Health in the 1970s, Michael Brown MD and Sidney Goldstein MD, to unravel much more of the path of this potentially deadly molecule in the human body. The man that did so much for the future understanding of heart disease[47] passed away in 2007 from heart failure.

The kind of research Gofman did with cholesterol helped to turn the focus toward prevention, but there were still plenty of people

---

47 In 1974, the American Heart Association named Gofman one of the top twenty-five researchers in cardiology for the twenty-five-year period prior. William Virgil Brown calls him the "Father of Clinical Lipidology."

who needed critical care at the last minute. Whether they would survive a quick strike by the Widowmaker would greatly depend on a new and seemingly impossible innovation.

CHAPTER 10

AN OUT-OF-BODY EXPERIENCE: THE HEART-LUNG MACHINE

The weak muscle, the irregular beat, the gaping hole, I take no joy in capitalizing on these weaknesses. For who can blame the victims for such hapless luck, to be born through no fault of their own, with a compromised heart?

Yet what would ever allow humans to mend these flaws?

THE MOST DIFFICULT OF DAYS

She was a young woman in her twenties who had a rare, mysterious, and often deadly tongue-twisting disease called thrombotic thrombocytopenia purpura. "TTP" is a blood disorder that causes the body's platelets to clump inside the blood vessels for no apparent reason, causing red skin lesions known as purpura, kidney failure, and brain cell death (strokes). The hematology experts had nothing to offer her. At the time, it was thought that removing the spleen, the abdominal organ that normally helps degrade blood cells and platelets, might help. It was a real shot in the dark, but there was no other treatment in 1975.

The surgery was going smoothly; we had opened the abdomen, dissected out the spleen, and carefully removed it. There was no excessive bleeding that we could see. However, several minutes after the spleen was out of the body, her heart rate unexpectedly slowed down, and then the heart just stopped.

We quickly injected medication to try to restart it. No response. We cracked open her chest and the surgeon took her heart in his hands and massaged it in an attempt to force blood to flow through it. Still, no response, and now we were out of options. Her time of death was called. A person in the prime of her life, who was alive just two hours earlier, now lay dead on our operating table.

A heavy hush filled the room. Everyone at the OR table stood motionless for several minutes. The only steady sounds piercing the silence were the respirator still blowing oxygen into the patient's lungs and the harsh blare from the cardiac telemetry monitor telling us what we already knew—there was no heartbeat. Mercifully, the anesthesiologist made the first move, muting the now-useless machines.

After about five minutes, life needed to go on. We sewed up the abdomen and the chest. The residents and I left the OR, leaving the attending surgeon to meet with the family and the nurses attended to the body. Although we knew that her disease was life threatening, none of us could escape the thought that we had hastened her death.

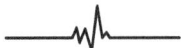

THE DAWN OF CARDIAC SURGERY: JOHN GIBBON'S IDEA

Decades earlier, John Heysham Gibbon Jr. (1903-1973) had a similar experience as a young trainee in an OR. The events of that day would transform his life and launch him on a quest for a machine that one of his colleagues would refer to as something from a Jules Verne science fiction novel.

Gibbon was born in Philadelphia in the first decade of the twentieth century and decided that he would follow in his father's footsteps and pursue becoming a surgeon. Surgical training in those days meant being mentored by a prominent surgeon, and Gibbon soon had the benefit of studying under Edward B. Churchill MD (1895-1972) at Harvard Medical School. In the fall of 1930, Gibbon and Dr. Churchill were called to see a woman with shortness of breath and a feeling of a "lump" in her right chest that quickly became a sharp pain. She had been on bed rest for two weeks following removal of her gallbladder. This lengthy bed rest was the standard of care at the time. Churchill knew immediately what was wrong: this woman was suffering from a pulmonary embolism, a blood clot that had traveled from her leg or pelvic veins. The clot had formed as a result of her prolonged immobility and the stagnant flow of blood in her veins. It now occluded the main artery carrying blood from the right side of the heart into the lungs to pick up oxygen.

The patient's options were very few. If she continued to worsen, there was only one treatment choice: to open up the chest and surgically remove the blood clot from the pulmonary artery. In the United States, on the rare occasions that this surgery had been performed, no one had survived. As a precaution, an orderly moved the patient to the OR in the event Churchill decided to perform an operation named the Trendelenburg procedure. Churchill described this surgery as the "prelude to an autopsy." Gibbon understood the seriousness of the situation and knew exactly where he was going to be for an unknown number of hours: at the woman's bedside measuring her blood pressure, heart rate, and respirations every fifteen minutes.

Sitting there for hours, the young surgeon's mind wandered and then settled on an extraordinary idea that could perhaps save patients like this. Suppose he could remove the blood from the veins before it reached the blocked right side of the heart by pumping that blood into some machine that provided oxygen outside of the body. He would then return that oxygenated blood back into the body. This theoretical pump would replace the function of the heart and the lungs: a heart-lung machine. While his idea for a heart-lung machine was not new, no one had developed the extraordinary technical skills to pull this one off. He thought about it all night. By the next morning, it was clear that the poor woman was dying. As Gibbon watched, Churchill opened her chest in seven minutes and removed the clots in the pulmonary artery. But true to past experience, the patient did not survive. This encounter solidified Gibbon's decision: the heart and lung replacement machine would be his research quest.

Fortunately, in medical school, Gibbon learned an invaluable lesson that would soon come to guide him for many years in the future. Working with a professor on research into the relationship between salt intake and high blood pressure, he came to appreciate the importance of the meticulous, repeated experiments necessary to take an idea to fruition, verifying its truth or fallacy. The engineering complexity of designing a heart-lung machine would dissuade all but the most daring and persistent inventors. To successfully operate on the heart, the entire volume of blood needed to be gradually drained from the veins, a risky endeavor from the start. Then that blood must be put through some type of "oxygenator" machine. What that was, the engineers had no idea. If the patient was still alive, the blood then had to be pumped back into the arteries. How to prevent the heartbeat from just stopping completely during this process was a hope and prayer in 1930.[48] And on top of all that, the idea that the organs could simultaneously receive enough oxygen to stay alive belonged only in a science fiction story.

Nevertheless, Gibbon knew others had already proved some key concepts. In 1812, a Frenchman engineer named Louis de Gallois (1775-1825) wrote, "If one could substitute for the heart a kind of injection of arterial blood, either natural or artificially made, one would succeed in maintaining alive indefinitely any part of the body whatsoever." A few decades later, investigators discovered that they could "oxygenate" blood by placing high concentrations of the gaseous element into physical contact with blood. The work of Charles-

---

48 Decades later, the heart was allowed to completely stop because it could be restarted with a defibrillator at the end of the heart surgery. Gibbon had no idea that this was possible when he started his project.

Édouard Brown-Séquard (1817-1894) was particularly useful but also ghastly. He used his own blood and its oxygen to perfuse the limbs of guillotined criminals to prove that the muscle tissues could remain viable for hours after being dismembered from their owners. He showed that the lungs were not necessary to keep tissues alive.

In the twentieth century, efforts began in an attempt to create a machine that could oxygenate organs. The closest anyone came to an effective extracorporeal perfusion machine was Alexis Carrel MD (1873-1944), a French-born surgeon who did remarkable work on the surgery of blood vessels and founded the field of vascular surgery. In the 1930s, he began to work with the American aviation hero Charles Lindbergh (1902-1974) designing a device that could perfuse the hearts and thyroid glands from animals. The pair performed almost one thousand experiments providing oxygen to organs outside of the body successfully for up to twelve hours. The Lindbergh-Carrel perfusion pump was a popular exhibit at the 1939 New York City World's Fair. Unfortunately, World War II ended their collaboration.

So by the mid-1930s, Gibbon, while encouraged by these advancements, was not interested in removing organs to keep them alive outside of the body; he wanted to partially empty the heart and bypass the lungs so surgeons could safely operate on the heart. He knew that the answer to successful heart surgery did not lay in the ability to quickly cut cardiac tissue and sew it up again. Meticulous surgery took time, time surgeons did not have if the heart continued to move and pump out blood as they tried to repair a damaged heart valve or sew up a hole in the heart of a child. Gibbon left Boston and returned to the University of Pennsylvania with a new idea and a new bride, Mary, who was just as dedicated to the endeavor as he was.[49]

The Gibbon family project had no chance of success unless they were able to overcome a fundamental problem: the challenge of removing a huge amount of blood from the body. Outside of its

---

49 Mary Gibbon would become John's primary collaborator on the heart-lung machine project for over twenty years.

internal environment, blood doesn't stay in liquid form; it clots. Within a few minutes, the blood supplied with oxygen that they wanted to return to the body would coagulate into a sticky mass of protein, platelets, and red blood cells. Without a way to prevent the coagulation, there was no reason to even pursue the project. But as luck would have it, they were at the right time to even dream about producing a machine that would work.

In the early twentieth century, the blood coagulation system was a fruitful area of research. William Henry Howell MD (1860-1945) was a Johns Hopkins Medical School Professor of Physiology who focused on this arena of discovery. In 1916, a medical student named Jay McLean MD (1890-1957) came to help out in Howell's lab. McLean isolated a strange substance from dog liver that actually prevented coagulation rather than caused it. Howell continued to look for other "anticoagulants." He found a second one in 1918 and named it "heparin," after the Latin word for liver, *hepar*. By the time John Gibbon had his moment of enlightenment in the OR in 1930, heparin was a commercially available anticoagulant. The new drug arrived at just the right time for the Gibbons to begin their work, and thus, heparin solved their first problem: they could keep blood liquid outside the body.

With that box checked, the engineering phase began. The Gibbons decided that cats were the right size animals to use. They planned to insert a tube into a large vein in the neck to drain the blood and have it fall by gravity into a bulb-like glass reservoir. The blood in the reservoir would then be pumped through the real "guts" of the device, the oxygenator. They knew that the best way to get the most oxygen into the blood was to create a thin film of blood and expose it to a high concentration of oxygen. The Gibbon team first tried using a revolving cylinder oxygenator with a goal of achieving ninety-five percent oxygen saturation in the venous blood. The pump allowed the blood to "stream" around the cylinder, maximizing the contact with the oxygen. The blood with its fresh supply of oxygen needed to be pumped into a tube that returned the blood to the femoral artery in the groin area of the cats and then pushed against the normal flow in the artery, which came from the heart, up to the aorta and the brain, and also down into the legs. The blood returning from the oxygenator needed to "swim against the tide." The Gibbons' first pump used a one-quarter horsepower engine that could oxygenate 500 cc of blood a minute, more than enough, they hoped, to supply the needs of a cat.

Their early experiments separated each stage, with the machine focused first on just bypassing the lungs. Gibbon partially occluded the main pulmonary artery of the animals but let the heart keep beating. In doing so, he was mimicking what had happened to the woman he saw die from a pulmonary embolism in 1930. Still, the process was an uncertain one with some, but not all, of the cats surviving the procedure, and building up stable time on the machines was a challenge.[50]

As with most bold new research endeavors, the Gibbons soon recognized unanticipated problems, and the most troubling one was anemia. It turned out that the walls of red blood cells, although strong enough to travel through the smallest blood vessels in the body, did not react well to contact with manmade surfaces, like the screens in the oxygenator that separated the blood cells from the oxygen gas. This process damaged many of the red blood cell walls, and they burst apart, a process known as hemolysis. For the heart-lung machine to stand a chance, this problem would have to be solved.

Fortunately for the Gibbons and the fate of their invention, a fortuitous meeting would provide the answer. Though known today as the greatest cardiac surgeon of the twentieth century, in the early 1930s, Michael DeBakey MD (1908-2008) was just a medical student focused on a challenge.[51] As a student in Tulane University School of

---

50 By 1937, John and Mary were able to use the lung machine for up to four hours.
51 His legendary achievements are documented in many books and countless medical publications.

Medicine in New Orleans, DeBakey worked in a laboratory trying to improve the efficiency of blood transfusions. DeBakey and his mentors were struggling with the problem of hemolysis of blood, and DeBakey developed a pump to help study pulse waves that could decrease the trauma to red blood cells outside the body. At a medical meeting in the late 1930s, DeBakey met John Gibbon, and they discussed Gibbon's dissatisfaction with the pump he used for his heart-lung machine. Naturally, DeBakey suggested that John try using his new roller pump. The rest is history—the hemolysis problem was much reduced.

By the late 1930s, John and Mary Gibbon, while convinced that their oxygenator pump would be a success, knew they needed to perform experiments in larger animals than cats before attempting to use the device in humans. Even with their impressive progress in the laboratory, many of their colleagues described their work as "fruitless, bordering on ridiculous." But John Gibbon kept the real prize in view: success was more than just a well-functioning, safe machine. He wanted the heart-lung device to make cardiac surgery possible and destroy another shibboleth from the nineteenth century; not only could catheters enter the heart as Werner Forssmann had demonstrated, but skilled surgeons could repair problems like inherited (congenital) heart malformations and heart valve disease. But just when the Gibbons were getting close to a great achievement, the events of the world stopped the heart-lung machine endeavor abruptly.

December 7, 1941, changed the world forever. The attack on Pearl Harbor jolted the United States into action, including the medical profession. Within months, almost all of the surgery faculty at the University of Pennsylvania volunteered to become military surgeons, including John Gibbon. By January 1942, he was on active duty as a surgeon in New Caledonia in the South Pacific. After more than three years at war, Gibbon came home in 1945.

In their new laboratory,[52] the Gibbons often had medical students work with them—the price was right (usually $0), and the students needed mandatory research experience in those days, and one in particular procured a fortunate connection. The Gibbons employed a Jefferson student, E.J. Clark, who was very enthusiastic about the heart-lung project and, through his father-in-law's business contacts, introduced the team to Thomas Watson (1874-1956), the CEO of International Business Machines (IBM). Watson was immediately struck by the implications of the project and offered Gibbon any help, both financial and technical, that IBM could provide, going so far as to assign his chief engineer, Gustave Malmros, to work with Gibbon. Malmros became a key member of the Gibbon team, helping them develop a larger oxygenator that could be used in bigger animals and then hopefully humans. In 1949, IBM shipped an improved heart-lung machine, the Model I, to Gibbon. It was so large and heavy that delivery to Gibbon's lab required the use of a crane to lift the machine several floors off the ground to maneuver it through an open window.

The animal experimental results from 1949 to 1952 were astounding. Using dogs this time, Gibbon experimented with total support of both the respiration and circulation, instead of only respiration. For the first time, the heart was completely stopped from beating and was then restarted. The data were impressive. Mortality dropped from a rate of seventy-nine percent initially to just twelve percent, with perfusion times up to one hundred minutes. The team even worked with surgical techniques "on bypass," creating in the animals common childhood heart defects and then devising surgery to repair the holes between the heart chambers they had artificially created. Encouraged, they continued to improve the device by using larger tubing to increase blood flow, and the Model II machine rolled out in 1952.

---

52 The Gibbons resumed their animal work at Penn, but within a few months, John was offered a position at Jefferson Medical College, not only as a Professor of Surgery, but also as the Director of Surgical Research. He and Mary moved their laboratory just a few miles away to the Jefferson campus in center city Philadelphia.

By early 1952, John Gibbon believed he could place a human being on his "bypass" device and correct a congenital defect in a child or teenager. If successful, this would open up a whole new area of surgery: surgery on the heart itself, a heart containing almost no blood and not beating at the time of the operation. Surgery on congenital malformations of the heart had already been done without the heart-lung machine, pioneered by the brilliant work of the pediatric cardiologist Helen Taussig MD (1896-1986), one of the few women in cardiology at the time, and the surgeon Alfred Blalock MD (1899-1964) and his African-American laboratory technician Vivien Thomas (1910-1985). But there were so many other children whose defects could only be corrected by stopping the heart first. Gibbon and his team rigorously prepared for those days.

The first opportunity arrived in February 1952. A very ill fifteen-month-old girl was dying due to a large hole between the right atrium and left atrium chambers of her heart, a disorder called an atrial septal defect. The team took her to the OR, successfully placed her on bypass, but then, oddly, could not find the suspected atrial septal defect.[53] Sadly, the young heart would not restart after removing the support of the heart-lung machine. John Gibbon was crestfallen, especially since there was no cardiac catheterization done prior the surgery that could have accurately diagnosed the exact problem that required surgery. Gibbon returned to waiting for the right patient to try to save.

By early May 1953, an eighteen-year-old college freshman from Wilkes-Barre, Pennsylvania named Cecilia Bavolok was dying from the effects of an atrial septal defect. She and her family had tried everything and came to Jefferson with only hope. A few days later, Gibbon and his team placed the young woman on total respiratory and circulatory support for twenty-six minutes, and Gibbon repaired her defect. Cecilia Bavolok survived the procedure without any

---

53 An autopsy revealed that she had a different congenital defect, not the suspected atrial septal one.

complications and went on to live a normal life. The unimaginable had finally happened.

John Gibbon had performed the first successful open-heart surgery using the heart-lung machine he and Mary had so painstakingly developed. The idea that a surgeon could have the time to repair a diseased heart, while the heart was dead-still, that an external machine could provide blood and oxygen to all of the organs of the body while the operation was proceeding, and that the flaccid pump of life could then be restarted to its normal function, and the patient would not only survive, but thrive—this was a medical and scientific miracle that few had dared even contemplate. *This was one of the greatest achievements of the twentieth century.*

The long-anticipated historic moment had finally arrived, and one would have thought that Gibbon would have been euphoric, celebrating with his colleagues and asking his team members to contact the newspaper and radio media about this stunning accomplishment. But he did not. Gibbon, ever the pure scientist, was skeptical; how could one make a conclusion about a new treatment or technology so soon? After all, the mortality rate was fifty percent—one out of two. Gibbon did present his data at a surgical conference but had to be convinced to publish a case report about his success. It was not until 1954 that the description of Ms. Bavolok's surgery finally appeared in an obscure medical journal named *Minnesota Medicine.*

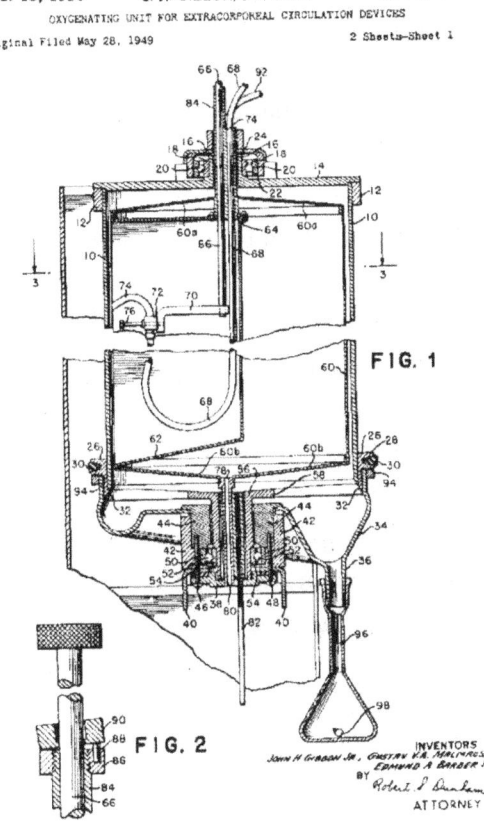

Figure 13. United States patent application for first heart-lung machine by John H. Gibbon Jr. MD, 1955. (Courtesy of United States Patent Office)

After using his heart-lung machine in humans only four times,[54] Gibbon surprisingly announced to the Jefferson faculty that he personally was not going to use the Model II heart-lung machine again, and he turned over the heart surgery program to one of his younger Jefferson colleagues, John Y. Templeton III MD (1917-2007). Sixty years later, it is still uncertain why Gibbon decided to stop using the pump that he invented. Performing surgery certainly carried an emotional toll. Gibbon likely hated seeing patients die

---

54 In the next case, the patient suffered a cardiac arrest even before Gibbon could place her on the heart-lung machine, followed by a case in which he used the machine, but the patient's heart did not recover when he removed the bypass support.

in the operating room. Perhaps he had been there too many times. One of his colleagues opined another view, that the decision was not that surprising; John had proven that his idea was viable and now turned to other ventures,[55] believing it was time for others to advance and perfect the heart-lung machine. He would have agreed with a quote from the great inventor Thomas Alva Edison (1847-1931): "The essence of great scientific work is that it is transitory, because, particularly with respect to technological inventions, it is linked to the course of progress."

Significantly, the news of Gibbon's one success sparked great enthusiasm in other medical centers, in particular the Mayo Clinic in Rochester, Minnesota. John Kirklin MD (1917-2004) and his colleagues pushed the technology much further. In their hands, the mortality from cardiac surgery dropped from fifty percent to ten percent. Within several years, most major medical centers around the world regularly used the heart-lung machine.

Although Gibbon retired in 1967,[56] the medical community did not forget him. In the last years of his life, as cardiac surgery flourished quickly, Gibbon received many honors, and much was written about him. In 2003, the fifty-year anniversary of the first successful use of the heart-lung machine, one of his colleagues, Harris Shumaker MD, summed up the man: "Some men are crushed by the mantle of greatness. Some find it so heavy that they must stand tall, erect, and arrogant. Jack wore his with easy grace, with no undue pride, but rather with pleasant, somewhat surprised satisfaction." Gibbon's work was a triumph of science and engineering, forged by over two decades of constant attention to detail and healthy skepticism before claiming success.

While John Gibbon had created a revolution, there was much

---

55   Gibbon pursued new interests in liver disease, thoracic surgery, teaching surgery, and served as the editor of a prestigious journal of surgery.
56   Gibbon continued to enjoy his tennis, his books, and even tried painting. However, throughout his retirement, Gibbon continued smoking heavily, but when he began to have chest pain, he refused to see doctors. In 1973, John Gibbon died suddenly from his heart disease while playing tennis.

more to come. The forbidden task of performing surgery on the beating human heart became a problem of the past, and as Michael DeBakey wrote about Gibbon, "He opened the door that had been locked for centuries." Yet neither Gibbon, John Templeton, nor John Kirklin envisioned in the 1950s that cardiac surgery could be used to treat coronary artery disease. Success came in the treatment of congenital heart disease and disease of the heart valves, but atherosclerosis was still not close to becoming a surgical disease. The Widowmaker was just hitting its stride in the 1950s and 1960s. It would take the work of a new generation of cardiologists and cardiac surgeons to spark new life into that fight.

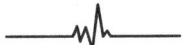

THE RIGHT MACHINE AT THE RIGHT TIME

"Hey, intern boy, let's go—the cath lab needs us STAT."

I had the temerity to ask, "What's going on?"

"You don't need to know, just get your ass moving and follow me up there—NOW."

I was in the second month of my surgical internship, with my operating room shoes still looking almost as white as when I took them out of the box. As we ran toward the cardiac cath lab, I was still totally in the dark as to what we were going to find. We entered the lab and saw a cardiology fellow doing chest compressions on a patient who had just undergone a cardiac catheterization.

I overheard the cardiac cath lab attending physician tell my obnoxious second-year resident, "We need to get this man to the OR immediately. We accidentally tore the inner lining of his left coronary artery with the tip of a catheter, and he had a cardiac arrest on the table. Get your attending on the phone—NOW! He needs to get over here and bypass that artery or we're going to lose him."

My resident turned to me and barked, "Intern, get up there and start pumping on this guy's chest." I did what I was told, jumping up on the cath lab table and straddling the patient. Leaning forward with both hands, one on top of the other, I began pressing on his chest and then rhythmically pulling back, over and over again.

The attending surgeon arrived quickly, looked at the cardiac cath images, and agreed that the patient needed bypass surgery immediately. So off we raced to the OR, with me riding on the stretcher, straddling the patient and getting fatigued from doing the strong, rapid chest compressions. I still remember the glances of other hospital employees as we went galloping down the hallway.

Once we got into the OR, the anesthesiologist and the nurses moved at lightning speed, and I noticed another man, who was scrubbed in and waiting for us, whose job it was to start the heart-lung machine, "the pump" that might save our patient's life. I knew what the machine did. With the man's chest already opened up, the surgical team was pulling the blood from this man's vena cava, the main vein in his neck, through a large plastic tube into a whirling pump, providing it with oxygen, and then pumping it back into the largest artery in his chest, the aorta. His heart would stop pumping altogether, so that the surgeon could place pieces of veins from his legs and sew one end into the aorta and the other into his coronary artery, but beyond the point of the blockage from the tear in his left coronary artery. During the surgery, the machine would keep the patient alive. Perhaps most amazingly, when the surgery was done, the surgeon would restart his heart.

Within a few minutes, the OR calmed down and the crucial part of the surgery began. The patient's circulation was supported, and oxygen was getting to all of his organs. I stood against the back wall of the OR staring and listening.

Before he began to scrub his hands to assist on the case, my resident got in my face—"What are you still doing here? Get back to the floor." But Dr. Junior Professor hadn't counted on having his words overheard by someone with more authority. Dr. T, the Chief Resident in Cardiothoracic Surgery, had heard this resident berate interns and other residents many times. From his position already scrubbed and ready to start surgery, without looking up, he calmly said, "No, let the kid stay. We'll put him to work and maybe he'll learn something." He followed up with a final zinger to my oppressor, "You go out on the floor." To a surgical resident, that's like telling a US Marine to leave the battlefield and do paperwork. Dr. Junior Professor stormed out of the OR.

That day, I learned how to help remove veins from the leg, how to trim them, and how to prepare them for the bypass grafts. I saw how the surgeon did his work, how he first stopped the heart with a tiny defibrillator and then restarted it when he was done. I learned how to sew up the chest wall when the procedure was over. It was a memorable experience for a new intern.

The patient did survive the surgery and was awake and eating dinner within thirty-six hours. He spent a week on our service until he finally went home. His heart had been damaged but not severely. The prompt surgery had saved his life.

His surgery was only made possible by the invention of a determined surgeon-engineer, a machine that took twenty years to perfect before it could be used in cardiac surgery and then another fifteen years until the idea of surgery on the coronary arteries became a reality. Chasing the Widowmaker was always a long process, but on this day in 1975, we caught up. By that time, we had other crucial tools that gave us a chance to save more lives. They were shocking inventions.

CHAPTER 11

IT'S ALIVE!: THE SHOCKING INVENTION OF DEFIBRILLATORS AND PACEMAKERS

More than muscle and structure, the heart has a rhythm to it. Often it is the smooth Bach, but at times it can be the arrhythmic Beethoven or the exuberant Mozart. the pattern lost to all but the trained ear.

For centuries, I have been heralded by this song, signaling me when to deal the final blow. But what if man finally learned to conduct the music of the heart and alter its course?

EMERGENCY ELECTRICITY—FALL 1994

James' chest pain began a few days prior and had come and gone. His wife Claire convinced him to see a cardiologist, but he was not happy about that. He was my age, forty-four years old, and although overweight, he had no history of any heart problem and no history of risk factors such as high blood pressure, diabetes, cigarette smoking, or elevated blood cholesterol.

James and Claire were headed from their suburban home to Philadelphia to see her father's cardiologist about James' chest pain when he had another bout of pain in the car. Claire was driving and said she had heard enough; they were going to the nearest emergency room. So on a Tuesday morning, instead of being at work, James was in the emergency room at a suburban hospital staring at his "worst nightmare" —a stranger who was a heart disease specialist charged with saving his life. He needed this stranger, however, because as it turned out, he had just had a heart attack.

I stood at his bedside in the ER, listening to him speak and thinking of the next thing I wanted to ask him, when I saw his eyes roll back in his head. My eyes immediately shifted to the heart monitor, where I could see his heart rate had shot up to 150 beats a minute from ninety, and the shape of the electrocardiogram tracing changed strikingly; James was in ventricular tachycardia, a rapid heart rate originating from the left ventricle. In a matter of seconds, things got much worse, and now his rhythm looked like just a quivering of electrical activity with no regular pattern. He now had no blood pressure and the blood flow to his brain was plummeting to zero. He was in ventricular fibrillation.

"VF!" I shouted, and in less than ten seconds, a crowd of nurses and the ER doctor burst in from behind the curtains in James' cubicle. They knew what came next . . .

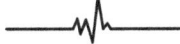

THE CHARGE OF LIFE: SHOCKING THE HEART

"Death may usurp on nature many hours, And yet the fire of life kindle again. The o'pressed spirits, I heard of an Egyptian That had nine hours lied dead, Who was by good appliances recover'd."

—*Shakespeare, Pericles, Act 3, Scene 2.*

In the 1931 film, the pivotal scene begins with Dr. Henry Frankenstein slowly raising his operating table with a strapped down cadaver through the open roof of his laboratory into a fierce thunderstorm. Dramatic lightning strikes every few seconds. With ominous music playing in the background, the camera pans the laboratory. The eerie machines cackle and throw sparks as the electricity from the lightning surges through vacuum tubes and into the electrodes drilled into the skull of the lifeless corpse. The witnesses cower in fear. After just a few seconds, Dr. Frankenstein carefully turns the wheel that lowers the table back into his laboratory.

The frenzied doctor quickly walks toward the corpse and the camera moves in for a close-up view of the cadaver's right hand. Frankenstein sees a flicker of the fingers and shouts, "It's moving, it's alive—it's alive, it's alive, it's alive, it's alive, it's alive, it's ALIVE. In the name of God, now I know what it's like to be God." The doctor's experiment had triumphed over death. At least in the movies.

In the *Frankenstein* film, the story fashioned after the nineteenth century classic tale of Mary Shelley (1797-1851), a bizarre procedure for restoring life is channeled by a phenomenon known for millennia—lightning strikes. The electrical machines capture their energy and pass them into the body of the previously dead but soon to become very much alive monster. When Universal Pictures filmed *Frankenstein* the possibility that electricity could be used to save someone was a belief held by almost no one. After all, how could electricity revive a human heart?

MIRACULOUS REVIVALS

For many years, the stopping and starting of hearts was relegated to the realm of animals. The Italian Giovanni Bianchi MD (1693-1775) approached his experiments using a Leiden jar,[57] a not uncommon device that stored an electrical charge delivering a shock capable

---

57   Named after the Dutch city where it was invented.

of killing small animals. Thus electrocution was born. He used the Leiden jars to shock dogs, causing seizures and respiratory arrest.[58] Bianchi then applied a *second* electrical shock to the animals' chests. The jolt of electricity restarted their hearts and brought the dogs back to life! Bianchi had just changed the course of medicine, and soon anecdotes about miraculous revivals from electricity followed. P.C. Abdilgaard (1740-1801), a Danish veterinarian, reported in the 1775 *Proceedings of the Medical Society of Copenhagen* that he experimented with chickens, "killing" them with an electric shock to the head and then bringing them back to life with another electric shock, the second time to the chest of the stunned animals.

Then in 1788 an English doctor named Charles Kite reported a story about a three-year-old girl who fell out of a window and struck the pavement, leaving her unconscious and apparently dead. One of the neighbors offered his assistance. His handy Leiden jar just happened to be at the ready, and he delivered several electric shocks to the child's body. After a few tries, he felt a faint pulse. The child survived and was acting normally in about a week. No one will ever know if the child had a cardiac arrhythmia or a concussion, but the tale impressed Kite.

Doctors in the late nineteenth century still did not know why many patients died suddenly hours after a heart attack (or without warning even years later), but the son of a Scottish farmer would solve a large part of the mystery. John A. MacWilliam PhD (1857-1937) became a physiologist at the University of Aberdeen in 1886 and began studies of the muscles of the heart, at first in eels. He outlined the path of contraction of the heart muscle and found out that the same pattern was found not only in eels, but also in mammals. His experiments on cats confirmed that electrical stimulation of the beating heart muscle would induce fibrillation. MacWilliam found that it did not take much electrical current to induce the "high excitability of the ventricular tissues." The fibrillation could be induced in just about

---

58 These animal experiments, considered unethical now, were not uncommon in the eighteenth century.

any part of the heart muscle of the ventricles but also could start up in the atrial muscle. He produced atrial fibrillation, recognizing that disorder in animals long before Einthoven's electrocardiogram made diagnosis much easier.

Using his research findings, John MacWilliam became a visionary of the first order. He sent electrical impulses through the chest wall to speed up the heart rate[59] and showed that gentle electrical shocks could sometimes restart the heartbeat in an organ that was not beating at all. Applying his work to human disease, he proved that different triggers could produce a "hypersensitive" state of the heart, such as exercise-induced changes in heart rate and blood pressure, the heart medication digitalis, the common anesthetic agent chloroform, and finally and most remarkably, the blockage of a coronary artery. In doing so, he discovered a clue to one of the Widowmaker's most dangerous effects.

MacWilliam's research demonstrated that an electrical current could induce fibrillation, but there were only a few scientists willing to pursue his work. The question remained: could an electrical shock both stop and restore a normal heart rhythm as the scattered reports of the eighteenth century suggested? In 1899, the Swiss physiologists Prévost and Batelli took up the cause and made two striking findings in animal hearts; shocks of 2,400 to 4,800 volts could arrest the normal contraction of the heart and bring on fibrillation, *and* a repeat jolt could stop fibrillation and restore the heart rhythm to normal in a matter of seconds. Electricity could both take life and restore it.

In spite of the remarkable finding that electricity could treat a major cause of death from heart attacks, treatment of arrhythmias focused on trying to find effective medications (with little success) and research using electricity waned. Then in the late 1940s, with attention placed on a few centuries-old observations and the inspiration for Mary Shelly's story of reviving the dead monster, there was an awakening.

---

59 A procedure later called transthoracic pacing.

REDISCOVERING SHOCKS

Paul Zoll MD (1911-1999), born in Boston, was someone who stepped in to fill a void in the fight against the sudden death of heart disease. His biographer Stafford Cohen MD described him as an "unlikely hero." He was slight and short, with prominent "jug handle ears." Though shy and reclusive, he was an exceptional student with a particular prowess in mathematics and science, a "cerebral scientific nerd." These traits would serve him well in the challenges he chose to tackle.

After graduating from Harvard College and its medical school and residency training in Boston and New York, Zoll returned to Boston to do research with Monroe Schlesinger MD (1892-1955). Their study compared patients' coronary artery anatomy at autopsy with the history of the symptoms of their disease. It must have been grim work, but at the time, it was the only way to collect the data. The research focused Paul's interest in heart disease, a field with few and largely unproven treatment options.

During his service in World War II, Zoll's connection and subsequent work with a former classmate, Dwight Harken MD (1910-1993), would have a lasting impact on Zoll and what he knew was possible in treating victims of the Widowmaker. Harken had the audacity to believe he could successfully remove bullet and shrapnel pieces from the hearts of wounded soldiers, saving these men from almost certain death. From 1944 to 1945, Harken successfully removed fifty-six foreign bodies from human hearts, and Zoll took careful mental notes of the surgeries. Most important to Zoll's future, he learned that "the heart responds to stimuli." He noticed that when Harken's hands or instruments touched the heart, the muscle would often twitch due to an abnormal heart rhythm, but it would not be long before the normal heart contraction pattern resumed.

After the war, Zoll returned to the Beth Israel Hospital in Boston, and with Harken's work fresh in his mind, he was inspired to pursue the idea of studying the electrical rhythm of the heart and what that research might do for patients. Zoll was also encouraged by another report in particular, one unique experience of a surgeon in Cleveland that fueled Zoll's obsession with electrical treatment of the heart.

In 1947, Claude S. Beck MD (1894-1971), the chief surgeon at Case Western University in Cleveland, Ohio, reported the resuscitation of a young boy undergoing surgery for a chest deformity, using medication, physical massage of the heart muscle, and then finally multiple electric shocks with electrodes applied to the surface of the heart. Beck's one case report held enormous significance; for the first time, there was concrete evidence of the presence of ventricular fibrillation and its eradication by electric shock. Beck had an electrocardiogram attached to the patient, and anyone who looked at the tracings could confirm the veracity of his story. The case, published in the *Journal of American Medical Association*, reached a wide medical audience, including Paul Zoll.

In 1948, Zoll treated a patient with a heart disease known as Stokes-Adams attacks, a disease of the heart's electrical system that causes the heart rate to suddenly drop without warning, resulting in low blood pressure and syncope, or passing out. Medication could help this condition at times but not consistently, and Zoll's patient died. There and then, Zoll committed the rest of his life's work to studying the use of electricity for treating heart disease. There had to be a better way.

By the time Paul Zoll tried treating patients with slow heart rates, the medical world already recognized another ominous problem with the heart's electricity highlighted by the epidemic of the heart attack. Through the widespread use of the electrocardiogram, doctors could see that many patients died quickly after a heart attack because of the sudden onset of abnormal cardiac rhythms. There was no treatment for these arrhythmias, and even if a patient survived the early hours of a heart attack, many were at great risk for these deadly rhythms to arise at any time. These distressing consequences of the Widowmaker's work left heart specialists with deep frustration. Zoll saw an opportunity.

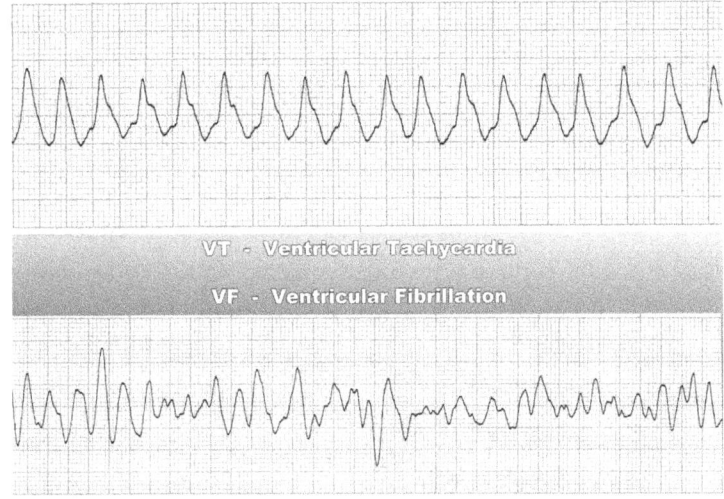

Figure 14. Malignant arrhythmias associated with acute myocardial infarction documented by EKG; usually result in total cardiac arrest if not treated with electric shock. (Copyright Shutterstock)

Zoll was convinced that the scientific concepts of using electricity for the heart were sound, that with the right technology one could both force the heart to beat when its electrical conduction system failed and the heart rate was too slow and also shock the heart out of the deadly rhythms of ventricular fibrillation and ventricular tachycardia, allowing the normal heart rhythm to return without any long-term damage to the heart muscle or the patient. These were remarkable assumptions in the late 1940s. Proof was necessary.

One key problem was that Zoll struggled to find a machine to serve as a stimulator for the heart but discovered a great clue at a surgical conference in Boston. Wilford Bigelow MD (1913-2005), one of the early pioneers in cardiac surgery for congenital heart problems, had used hypothermia (very low body temperatures) to try to decrease the heart's metabolism and preserve its function during the operation. Bigelow presented results that were pretty dismal, but he described something of significance to Zoll. As Bigelow waited for the heart to be re-warmed after the surgery, he would sometimes inadvertently tap the heart with a surgical instrument. As the heart got warmer, Bigelow noticed that the heart rate increased with the physical stimulation. Zoll remembered he had seen something similar when he worked with Harken in the war.

Bigelow's research and experiments seemed particularly relevant to Zoll's problem. Significantly, Bigelow thought that perhaps electricity could replicate the effect of his physical stimulation of the heart and control the heart rate of someone whose heart rate was too slow, just like with Stokes-Adams attacks. He set his team to work, asking John Hipps, an engineer, and John Callaghan MD, another surgeon, to work with him. Hipps fashioned a thin sleeve that contained two electrodes that had been twisted together. The device was so thin he thought he could use it in a new way. Copying what Werner Forssmann did in 1929, Hipps inserted the electrodes into an arm vein and slid them up over the shoulder and down into the right side of the heart. A gentle push would then allow physical contact between the electrodes and the inner wall of the heart muscle. Hipps turned on his electrical stimulator machine connected to the electrodes inside the heart. Would the electrodes be able to "capture" and control the heartbeat when the current was turned on? Yes, indeed, they could; the first use of "transvenous" pacing was in the history books.

When Zoll heard about this he wanted to see if he could also "pace the heart" with electricity. He located one of Hipps' machines, sold by the Grass Stimulator Company, and began work. Instead of using transvenous pacing, he used the stimulator to successfully pace the hearts of dogs by passing current between the chest wall near the spine and the esophagus, "trans*thoracic* pacing." Satisfied that he could consistently pace the dogs' hearts, he turned his attention to using the procedure on humans.

In the days before institutional review boards[60] carefully examined the ethics of any new procedure, doctors had almost free rein to try out new ideas, especially in desperately ill patients with no other viable treatment options. Paul Zoll was also desperate to try out his pacemaker, and his opportunity came in 1952 when he was called to the bedside of a dying man. The patient had an accumulation of blood around the heart, inside a thin layer of cells called the pericardial sac. Despite several injections of adrenaline, his heart failed to restore a consistent heartbeat. When his heart stopped completely, Dr. Zoll reasoned there was little to lose by trying out his electrical pacemaker. He attached the two electrodes to long hypodermic needles and placed the needles under the skin on opposite sides of the front of the patient's chest. He cranked up the Grass stimulator—electricity flowed, and he saw a heartbeat on the electrocardiogram! Remarkably, the device paced the man's heart for twenty minutes before he ultimately died.

It was Zoll's second patient, however, that created the "buzz" in the medical world. This man had Stokes-Adams attacks causing him to pass out without warning. Mr. A had little hope for survival, and as a last resort, his personal physician called Dr. Zoll, who agreed to help. The Zoll pacemaker worked consistently in Mr. A for fifty-two hours! His Stokes-Adams attack abated for unknown reasons, and he was actually able to leave the hospital conscious.

The response to this miracle machine was mixed. As marvelous as this success was, that an external electrical stimulator and electrodes could control the heartbeat, the first transthoracic pacemaker had a major downside. The "therapeutic" electric shocks intensely stimulated the major muscles and nerves, causing discomfort so severe the patient required strong pain medication or sedatives, and sometimes anesthesia, to induce sleep. Many patients called the device "the torture machine" and wanted it removed, even with the

---

60 The purpose of an institutional review board (IRB) is to have other researchers not involved with the study evaluate new projects before they begin to make sure that the rights and welfare of human subjects are protected as much as possible.

understanding that their lives would likely end without it. The patients may have rebelled, but the public was fascinated. A headline in the *Boston Evening Post* in February 1953 read "Three Dead Brought Back to Life," the story recounting the successful resuscitation of patients with slow rates using the Zoll pacemaker. Over the next few years, doctors used Zoll's pacing system more often, but given the painful drawbacks, the medical world held great skepticism that the Zoll technique would work in the long-term.

When Zoll met Alan Belgard, an engineer and co-owner of the Electrodyne Company, a longtime collaboration began, and together they produced new devices intended to tackle the most pressing problem of how to deal with the sudden death from ventricular fibrillation. When Zoll and Belgard began studying how to use electricity to convert ventricular arrhythmias, they ran into an already brewing controversy about how to best deal with the problem. Claude Beck, the first to present irrefutable evidence that electric shock could eradicate ventricular fibrillation, used an "open-chest" approach. This massively invasive intervention required a thoracotomy, a procedure that starts by taking an electric-powered saw to cut the breastbone, spreading the chest by forcing the ribs on both sides of the body apart, and then using a scalpel to cut through layers of tissue to expose the heart, all in the hope that the patient did not bleed to death before the heart could receive the shock.[61] On the other hand, Zoll's idea of defibrillating the heart from the surface of the body, the "closed chest" approach, had much greater appeal if it would work consistently.

Zoll and Belgard kept up their pursuit of an effective heart defibrillator and in the process thought of another useful idea: they created heart rhythm monitors connected to electrodes on the patient's chest so that their heartbeats could be monitored constantly while in their hospital room beds. The monitors had alarms that alerted the nursing staff to abnormal heart rhythms. The Zoll/Belgard

---

61 From the perspective of over sixty years later, how Beck thought that this technique would become widely applicable is more than astonishing.

monitors just kept getting better and better; the team attached a pacemaker to the monitors so that when the heart rhythm got below a certain rate, the pacemaker would shoot current through the chest electrodes to force the heart to beat.

By late 1955, Zoll was confident his new stimulator machine could generate enough voltage to defibrillate a human heart. He and his team reported their first four cases in the *New England Journal of Medicine* in April 1956. Details of the individual cases were demoralizing; only one of the four patients survived. Two of the patients had severe coronary artery disease and the Widowmaker's work had severely damaged their heart muscles. Even when the defibrillator worked to convert the ventricular arrhythmia, new abnormal rhythms recurred, followed by another fibrillation, requiring multiple shock procedures over a short period of time. At first glance, the success rate seemed dismal, but from the perspective of medical history, successfully stopping ventricular fibrillation in even one patient was a monumental achievement in cardiology.

The twenty-five percent success rate brought to light important observations that would stand the test of time. *The man who survived received his defibrillation treatments in two to four minutes after the doctors saw the arrhythmia on his cardiac monitor.* The three casualties had to wait *over seven minutes* until the current shocked their hearts, suggesting that the sooner the heart rhythm could be restored, the better the outcome. The team also observed that when ventricular fibrillation occurs in a badly damaged heart many hours after an acute heart attack, it was an ominous sign that the heart muscle would soon die. A shock could restore a better rhythm temporarily, but the fibrillation and then "cardiac standstill" would follow. A very bad heart simply had a limit to how much it could respond to treatment, defibrillation, pacing, or medication.

Paul Zoll had done something revolutionary, but he was not

alone.[62] and his future success would depend heavily on the work of others around the world.

THOSE RUSSIANS AGAIN

On the other side of the world, in Stalin's Soviet Russia, Naum L. Gurvich PhD (1905-1981) was also exploring how to stop ventricular fibrillation. He experimented with two types of electricity, alternating (AC) and direct (DC), to start and then stop the arrhythmia. In 1945, Gurvich published his work from the 1930s in English. His experiments in 650 animals showed that the DC current was the better form of electricity. DC used less energy than AC and, more importantly, was safer; the scientists weren't getting shocked or electrocuted doing their experiments. The animals shocked with DC survived much more often and without damage to their heart muscle. Their heart rhythms returned to normal more often as well. It was no contest—DC was the right choice for the job.

In addition to his experiments comparing the two forms of electricity, Gurvich greatly expanded the science of the field and used all he had discovered about electricity and the heart to invent a safer way to stop arrhythmias. The technique, called a biphasic shock, decreases the energy needed to break up the reentry circuit. When timed properly, this two-part shock is very effective and requires sixty percent less energy than the older monophasic shock. Based on this technique, Gurvich produced the first commercially available defibrillator. His device went to market years before Zoll and anyone else manufactured their own models. Perhaps, had everyone known about each other's work, their medical advancements could have come sooner. But world politics once again played a role; Soviet

---

62   William Kouwenhoven (1886-1975), a PhD engineer, became a strong competitor for Zoll's designation as the first pioneer to use electricity to shock a heart rhythm back to normal. In addition, Kouwenhoven and his colleagues studied a nonelectrical technique that might save lives—chest massage. In years to come, Kouwenhoven's work would lead to the development of now-established protocols for cardiac resuscitation using external chest compression and ventilation of the lungs.

Russia, with its strong medical and scientific traditions dating back to Pavlov and Anichkov, kept their research to themselves. The western scientists doubted what little data the Russians provided, and during the Cold War between the US and the USSR, they feared collaborating with the communists.

Hubert Humphrey (1911-1978), a senator from Minnesota, helped break the scientific silence from the USSR.[63] In 1958, he visited Soviet Premier Nikita Khrushchev (1894-1971) in Moscow and met Naum Gurvich while touring the Moscow Institute of Reanimatology (Resuscitation). Returning to the United States, Humphrey became a strong advocate of governmental support for medical research. In 1962, he urged the establishment of a National Institute of Health project to investigate the nature of death and resuscitation. On the floor of the United States Senate, he said, "I urge that the United States compete with the USSR in bold research toward at least partial conquest of death." This was music to the ears of people like Paul Zoll.

UNPLEASANT SCIENTIFIC CONFLICT

Zoll was predictably dismissive of the Russians' data, insisting that the best treatment for ventricular arrhythmias was his AC device, but not everyone in America agreed. It was another Harvard professor, Bernard Lown MD (1911-), who finally convinced the medical world that direct current was the best answer to this life-threatening problem. By the early 1960s, Lown had already made major contributions to improving the care of the heart attack patient. He was also obsessed with treating ventricular arrhythmias. He believed that there were many patients with hearts not severely damaged by a heart attack, and yet they died from abnormal heart rhythms. Lown was eager to get his hands on a DC machine like the one that Naum Gurvich used and find out why.

---

63 Humphrey served as Vice President under Lyndon Johnson from 1965 to 1969, and lost a very close US Presidential election in 1968 to Richard Nixon.

Fortunately, Lown was a brilliant physician-scientist but unfortunately not much of an engineer. Luckily, he knew someone who was, Barouh Berkovits (1929-2012), a Jewish immigrant from Czechoslovakia, the only member of his immediate family to survive the Holocaust. He worked for a company producing AC defibrillators, but he had his doubts about the effectiveness of that type of current. By the early 1960s, Lown and Berkovits had the data to show that a DC defibrillator was smaller, used less energy, and was safer than the Zoll AC unit, just as Gurvich's work had shown.

To put it mildly, Paul Zoll did not take Lown's results kindly. For several years, he continued to insist that AC was the preferred method of defibrillation, at times engaging in aggressive verbal battles with Lown at national cardiology meetings. When others confirmed the Lown data, Zoll grudgingly had to agree. Paul Zoll was a brilliant, proud, feisty, and stubborn man given to fits of pique with other researchers. He was also very concerned about his reputation and being right all the time. Great scientists become greater when others use their work to build upon for future advances. Zoll too often was not able to recognize that. For all of his achievements, his legacy is a bit tarnished.

Nevertheless, by the dawn of the 1960s, conclusive evidence proved that electricity could not only start but also stop both ventricular tachycardia and fibrillation. Pacemaker wires inserted into the right side of the heart could speed up the heart rate when necessary.

Still, the heart attack epidemic flourished, and there was a very high incidence of patients who looked like they were going to survive a heart attack and then died suddenly, often found in bed in the morning. There had to be a better way to use this technology that seemed so promising. Maybe hospitals and emergency rooms needed more laboratories like Dr. Frankenstein's. Or just maybe doctors needed to find a way to let the heart fight for itself.

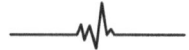

THE JOLT TO RECOVERY

... "Get the paddles—crank it up all the way!" I shouted. A nurse hurriedly wheeled in the defibrillator, the machine's cartwheels clattering on the floor. She plugged it into the wall socket and turned on the "juice," while I tore open James' hospital gown, exposing his burly, hairy chest. He was so large that I wondered if the shock would have enough energy to convert his heart rhythm back to normal. I grabbed the tube of lubricant, reached for the defibrillator paddles, and squirted the gooey liquid on the two paddles, as James' stunned wife was escorted out of the room.

The nurse yelled "charging" and then "charged," meaning the defibrillator was ready to deliver its life-saving shock. I looked up at the monitor again, and I still saw VF. "Clear!" I shouted so no one would touch the bed and get shocked. I pushed the paddles on to James' chest, one in the center and the other under his left armpit.

"All clear," said the head nurse. "Go!"

I pushed the button, and for a few seconds that seemed like an eternity, nothing happened—then the jolt of electricity hit James' chest. He groaned and tried to turn over. We grabbed him and pinned him to the stretcher. I turned my head up to the left to see the monitor—normal rhythm! No more VF, the left ventricle was now pumping blood normally. The scent of singed chest hair filled the air.

James struggled for a few more seconds and then calmed down. He was awake, staring at the ceiling, his mind in a daze. "James, you're all right, doing fine," I said softly in my practiced calm voice. I had been here before. We had a lot of work ahead of us, but the first barrage from the Widowmaker wasn't fatal. I wrote orders, and James was taken up to the ICU. I spent some time with his shaken wife, explaining what happened, and assured her that we'd take good care of him.

In the space of less than an hour, a wife's decision to change direction saved her husband's life. If he'd had his arrhythmia in his car, the outcome would have been very different. James recovered quickly, without complications. He returned to work, took his medications, and came to see me on a regular basis. He never did lose that weight, however.

The idea that an electric shock could save the life of someone suffering from the work of the Widowmaker doesn't make sense. Of all of the treatments that doctors could think of to treat heart attacks, why did this one work? It would take centuries to make this common treatment a reality.

Certainly, the defibrillator was saving lives, but you needed to be at the right place at the right time, with trained doctors and nurses available in seconds. The best way to get this tool to be used more often was still in progress in the 1960s. By the time James needed his shock, progress had been made for many more victims of the Widowmaker, but at the same time, Zoll and Lown were yelling at each other at scientific meetings. New ideas were just beginning.

CHAPTER 12

PRELOADING AND AFTERLOADING: HELPING THE HEART FIGHT BACK

The heart itself is a worthy adversary—born into perfection, 20 grams of muscle pumping at 70 beats per minute, the whole working like a well-oiled machine.

Like gladiators in a ring, we are pitted against each other; yet the favors these doctors throw at the heart may tip the scales and allow it to fight another day.

A SHORT-TERM RESCUE—2014

A rule of critical care: if you think that your patient might need a ventilator, do it; things will only get worse. But like all rules there are exceptions.

Mr. J was in his sixties, a thin African American man from the inner city of Philadelphia. His shortness of breath began just a few hours earlier followed by worsening chest pressure. His blood pressure was 200/120, dangerously high, and his heart rate 120 beats a minute, very fast, both indications that his body was pouring buckets of adrenaline and noradrenaline into his bloodstream. His heart sounds had an extra sound called an "S3," a sure physical exam finding of congestive heart failure. In addition, his lungs were full of fluid and he had some minor swelling of his legs. His EKG was very abnormal; there was evidence of an old heart attack affecting the front wall of his heart. He had already survived a Widowmaker lesion sometime in the past. More worrisome, the EKG also showed that his left ventricle, at least the part not damaged from the heart attack, was very thick, a condition called left ventricular hypertrophy, certainly due to long-standing and badly treated high blood pressure.

First, we had to focus on what we knew. He couldn't remember when he had the heart attack or the last time he had seen his family doctor and denied ever seeing a cardiologist. I asked him if he was taking heart medicine; he said yes, but not in the last few months. My residents and I were clear that his chest pressure resulted from his high blood pressure and the high pressure inside of his heart, increasing his diseased heart muscle's demand for oxygen. The inside of his left ventricle was being stretched tight like an inflated balloon. His congestive heart failure was a complication from the damage done by the previous heart attack and his high blood pressure.

Fortunately, the blood tests showed that he was not having an acute heart attack. We gave him oxygen to ease his shortness of breath and some morphine to relieve his chest pain and anxiety. The morphine had another effect; it increased the size of the veins in the lower part of his body, and that decreased the amount of blood being forced into the heart. Then we followed up with a very large dose of an intravenous diuretic, furosemide, stimulating the kidneys to increase his urine output, which would drop his blood volume.

These interventions had allowed me to successfully break the "ventilator rule." Within ten minutes, my patient was much calmer, breathing easily, and his kidneys were doing their job to get rid of the excess fluid. Nevertheless, he was not yet stable; his blood pressure was still sky high, so his heart was working really hard to push oxygenated blood to his organs. He needed his blood pressure and heart rate lowered. To do that, we chose two drugs, one called lisinopril and the other known as labetalol. In an hour, these medications lowered the pressure and decreased his heart rate as well. We had succeeded in decreasing his damaged heart muscle cells' demand for oxygen.

There was still more to do. We had to do more things to let the heart fight back. We started an intravenous infusion of nitroglycerin to relieve his chest pain and also further drop the pressure inside of his heart. The chest pain dissolved, and our patient was headed in the right direction. His next stop was the CCU for close monitoring . . .

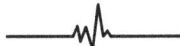

THE HEART REVEALS ITS SECRETS:
FROM THE ANIMAL LAB TO THE BEDSIDE

The President of the United States, Dwight Eisenhower, had his first major myocardial infarction while playing golf in Denver in 1955. His doctors, the premier specialists in the country, flew to his bedside, gave him morphine for his chest pain, and put him in an "oxygen tent." Then the only thing the experts did was talk and ponder the man's future. No wonder the US stock market tumbled for a few weeks. But the President's heart surprisingly recovered, and Eisenhower went on to complete his term in office in 1960 and lived another nine years. That his heart could heal after the serious blow of that heart attack seemed miraculous. In the sixties, the survival rate of a first heart attack was only slightly better than fifty-fifty, and no doctor could figure out why some hearts healed and others did not.

At the time of President Eisenhower's confrontation with the Widowmaker, there was a young man named Eugene Braunwald MD (1929-) who was beginning to lead the charge to uncover the secrets of the normal heart's behavior and then how the heart changed in response to the injury of the heart attack. Eventually, his work would lay the foundation for dramatic improvements in treatment. Yet years before any of this would happen, Braunwald's fate hung in the balance.

DESPERATE TIMES—VIENNA, AUSTRIA, SPRING 1938

Clara Braunwald's mind was racing that morning. The Austrian Nazis had arrested her husband Wilhem, a successful businessman, the night before for the crime of being Jewish, and she knew they would come soon for her and her two sons, Eugene and Jack. Clara thought she had only one ploy that might change the fate of her family. The authorities had already been to the Braunwalds's home before Wilhelm's arrest; the Nazis sent an officer to arrange for the sale of their business. All Jewish enterprises were scheduled for "liquidation," the proceeds turned over to non-Jewish Austrians and a good chunk of cash and ownership commission given to the Nazi officer assigned to the case. Sure enough, the Nazi business liquidator showed up at Clara's home the morning after her husband's arrest. She told him about Wilhelm's arrest and bravely explained to the man that without her husband's knowledge, it would be difficult to locate and assess the value of his business. The SS man might not get as large a "cut" of the sale as he should, she argued, which quickly convinced him to insist that Wilhelm be found and returned to his family. Only a few months later, the family fled Germany to England and finally to the boys, one of whom would grow up to join the ranks of those pursuing the Widowmaker.

Eugene Braunwald grew up to attend medical school in New York City and began work in the cardiac catheterization laboratory at Bellevue Hospital, then directed by André Cournand, the Nobel Prize winner for his work studying the heart using catheters, the idea of Werner Forssmann from 1929. This was a time of exciting advances as well as plaguing questions. Cournand and his colleagues were already able to obtain x-ray images of the heart and its chambers, which were incredible advances but only in anatomy. The function, the how and why, the physiology of the heart engine and its interaction with the circulation as a whole, that information was sketchy. Braunwald was in the right spot with the right people to try to uncover the details of the marvelous adaptability of the human heart. The heart pump could deal with changes in oxygen demand for exercise or hard work by adjusting the heart rate up and down and the body's blood pressure could rise and fall. Studying normal hearts was one pursuit. But what happened in a diseased heart? How did President Eisenhower and others survive their heart attacks? How did the human heart "compensate" for its shortcomings?

"YOU DON'T THROW A WHOLE LIFE AWAY JUST BECAUSE HE'S BANGED UP A LITTLE"[64]

Braunwald's interests were not just intellectual; he was a scientist *and* a doctor and, therefore, someone who wanted to help his patients heal and recuperate. He wanted to understand normal physiology, but more importantly, pathophysiology. How does the damage from a myocardial infarction change the heart? What explained why some patients did well and others not? He didn't just want to become a mechanic—he wanted to become an engineer. He wanted to understand what was going on inside of the heart and its effect on the circulation. The mystery of how a damaged heart was able to change its output of blood was unsolved. How did the heart cells respond to injury, and at what short- and long-term cost to the heart? What was driving this response? The end result was clear: the remaining living heart muscle cells needed to generate more force or they needed to beat faster, or they needed to do both at the same time. How the cells did that was complicated.

Braunwald's hope was that learning these determinants of how the heart engine changed its output would become the "levers" to

---

[64] Actor Chris Cooper referring to the champion racehorse Seabiscuit, as Tom Smith, the horse's trainer, from the film of the same name, 2003.

adjust the heart's function. Only with that knowledge could doctors even imagine how to assist a scarred heart in its recovery. Medications might well increase or decrease the heart's output. The cardiologist at the bedside might truly become an engineer driving the heart.

Using animal and human samples of heart muscle, Braunwald and his colleagues at the National Institutes of Health (NIH) in Bethesda, Maryland, established that two of the main drivers of the output of blood by the heart were the heart rate, how fast it was beating, and something called "contractility." His analogy was to think about a team of horses pulling a stagecoach; if you want the stagecoach to move faster, either you can add more horses or whip each horse harder. There are two hormones that can increase heart rate and contractility. Adrenaline and noradrenaline come from the nervous system and the adrenal glands, chemicals released when the brain sends a signal that more cardiac output is needed to perform work or exercise. And these molecules were also likely candidates to become activated during and after a heart attack. These hormones create "chronotropy," a faster heart rate, and "inotropy," the ability of the heart muscle cells to generate more force with each beat.

In addition, the heart muscle cells, called sarcomeres, push blood forward using two key molecules called actin and myosin. The molecules form chemical bonds with each other and, using energy from the molecule adenosine triphosphate (ATP), slide back and forth, forming and then breaking apart their bonds. The more the actin and myosin overlap each other, the more force generated. The heart muscle cells resemble the complex gears of an engine transmission that allow your car to work harder going up a hill and "downshift" when you slow down around a curve.

The motivation behind Braunwald's work was to see what happened to the heart muscle when it had a normal blood supply and then try to understand what happened to heart muscle damaged by lack of blood supply. Molecules like adrenaline and noradrenaline did increase the contractility of the heart overall when they were used in the experiments. These chemicals, which were starting to be used to increase blood pressure in patients with severe heart attacks, are appropriately called "inotropes." In addition to providing more force-generating ability to each heart muscle, some of these medications also increased the heart rate; they did "double-duty" as chronotropes.

A major heart attack that damages a good portion of the muscle of the left ventricle puts an immediate huge burden on the heart muscle cells, the sarcomeres that still had normal blood supply. The normal cells needed to beat faster and harder. For decades, doctors noted the increased heart rate seen in heart attack patients. It was also clear that they had signs of too much adrenaline in their blood; the sweating and the anxiety this powerful molecule causes is usually obvious. It certainly looked like the release of adrenaline and noradrenaline by the body, or doctors giving adrenaline to heart attack patients, was the logical and right thing to do to try to support the blood pressure and heart rate while the heart healed.

Braunwald and his NIH researchers for the first time put some real numbers on the effects of a variety of medications on the heart's output and use of oxygen. But they knew that there was a second part to the story of how the normal and injured heart interacted with the other blood vessels, that is, how the entire system of the circulation functioned.

In 1968, invigorated by a new facility on the West Coast, Braunwald and his team[65] did meticulous research on the effect of the blood pressure on the function of the normal heart and a heart damaged by a heart attack. The blood pressure is the resistance in the arteries that the left ventricle needs to pump against to push the blood to reach the tissues; the higher the resistance, that is the more constricted the blood vessels, the harder the heart muscle cells need to work. The resistance to blood flow is named "afterload." The lower

---

65   Braunwald agreed to move to San Diego, California, to lead the Department of Medicine of a brand-new medical school. Many of his key collaborators followed him to the West Coast.

the afterload, the blood pressure of the arterial side of the circulation, the easier it is for the left ventricle to pump more efficiently. But the research showed that there was a range of blood pressure that was optimal for the performance of the heart. If medications dropped the resistance in the arteries too much, then the heart could not deliver enough blood and oxygen to the organs.

What about the other side of the circulation? The veins empty blood into the right side of the heart where it is pumped through the lungs and returns to the left side. Braunwald knew that the pressure in the veins and the right side of the heart must have a significant effect on how much blood could be "loaded" into the left side of the heart to be pumped forward. If there was not enough blood and pressure in the right heart, there was less blood to "prime the pump" on the left side of the heart and then less output of the heart. Here again is the engine metaphor—the cylinders of the engine might be fine, but if the fuel pump is faulty, the cylinders can't do their job well. This influence of the veins on the heart is called "preload." Preload, just like afterload, is tricky. The right amount of blood entering the heart from the vein will stretch the heart muscle cells a bit more and create more actin and myosin bridges.[66] The heart is like a rubber band—stretch the right distance and it will snap back more with more force. But don't over-stretch it.

If the heart muscle is weak from disease, often there is too much blood or liquid in the veins. In the short term, this retention of fluid is beneficial; the heart muscle stretches and the effect helps improve the heart's function. But this improvement in function comes at a cost: as the left ventricle expands, the inner lining of the cells of the ventricle use more oxygen. The ventricle is like a plastic balloon; the larger it gets, the more pressure is placed on its cells. This "wall tension" was the third key driver of the demand of the heart for oxygen. The demand was not just from the heart rate and the intrinsic contractility of the

---

66 This effect of the volume of blood on the heart is called the Frank-Starling Relationship, first discovered by physiologists of the late nineteenth century.

sarcomeres. In people with damaged hearts, too often the right and left sides of the heart reach their limit of adaptation, and excess fluid ends up in the lungs as "pulmonary edema" or in the lower part of the body as "edema," swelling of the legs and abdomen. Doctors were aware of this effect of all types of heart disease for centuries, but now with sophisticated animal experiments, Braunwald and his colleagues demonstrated how and why these physical findings arose.

By the early 1970s, Braunwald's epic volume of discoveries included maneuvers to change the heart's response to damage to part of its pump from a heart attack. Researchers also realized that using these new strategies of treatment, like using medications to increase the heart rate, the blood pressure, and the volume of fluid in the heart, was very delicate. In a heart suffering a myocardial infarction, there were three kinds of cells: undamaged cells, dead cells, and an important group of cells that were injured and could recover. The extent to which these latter cells recovered greatly affected the outcome. It logically concerned doctors that if they prescribed medication to try to get those cells to beat harder and faster and use more oxygen, perhaps the drug would further damage them, maybe to the point where they would surely die.

The ideas of inotropy, chronotropy, afterload, and preload had immediate effects on treatment of congestive heart failure, the dreaded heart attack complication. By the 1960s, cardiologists for the first time had a clear scientific basis for medications that had been used for years. Digitalis, the drug made from the foxglove plant since the eighteenth century,[67] had inotropic properties similar to adrenaline; diuretics caused the rapid elimination of excess fluid and decreased preload; medications that lowered the blood pressure lowered the afterload; and medications that raised the blood pressure increased the afterload.

---

67 William Withering MD (1741-1799), an English doctor, first described the use of digitalis for heart disease in 1785. He discovered that local women were using a plant extract for palpitations and leg edema. Foxglove is a common plant native of Europe, Asia, and Africa.

These might all be beneficial for the slow-burning, heart-disease patients, but what about the dire, massive heart attacks? To this end, in the late 1970s, Braunwald and his colleague Peter Maroko MD embarked on ambitious experiments in dogs. The purpose of their study was to address their chagrin about the treatment of the sickest heart attack victims. Their article in the journal *Circulation* begins with a regret and a hope: "The classical treatment of power failure of the heart[68] consequent upon myocardial infarction is relatively ineffective . . . a possible therapeutic approach to this syndrome would be an attempt to limit the size of the infarction." Quite simply, the treatment at that time for a major heart attack was very poor; doctors needed to figure out how to save as much heart muscle as possible from permanent damage if prognosis was going to improve.

Using an elaborate experimental model, Braunwald and Maroko occluded the left anterior descending coronary arteries of dogs and observed two data points over time: how much EKG change of severe damage to the heart cells was seen in different locations in the heart and how much of a "biomarker" molecule was released into the dog's blood because of the death of heart muscle cells. The two values would indicate how much heart muscle was damaged by the occlusion of the artery. Then they would try different medications to try to increase the heart rate and the output of the heart: four that were inotropic drugs, and one, propranolol, that had the opposite effect of decreasing both contractility and heart rate. The overall results of the study were very upsetting and discouraging. The four inotropic medications, the ones that made the heart beat faster and harder, all increased the destruction of the heart cells, even compared to cells of dogs that were not treated at all after their main heart blood supply was cut off and a heart attack created.

In experimental animals, Braunwald and Maroko demonstrated the great paradox in treating major heart attacks; the necessary "first

---

68   Power failure meaning congestive heart failure from the death and damage to heart muscle cells.

aid" treatment might do more harm than good in the long run. As the undamaged sarcomeres struggled to assume their increased load, the assistance of the body's own chemicals like adrenaline were only very short-term aids; these chemicals, and the medications that Braunwald and Marako used in their experiments, were forcing those cells to use too much blood and oxygen and creating even more damage. Although these medications will transiently increase blood pressure and heart rate, they were actually toxic to an injured heart. But often a cardiologist treating a patient had no choice but to use these drugs while trying to save someone with a low cardiac output in the first hours after a heart attack.

But there was one important hopeful lesson from this research: *The propranolol reduced the extent of heart muscle damage.* This was a great clue to a new approach to the treatment of the heart attack. Perhaps by turning down the heart's demand for more blood and oxygen with a medication like propranolol, cardiologists could save many more damaged heart cells and let them recover. Coupled with the knowledge that the amount of fluid in the body also affected the damaged heart's need for oxygen, a new treatment strategy could improve the outcome for many more people with heart attacks. There was much more that cardiologists could do besides stand around and just observe, as Eisenhower's doctors did in the 1950s. In an era where the best treatment, opening up the blocked artery and restoring the blood supply, was just a dream, management of heart rates, fluid volume, and blood pressure were the keys to improved outcomes. It would take another decade until a radical form of medical treatment would open up arteries.[69]

Dr. Braunwald barely survived his youth but would go on to advance the care of patients with heart disease in so many ways that

---

69 When this revolution in heart attack care exploded in the early 1980s, Eugene Braunwald had moved back to the East Coast and was the Chairman of Medicine at one of Harvard Medical Schools flagship hospitals, the Peter Bent Brigham Hospital, later renamed Brigham and Women's Hospital. If Dr. Braunwald's contributions to Medicine ended then, his accomplishments would still have established his position as one of the greatest cardiologists of the twentieth century. But he was not done.

it's difficult to summarize his accomplishments, as well as those of his many protégées; their contributions to medical science and cardiology continue to this day. Dr. Braunwald has set the standard in academic medicine for the "Triple-Threat" physician—a researcher, a clinician, and a teacher. His career came so close to not even starting.

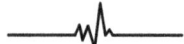

AFTERMATH: THE REAL PROBLEM

... When Mr. J was able to talk in full sentences without gasping for air, we did get more medical history. He wasn't sure, but he thought his heart attack had been within the last five years, and in that time, he had gone to several other Philadelphia hospitals for the same problem. His echocardiogram, the sound wave images of his heart, confirmed what his EKG had suggested. His heart's badly scarred front wall barely moved. His undamaged heart muscle was very thick because of his blood pressure.

Mr. J could not recall the names of his prescription medications. He had run out months ago and just didn't want to pay for the refills. He lived alone but had some close friends in his apartment building. He smoked cigarettes when he could afford to buy them. He did use alcohol on the weekends, sometimes with cocaine. But he insisted he never used these during the week. I found it sadly ironic that he was willing to pay for cigarettes, alcohol, and cocaine, but not his heart medications.

By forty-eight hours in the hospital, Mr. J was feeling so well that he wanted to go home, but I insisted that he stay another day. As I always do when sick patients feel better, I asked him about his diet—what he ate for breakfast, lunch, and dinner. He admitted he often had fast food loaded with salt, meat, and fat; where else in the inner city could you eat all of your meals so cheaply? He admitted he was more of a fan of salt than sweets. I discussed the consequences of eating too much salt when you have a damaged heart muscle, explaining that salt makes you thirsty, and then you drink too much water that eventually ends up in the lungs and you become short of breath. He said he understood.

We prepared his medication list for discharge the next day and included oral doses of furosemide, lisinopril, and labetalol, as well as aspirin to reduce his risk of another heart attack and a statin to try to keep his cholesterol low. We discussed the possibility of having a surgically implanted personal defibrillator, explaining that because his cardiac function was so poor, he was at great risk of sudden death from an arrhythmia. The resident made an appointment for him to come to the Cardiology Clinic as an outpatient in about a week. We even arranged for a visiting nurse to check on him twice a week for a few weeks. Mr. J was ready to go home the next morning.

The residents and I were in a good mood the next morning. Our patients were doing well, and several were ready for discharge. We had done our job well, we thought. The team led me into Mr. J's room to just do a quick exam and say goodbye. He was sitting on a chair next to his bed, slumped over and hungrily munching on something, stuffing one after another into his mouth. As I walked closer, I saw the package—the colorful yellow outside and the shiny aluminum foil on the inside: a huge bag of potato chips. I knew Mr. J would be back to a hospital in short order.

CHAPTER 13

DISPELLING THE SECOND SHIBBOLETH: THE CORONARY ARTERY CATHETER

Though they now hear the message of the heart,
I have confidence that they
are barely learning to interpret its signals.
I am still many steps ahead.

There is talk, however, of peering inside, of tracing
the destruction before it's too late.
Are these rumors, or do they signal that I
will have to double my efforts?

SHOOTING DYE IN THE DARK—AUGUST 1979

You never forget your first experience in the cardiac cath lab. I was a first-year cardiology fellow when I walked into the cold room that reeked of Betadine antiseptic, the darkness broken only by the greenish glow of the monitoring screen in the corner of the room. I was completely overwhelmed and appropriately intimidated by the task at hand and remembered a heart surgeon's admonition, "If you give young people sharp tools, bad things can happen."

In preparation, I put on the required paper shoe covers, cap, and facemask over my scrub pants and shirt and then donned the heavy lead apron to shield my gonads from the radiation. I turned to the "circulating nurse," whose role it was to manage the necessary care outside the sterile area, and her expression told me she had seen numerous frightened trainees like me. Impatiently, she helped me put on a sterile gown, spun me around, and briskly tied the back, stopping just short of choking me. She jammed on my sterile gloves so quickly that if I hadn't been ready, she could have dislocated one of my fingers. While I was nervous, I knew the real action was not going to begin until much later, when (and if!) I finally gained the trust of the attending doctors.

By my second month working in the cath lab, I was beginning to understand the sequence of the procedure, learning what syringes to fill, what packages of "guidewires" to open, and what catheters to prepare. The attending cardiologists had previously observed my work and deemed me "not all thumbs," so by then, I became the "primary" operator on all of my cases. I was going to place a plastic catheter tube into a live person's coronary artery.

And then, I was going to shoot dye in the dark...

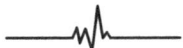

POISON INTO MAGIC AND SEIZING THE MOMENT: THE GENIUS OF MASON SONES

> "I take off my shirt and my pants and I hang up my balls.
> I am not going to carry my balls around all day for him to kick them.
> I put my balls back on when I leave."
>
> —*Arnoldo Fiedotin MD, cardiology research fellow of Mason Sones, MD*

"Cough, goddamn it!"

That may be the best-known quote in the insulated world of cardiologists.

October 30, 1958, was just another day in the cardiac cath lab at the Cleveland Clinic. The lab director, the irascible F. Mason Sones Jr. MD (1918-1985) was performing a standard heart catheterization on a twenty-seven-year-old man who had heart disease of the valves of the left side of his heart, the aortic and mitral valves. Sones and his assistant pushed a catheter from the patient's arm artery back over the shoulder and toward the heart, just as Werner Forssmann had instructed twenty-nine years earlier.

But Sones would go a step further than Forssmann; he would inject contrast dye a few centimeters above the top of the heart into the aorta. The dye would then eject forward to create a white image of the aorta on the fluoroscopy screen, a form looking just like part of a curving garden hose. If the aortic valve at the top of the left ventricle was damaged and leaked, some of the dye would flow back into the left ventricle. Sones could see the defect by filming the dye sequence.

From his "pit of revelation," a "duck blind" of a four-foot hole in the floor that he had built below the large x-ray tubes so that he could focus his eyes on the screen without needing to strain his back and neck all of the time, Sones watched the image on the small fluoroscopy screen take shape. What he saw terrified him. The pupils of his eyes must have grown to saucer-size in just a few seconds. Immediately, he screamed his infamous instructions at the patient, "Cough, goddamn it," as he briskly yanked the catheter out of the coronary artery.

What had just happened?

When Sones had advanced the catheter, it dove down toward the aortic valve, and instead of resting just on top of the aortic valve, it unexpectedly plunged into forbidden territory: the small opening of one of the two main coronary arteries. The catheter tip, continuing to eject dye, sat inside of the artery, while the dye created a very clear x-ray image of the inside of the young man's coronary artery. The man's heart rate immediately slowed down, and Sones thought for sure the patient was going to die within seconds.

Many shibboleths about touching the heart had been destroyed, but the last holdout in the 1950s was the prohibition against injecting contrast dye into the small coronary arteries. Most doctors, including Sones, believed the dye would suddenly cut off the supply of blood and oxygen to the heart muscle, leading to sudden death. The dye for sure would poison the artery and the heart muscle. So Sones acted quickly, using the only way he could think of to clear the dye from the coronary artery rapidly, by moving it into the heart muscle cells and then allowing it to drain through the heart's veins and back into the circulation. The force from the cough worked! The patient was in no distress, the heart rate picked up to normal, and the dye disappeared from the image screen.

By accident, Sones had just performed the first coronary artery angiogram. The ecstatic cardiologist now had a treasure—a film of the detailed image of the inside of a human coronary artery. He understood the significance. Sones had been frustrated for years that there was no procedure to look inside of the coronary arteries. Though he performed catheterizations mostly in children, he was also very aware of the epidemic of coronary artery disease and the implication his accident might have on fighting heart attacks. Returning to his office, he told his secretary, "We just revolutionized cardiology." After that unforgettable October day, he knew he had lots more work to do, and there was no one better prepared for the challenge.

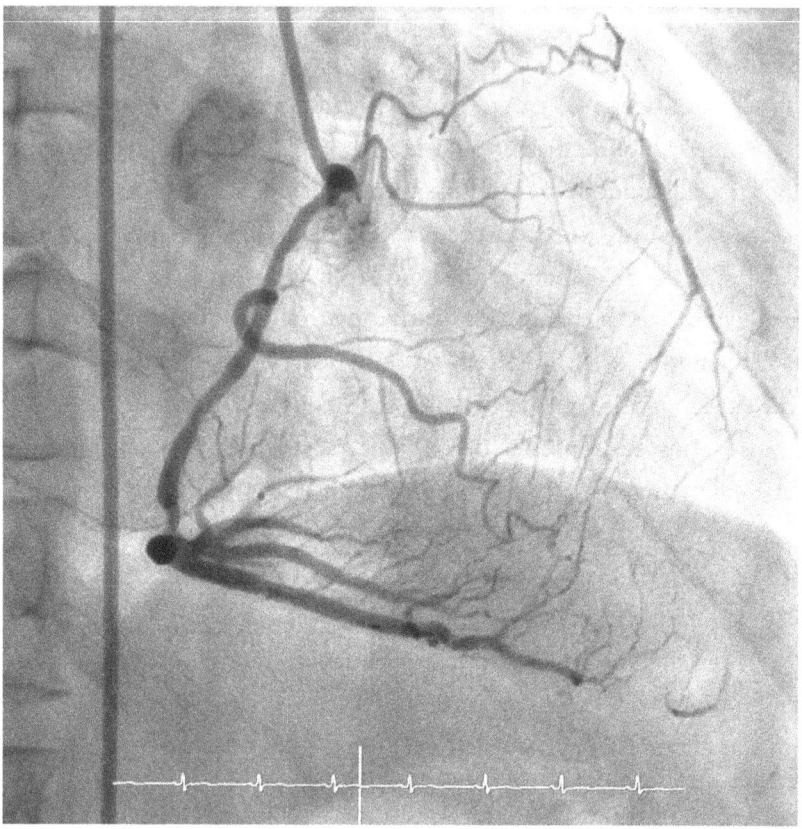

Figure 15. Example of imaging of the right coronary artery with contrast dye injection, accidentally discovered by Mason Sones MD in 1958. (Copyright Shutterstock)

Mason Sones was born in 1918 in Mississippi. During medical school, he expressed his interest in cardiology to one of his professors, who replied it was a "nothing specialty," but Sones ignored the discouraging advice, pursuing a career in cardiology at the Cleveland Clinic in 1950. Within a few years, he became the director of the cardiac catheterization laboratory at the world's leading heart hospital.

He made life quite difficult for those around him. Sones was a disagreeable workaholic and expected all of his colleagues and trainees to live in the hospital fourteen to eighteen hours a day, seven days a week. He chain-smoked and walked around the hospital in a stained T-shirt, looking more like a vagrant than the head of the cath lab. In the lab, he continued to take puffs on his cigarettes, using sterile forceps to hold the butts. He talked constantly, which his colleagues described as "exuberant, endless, and exhausting," and he cursed extensively. Those working with him said his lab was a "three-ring circus played out every day." His nickname, Little Napoleon, was well deserved.

Despite his many personal deficits, he was as focused on advancing cardiology as any human being could be. After he accidentally shot dye into that young man's coronary artery, he felt confident he could do this procedure safely on the many patients suffering from the life-threatening chest pain of coronary artery atherosclerosis. The ramifications of his procedure were immense; for the first time, doctors could see the actual anatomy of the plaques of LDL inside the coronary arteries of live human beings, providing the necessary data that could lead to possible treatments. Within days of his discovery, Sones asked colleagues to refer their patients with chest pain or a history of a heart attack to him for his new procedure.

The response was overwhelming, and the Cleveland Clinic cath lab patient volume exploded. They quickly enjoined physicists and engineers to develop new and better catheters. Sones and his colleague, Earl Shirey MD, worked like high-performance machines, impressively completing the tricky new coronary angiograms. Even with better tools, safely slipping the end of a catheter into the petite orifice of a coronary artery was part skilled dexterity and part art form.

Sones and Shirey recognized that they were exploring unknown realms of knowledge. The two researchers were pretty sure that a heart attack, one confirmed by the typical changes on an electrocardiogram, was caused by a one hundred percent blockage, but even that remained just an assumption. But almost nothing was known about the relationship between the symptom of chest pain and the severity and location of atherosclerosis in the coronary artery. What degree of blockage would cause chest pain? Does everyone with chest pain have atherosclerosis in the coronary arteries? Are there people with chest pain who did not have atherosclerosis, and therefore something else was causing the chest pain?

The Cleveland Clinic team practiced first and did not report any data to the outside world on their first one thousand patients with chest pain that their doctors thought might be due to atherosclerosis; they wanted to be sure they had done the procedures correctly and had collected reproducible and consistent information. Only when they had completed their next one thousand patients did Sones and his colleagues write up the data for publication, correlating the diagnosis made by the patient's doctors with their cath lab anatomy findings.

The data exceeded everyone's expectations and contained three key results. Ninety-nine percent of the patients whose electrocardiogram demonstrated "Q waves," the classic signs of a previous myocardial infarction in the patient's past, had a severe obstruction of at least one of the three major coronary arteries. The first result: Q waves on the EKG equals major atherosclerosis. What was even more interesting were the patients who experienced chest pain with exertion. The data would answer the question: how good were doctors in taking histories? Even in the age before effective treatment, this vital historical information revealed much about lifestyle and employment. The angiograms confirmed the doctors' judgments; ninety-five percent of patients with exertional chest pain had significant coronary artery blockages. The second result: exertional chest pain equals major atherosclerosis. What about the patients whose chest pain didn't resemble angina at all? The details are not in the publication, but it is likely that these people had sharp chest pain that came and went, was not related to physical exertion, and lasted only for seconds. The data left no doubt; ninety-six percent of the time, these individuals had no significant coronary artery obstructions. The clinical history was again very accurate. The third result: all chest pain does not equal atherosclerosis.

The data also revealed other surprises as well as confirming some suspicions. What about the people in the "gray areas" of clinical judgment, such as chest pain only at rest, and not with exertion? In those patients, sixty-five to eighty percent of them had some degree of coronary artery disease, and although it was likely that the chest pain was due to this disease, there was less certainty.[70] In addition, the overwhelming number of his patients were male, which supported the belief that the Widowmaker preferred men but did not explain why. Was the incidence of women with coronary artery disease lower at that time, were their symptoms different from those in men, and were they too often dismissed by the male-dominated medical profession? Was Sones guilty of "selection bias" in his work? Future generations would delve into these questions.

Sones and his colleagues became true investigators, like an FBI team trying to solve a crime. They collected so much data and then took the time to think carefully about what they had found. They did not want to offer just individual opinions but rather sound conclusions based on their newfound obsession with statistics and large numbers of patients. This was a far cry from the last century, when the advice of a lone "thought leader," like a surgeon who believed that he should never touch the heart, could convince the rest of the doctors that one man's opinion was the ultimate truth.

Mason Sones worked and lived for another twenty-seven years after 1958 and helped drive the remarkable advance of coronary artery bypass surgery as well as coronary angiography. Unfortunately, his love of cigarettes claimed his life: he died of lung cancer in 1985. His surgical colleague at the Cleveland Clinic, René Favaloro MD, summarized Sones' work aptly, "Without the work of Dr. Mason Sones Jr.—the most important contributor to modern cardiology—all of our efforts in myocardial revascularization would have been fruitless."

---

70   This controversy still rages today and often requires other tests, such as nuclear imaging of the heart blood supply with exercise, or the measurement of how the flow in a coronary artery responds to medication given at the time of the catheterization, to resolve the question.

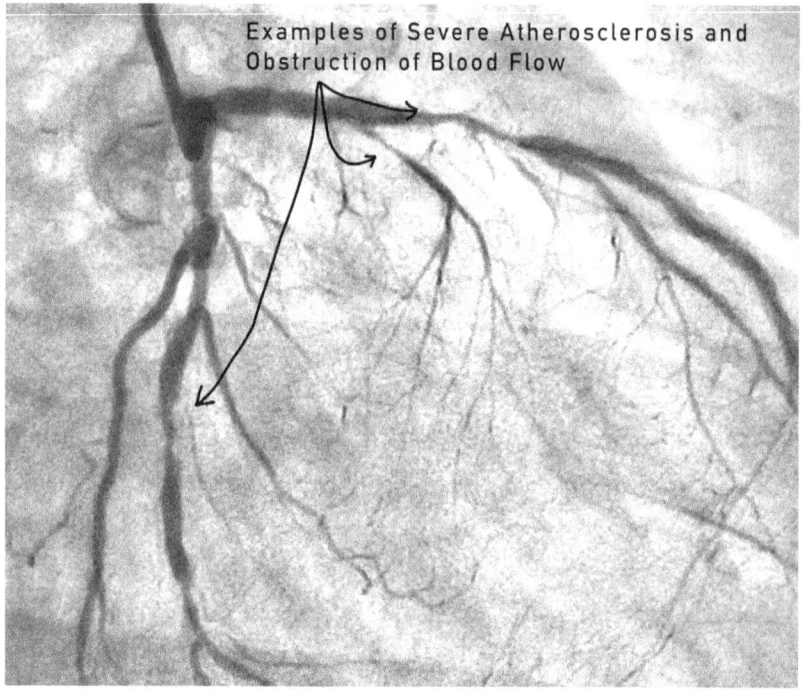

Figure 16. Coronary angiogram demonstrating multiple areas of significant atherosclerosis of the coronary arteries
(Copyright Shutterstock)

A BETTER PATH

The Sones' method was a crucial breakthrough in trying to defeat the Widowmaker, but it had serious drawbacks. The procedure required an incision in an artery, sometimes causing major trauma with nasty vascular complications. Would it be safer to perform the catheterization in a "percutaneous" way, through the skin into the artery rather than making an incision? If this worked, catheterization would no longer be a surgical procedure. A percutaneous entry would involve finding the artery by feeling the pulse and then placing a good-sized needle into it, which would provide access to the vascular system. But then what? How does one thread a catheter from the skin through an artery and then into the heart without making a major incision?

In 1953, Sven Ivar Seldinger MD (1921-1998), a Swedish radiologist, had an idea and devised a several step process to address this question. First, he developed a very thin metal wire that he called the "guidewire," much like the line on a fly-fishing rod. He inserted it through a needle into the artery. The wire was so flexible he could see, using x-ray guidance, that by simply pushing it forward he could move the wire through the peripheral arteries and into the chest arteries, just above the heart, giving him a foothold. He then slid the needle back and out of the skin without risking damage to the artery in the arm.

The real genius was the next step. Seldinger constructed a plastic catheter that fit snugly over the top of the end of the guidewire that was still out of the patient's body as it entered the arm artery. Using both hands, he pushed the catheter forward with his left hand and pulled the guidewire back and then out of the patient with his right hand. The amazing had just happened: Seldinger had a plastic tube, one very similar to the one Sones used, in an artery without a skin incision. The radiologist used the end of the catheter that was outside of the body to inject dye into the artery. Seldinger's three-part system, a needle, a guidewire, and a catheter, made it possible to image arteries throughout the body, including the kidneys, brain, and blood vessels of the legs. He did not, however, attempt to image the heart's arteries. Perhaps Seldinger thought that someone braver than he could try that one.

Seldinger's success did inspire others to go even further. Herbert Abrams MD (1920-2016) and his colleague Howard Ricketts MD from Stanford University in Palo Alto, California, expanded Seldinger's idea and his guidewire technique by accessing the heart through the blood vessels of the abdomen. While Abrams and Ricketts did have some success with this technique, in the early 1960s, the catheter design held back their progress because the plastic was too often too stiff for the fine movements necessary to place them into the openings of the coronary arteries. Melvin Judkins MD (1922-1985) believed he could do a better job with the catheters.

Judkins was born in Southern California and after graduation from medical school moved to a small town in Washington State to open a general practice in 1946.[71] But Mel Judkins did not want to be a general practitioner; he wanted to become a radiologist. And he wanted to do more than interpret images. He had set his sights on discovering how to combine imaging with other new tools that could turn the field of radiology into one with much better diagnostic capabilities. So Mel applied for training in radiology. In 1961, the University of Oregon took a chance on the thirty-nine-year-old general practitioner, and the gamble paid big dividends. Judkins aggressively pursued improving the field of arterial catheterization, traveling to Sweden to work with Seldinger and to Cleveland to watch Mason Sones' techniques.

His persistence would eventually be highly rewarded. Experimenting with different forms of plastic, by the late 1960s, Judkins had developed a nearly perfect polyurethane catheter to insert into the coronary arteries. He created catheters with pre-formed ends, manufactured in a series of sizes and curves. If the right shape and size was used, the catheter would just fall into a coronary artery opening. Judkins' technique quickly became the most commonly used way to perform cardiac catheterization. It was far easier and safer than Sones' method. Perhaps even more importantly, the Judkins' technique was much easier to teach than the Sones' method and allowed thousands of cardiology trainees to ply their trade in community hospitals worldwide, not in just a few select academic medical centers.

The work of these pioneers continues to evolve today,[72] and thanks, in large part, to Sones, Seldinger, and Judkins, the cath lab table became the "table of truth." Cardiac catheterization made it

---

71 Reportedly, Judkins' first patient was a dog, and as a courtesy, he did not charge the owners a fee for his services.
72 In the last ten years, the resurrection of a method first employed in 1989 has gained great traction. The heart catheterization begins at the radial artery, one of the two arteries supplying blood to the hand. With the development of smaller and more flexible catheters, this procedure punctures the radial artery and then by manipulating the catheter through the arm, just like the Sones' technique, it enters the aorta and the opening of the coronary arteries.

possible to define the anatomy and pathophysiology of coronary artery disease. Without knowing the anatomy of diseased arteries, treating this life-threatening problem is like trying to fly to the moon without understanding Newton's laws of gravity. The lessons learned from that accidental discovery of angiography led us to even more important discoveries.

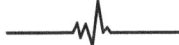

A LUCKY DAY IN NEW HAVEN

... It was a hot Friday in August that day when I came to work and headed straight to the cath lab to look at the schedule on the chalkboard. I had seen several patients the night before to obtain their history and have them sign a consent form, but I didn't know which cases I was going to be assigned to. It would be another day spent in a dark room injecting dye into someone's coronary arteries to see if they had atherosclerosis or not.

My eyes darted from the top of the board to the bottom searching for my initials. I saw three cases for me in the morning and only one in the afternoon, typical for the day before the weekend unless there were emergencies to add to the schedule. Then I looked to see which attending cardiologist I would be working with, and when I saw the name next to the afternoon case, my heart began to palpitate.

The name said "Fearon." I had already worked with all of the other cath lab attendings by then but not Richard Fearon MD. Dr. Fearon was one of the first cardiologists to perform cardiac catheterizations at Yale, a very skilled clinician and technician in the lab. Unlike all of the other cath lab attendings, Dr. Fearon did his procedures the first way they were ever done; he was a Mason Sones devotee.

The Sones technique is surgery, no doubt about it, and I had never done one. I had been a surgical intern, so I had some experience with blood vessel surgery (more than most cardiology trainees!), but that had been four years earlier. I had seen a Sones case done as an assistant, so I knew the sequence, but now I was going to the "primary operator." I had my other cases to do, but I kept reviewing the Sones method in my mind all morning. The morning procedures, all done through the artery of the upper leg using Drs. Seldinger and Judkins' methods, went smoothly.

Although my heart rate had slowed down, I did feel sweat around the back of my neck begin to soak my scrub shirt as I waited for Dr. Fearon to appear in the lab. I double checked all of the equipment and mentally reviewed for the fifth time the patient's history; he was a man in his fifties with chest pain, but a stress test that hadn't given a conclusive result as to whether or not the pain was from a blocked coronary artery.

Dr. Fearon showed up precisely at two p.m. He was a thin but muscular man of average height, looking as if he had been a competitive athlete, perhaps a tennis player or a runner. I knew he was a man of few words and his eyes, especially prominent over his surgical mask, were fierce. Thinking about him years later, Vladimir Putin comes to mind. He glanced around the room and said sternly, "Let's get started."

The patient was nearly asleep from the sedative I gave him, and I quickly numbed the skin of his right elbow. I made a smooth two-inch incision over his brachial artery and went to work, isolating the artery from the other structures in his arm. I took a deep breath and glanced at Fearon. He was still silent. I asked, "Are we ready to open the artery?" He nodded.

I carefully cut a small slit in the artery and was quickly able to advance the catheter into the hole and push it up toward the man's shoulder. Often it was difficult to manipulate the catheter through the artery of the arm to the shoulder and then down into the aorta of the chest, but the gods were with me that day—the catheter sailed smoothly "downwind" toward the heart. I could see the catheter bouncing with each heartbeat, and the pressure transducer hooked up to the end of the catheter was transmitting a beautiful normal pressure curve. The patient was snoring in rhythm with his heartbeat. It was still very cold in the room, but I was feeling calmer and had stopped sweating.

Quickly, I advanced the catheter into the heart, and we injected the contrast dye so that we could film the function of the man's left ventricle. The dye slammed through the catheter, and we could see the outline of the heart. The heartbeat sped up, and the front and back walls of the heart had a head-on collision with one another. This was a good thing; there was no evidence of a previous heart attack. His ejection fraction was normal.

Now with the easy part done, I pulled the catheter out of the left ventricle as Fearon removed the "power injector" of dye and re-attached a syringe filled with more contrast dye. The time had come to look at the coronary arteries.

The openings to the coronaries, one on the right and the other on the left, are just above the aortic valve. I maneuvered the catheter toward the left coronary artery, and Fearon "puffed" a bit of dye. I tried a few times, and I could see I was getting close. With one more subtle twist, a push forward on my end, and another puff of dye, the left coronary was outlined all the way to its end! More good news: there were no major blockages in the left coronary artery. It was clear of significant atherosclerosis. My first shot of dye in the dark with Dr. Fearon!

I pulled the catheter out of the left coronary and twisted it toward the right coronary artery opening, sliding it up and down the aortic wall. Fearon continued to puff the dye. Finally, some of the dye trickled into the right coronary, and I could see where to put the catheter. He handed me the syringe, and I pushed in the dye. As the dye flowed into the artery, we had our diagnosis—there was a ninety percent blockage in the top portion of the right coronary artery. This plaque of atherosclerosis was the cause of this man's chest pain, his angina pectoris. Sones' procedure made the diagnosis. The accuracy of his stress test just wasn't good enough, especially since only one artery was blocked.

As I removed the catheter, I tightened a suture above the hole in the arm artery. In less than five minutes, I placed nice-looking sutures into the artery itself then held my breath and loosened the suture I had previously placed further up the arm on the outside of the artery wall. The artery was pumping, but no blood was leaking out. I took my finger and felt the pulse over the incision, and it was strong and steady. Closing the skin was easy and my adrenaline high was wonderful.

Dr. Fearon said nothing to me. He left the room, and we took the patient to the recovery holding area, but the rest of the day I was smug and almost euphoric. Yes, I had passed the test of working with Dr. Fearon after only a few months of fellowship, but I also marveled at the procedure, of how we were able to do this, put a plastic tube into a man's artery, push it into his heart, takes x-ray images using a powerful substance like contrast dye, make a very specific diagnosis, remove the catheter, sew up the artery, and have the man go home the next day.

In spite of all our other sophisticated imaging techniques, the cath lab often remains the best place to make a diagnosis. There is great power in being able to image the inside of an artery, images that so often lead to the right decision about treatment. The cath lab findings continue to be a crucial clue in the Widowmaker chase and a major accomplishment for its time. Yet far greater advances were still in the offing for cardiologists, specifically one that might allow them to reach the victims of the Widowmaker just in the nick of time.

CHAPTER 14

BACK FROM THE BRINK: THE INVENTION OF THE CORONARY CARE UNIT

My prime advantage is the power of surprise.
For knowing that something is likely to happen,
is not the same as being there the minute it does.

With all their discoveries, the doctors may be able to
predict whom I am likely to revisit,
but often they cannot get to them in time.

A GOOD LESSON—FALL 1977

I stood outside the patient's room and peered in. She was sitting in her bed looking very comfortable, having skillfully opened up both sides of her newspaper, her reading glasses precisely engaged on the edge of her nose. The window shades were drawn open, bringing in the bright sunshine of a fall day. It was my first morning as an internal medicine resident in the Coronary Care Unit—the CCU.

I had learned from the "overnight" resident's morning report that this woman in her sixties came into the hospital the night before complaining of chest pain. Her electrocardiogram revealed that she was having a heart attack, confirmed by blood tests showing elevation of specific markers that indicated she had suffered heart muscle damage.

Her chest pain responded well to morphine, her blood pressure was now stable, and she had no fluid in her lungs or any other complications. Within a few hours, she was feeling fine, cared for in our small four-bed Coronary Care Unit. Only a decade or so earlier, she would have been cared for in a regular hospital bed without a cardiac rhythm monitor.

The resident had also reported that he had seen a few "extrasystoles," abnormal heartbeats from the left ventricle, on the heart monitor, but that there had only been single beats, not many in a row, before the normal heart rhythm returned. I knew that those extrasystoles could sometimes be harbingers of a potentially ominous future, the development of ventricular tachycardia, that converts to ventricular fibrillation, and then "asystole" —no heartbeats at all. Regardless of how severe a heart attack is in terms of killing heart muscle cells, the initial damage to the heart disrupts its electrical system and the consequences can be fatal . . .

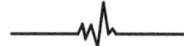

COUNTERATTACK ON THE WIDOWMAKER: SAVING LIVES IN SPECIAL PLACES

By the early 1960s, so much more was known about the causes of the heart attack and its complications. Nikolai Anichkov and John Gofman showed that atherosclerosis was caused by the buildup of cholesterol and LDL particles. Mason Sones had visualized the atherosclerosic blockages in the coronary arteries. The electrocardiogram and Paul Zoll's cardiac monitor illustrated the arrhythmias of the left ventricle that caused sudden death. Then Zoll and Bernard Lown demonstrated to the world that an electric shock could revive a damaged heart and that pacemakers could correct slow heart rates. Eugene Braunwald was investigating how the heart could survive heart attacks and possible treatments to preserve the heart muscle. Stress tests were available, and the data from Framingham was starting to emerge about how prevention might be possible. With so much progress, one might have assumed that we were nipping at the heels of the Widowmaker.

However, despite these amazing technical advances, the epidemic raged on without effective treatment for patients after they had suffered the Widowmaker's blow. Four out of ten patients did not survive their first heart attack. The meager treatment plan was pain relief with morphine or nitroglycerin if necessary, bed rest for weeks, and a big dose of hoping for the best. Even a guess at prognosis was just that, only a possible educated estimate. Too often patients were resting comfortably in the hours or few days after their attack, only to be found during morning nursing rounds to have died quietly overnight. There had to be a better way to deal with this sudden death problem.

Although Paul Zoll, the pioneer in the use of the defibrillator, had had only a small number of cases, his limited experience with shocking the heart revealed a key fact: the sooner the patient received the defibrillation, the greater the chance he or she would survive. In Boston, a few knowledgeable patients insisted that Zoll take care of them because they knew about his heartbeat monitor and protested when after some days in the hospital the monitor was taken away from them. Maybe these patients had the right idea. The monitor itself didn't save lives, but rapid defibrillation might. The patients had to be in the right place at the right time. Waiting more than just a few minutes would be too long.

In 1959, a young British cardiology trainee named Desmond Julian MD (1926-2019) witnessed many patients with myocardial infarctions have sudden cardiac arrests and knew there must be a better way. While he managed to save a few by performing open-chest cardiac massage and defibrillation, Julian knew many more died because help had arrived too late. To make matters worse, when most of the doctors and nurses arrived on the scene, they simply didn't know what to do. The answer to the problem of caring for the heart attack patient seemed obvious to Dr. Julian.

After completing his training in 1961, and unable to find a position in England or Scotland, he packed up and headed to Australia with a new idea. That same year, Julian crystallized his notions in an article published in the prestigious British medical journal *Lancet*. He wrote, "All wards admitting patients with acute myocardial infarction should have a system capable of sounding an alarm at the onset of an important rhythm change and of recording the rhythm automatically on an ECG . . . Such units should be staffed by suitably experienced people throughout the twenty-four hours." He was convinced that in a special place like this, the defibrillator could save lives if the machine was close to the patient and used very quickly.

Julian's idea for heart attack patients was just a proposal when he first wrote about it, but it was not without precedent. The idea of a designated hospital area that cared for patients with a specific problem that required special expertise was not brand new. For example, after major surgery, patients went to a "recovery room" area before going back to a regular hospital floor. The close care from nurses, surgeons, and anesthesiologists made a large dent in the complication and death rate in those people. The doctors at Sydney Hospital were intrigued. By early 1962, that medical center committed the resources to start a Coronary Care Unit (CCU). Here was a possible solution to the problem of sudden death from arrhythmias after heart attacks, and within three years, CCUs became a reality in Kansas City, Philadelphia, Toronto, New York, and Miami. However, Julian and his Australian friends ultimately lost the coveted "first to publish" war about the use of the CCU for heart attack patients to an unlikely group[73] from mid-America.

In 1962, a cardiologist named Hughes Day MD convinced Bethany Hospital in Kansas City, Missouri, to build a special four-

---

73 Bethany Hospital had no national or international fame nor a university affiliation.

bed area for "intense" coronary care. The unit had unique features; all the patients were attached to three electrodes placed on the chest to record their heart rhythm continuously. The monitoring stations had both visual and audible alarms, and a loud noise sounded to alert the nurses to any major change in the heart rate that lasted for more than ten seconds. The intense nursing care was beloved by the patients.

At the time, the average length of stay in a hospital after a heart attack was approximately twenty-eight days. Day's "intensive care" unit cut the average length of stay in the special unit to twelve days, a very long time by modern standards, but much shorter than the standard of many weeks of bed rest. Perhaps not surprisingly, many patients were unhappy with the shortened stay. They felt safe in this highly attentive cocoon and feared the complications of a heart attack in the absence of this individualized care. But Day and his colleagues realized that almost all of the major complications happened in the first few days after admission and that after that time period it was safe for patients to get out of bed, move around, and then go home to rest. The question remained: would the unit save lives in the end?

The intensive care unit for cardiac patients was a big success. In 1961, the death rate of heart attack patients at Bethany was thirty-nine percent, right in the predicted range for the time, but between May 1962 and May 1963, of the sixty-two patients in Day's special unit, only twelve died—nineteen percent! They had cut the death rate in half in just a year. In ten of the patients who did not survive, their cardiac condition was dire, with complications of low blood pressure (shock) and fluid in their lungs from congestive heart failure. These unfortunates had no expectation of a good outcome. Only two patients died unexpectedly. In contrast, during that year when Day's unit was first operational, of the forty-two patients whose doctors did *not* want them cared for in this special unit, eighteen did not leave the hospital alive, a mortality rate of forty-three percent, right in line with historical percentages. Day estimated the special coronary care units would save forty-five thousand lives a year in the United States.

The CCU movement was off to a rousing start. But how exactly were these deaths prevented? There were eleven episodes of a sudden cardiac arrest, eight from slow heart rhythms, which responded to medication or pacemakers, and three episodes of ventricular fibrillation, quickly reversed by defibrillation. There were also five episodes of ventricular tachycardia that the defibrillator eradicated. Not only did the defibrillator save lives but other treatments helped as well, such as newer medications and temporary pacemakers used to treat slow heart rates, a problem which usually resolved in a few days. Closer and quicker worked. Would others around the world find similar dramatic improvements for patients?

Back in Sydney, Julian's team "set up shop" in Sydney Hospital where their initial results with heart attacks were poor—thirty to fifty percent mortality rate depending on the year, but they still reported what they found. His monitoring technology also consisted of chest electrodes, this time connected to a three-lead "oscilloscope" (a "ratescope") as well as a recording device that could print out the tracings from the oscilloscope on demand. He used an eight-second delay to initiate an alarm, and to allay patient anxiety, he attached the oscilloscopes to the head of the bed, outside of the view of the patient. The Australians collected their data on seventy-five patients. Just short of fifty percent of the patients (thirty-seven of seventy-five) developed what Julian termed "significant arrhythmias" within forty-eight hours of admission to the special unit. He saw an array of different arrhythmias confirming Day's observations about the electrical complications of heart attacks.

Some patients had sustained a heart attack affecting the bottom and back wall of the heart, in the area where the heart's "conduction system" lies, the special cells that transmit electrical impulses from the top of the heart on through to the ventricles below. When these cells were damaged, they blocked the electrical impulses traveling to their destinations. As a result, the ventricles had to beat on their own, usually at a very slow rate. This phenomenon, seen on the heart monitor tracing, is called "complete heart block." If recognized and treated, this temporary problem resolves and has no effect on long-term survival. This was a clear demonstration of the benefits of a special unit and continuous heart rate monitoring.

Though Julian did recognize ventricular tachycardia or ventricular fibrillation in nine of the patients (twelve percent), in the end, twenty-four of seventy-five (thirty-two percent) of his patients died, and therefore he was not able to reproduce Day's astonishing results. Julian wasn't certain why, but he had some ideas about that. First, he considered that maybe he and his colleagues had admitted "the sickest of the sick," patients with heart attacks who were likely to die no matter what treatment was available. Next he took into account that he was using an AC defibrillator (just like the model that Paul Zoll had built) and that sometimes it just didn't work, and the ventricular tachycardia or fibrillation went on to its natural end—death. He desperately wanted that superior DC unit invented by Berkovits and Lown. Julian was still not deterred in his efforts to develop his CCU idea and understood that chasing the Widowmaker would be a long-term struggle.

Bolstered by the information gained from the early adopters, in the mid-1960s, the "big hitters" in academic medicine were bitten by the CCU bug. In early 1965, a CCU opened at New York Hospital, the major teaching hospital of the Cornell School of Medicine. The Cornell CCU was similar to Julian's but this time with a DC defibrillator at each patient's bedside. Their nurses received a minimum of forty hours of training in the recognition and treatment of the deadly complications: arrhythmias, heart failure with pulmonary edema, and complete cardiac arrest. Cardiology residents were in the unit, 24/7.

The Cornell project also did something revolutionary. Like other centers, they admitted patients to their CCU who had definite heart attacks, but they also admitted people whom they suspected had a heart attack but did not have a confirmed diagnosis when they arrived in the unit. These patients had the typical chest pain of coronary artery disease and often had some with electrocardiogram changes but not the classic changes of a heart attack. The Cornell team changed these criteria for CCU admission in the hope that earlier recognition of a heart attack would allow quicker treatment of the life-threatening complications. They simply could not justify delaying the monitoring while waiting for a blood test to come back indicating heart damage or for the EKG changes of a definite heart attack to evolve over time.

At first, the Cornell results were disheartening but would eventually improve. For the first one hundred patients, the mortality rate was still high at thirty percent, essentially the same as another one hundred patients cared for outside of the CCU. But for the next 150 patients, the chance of surviving rose to ninety-three percent, a mortality rate of only seven percent. The team at Cornell was getting much better at the prompt recognition of heart rhythm and blood pressure problems. The subsequent CCU research focused on both the diagnosis and treatment of the heart attack, attracting most of the young enthusiastic talent in cardiology. The CCU was here to stay.

The early observations in the CCUs brought out in bold relief some of the important but scattered clinical facts from years gone about the fact that there were dramatically different types of heart attack patients. First, there were the fortunate ones who, once the chest pain resolved, were left with little heart damage and a good prognosis. Second, there were those who had electrical system problems (the original scenario driving the CCU idea) who could develop the rapid heartbeat problems that would lead to ventricular fibrillation and death if not shocked back to normal by a defibrillator. They could also develop slow heart rates that could be treated with a temporary pacemaker.

Then there were the more dire patients. The patients in the third group had much more severe heart muscle damage, leading to high pressure in the left ventricle and fluid in the lungs. Many times, these patients had blockage in the heart's largest artery, the left anterior descending branch that supplies most of the left ventricle's blood. These blockages are classic Widowmaker lesions. This "acute heart failure" also became a treatable problem in many cases using newer medications, especially diuretics that allowed the kidneys to excrete fluid quickly. Nevertheless, this group still carried a "poor prognosis" label. Lastly, there were also the most unfortunate victims of the Widowmaker, those whose heart muscle was so damaged they could not produce an adequate level of "cardiac output," leading to kidney failure, among other problems. Often these patients also had fluid in their lungs. The term "cardiogenic shock" entered the lexicon. Most of these people could not be saved.

MORE TO DO: WHY WAIT FOR ARRHYTHMIAS?

Attempts to solve the problem of ventricular arrhythmias pushed the CCU movement. For sure the defibrillator was a lifesaver, but was there a way to either prevent or treat these deadly arrhythmias with new medication? Although antiarrhythmic drugs had been available for many years, their poor results and high side effect incidence explained the doctors' hesitance to use them in heart attack patients.

However, in the early 1960s, a drug from dentistry caught the fancy of cardiologists. Dentists commonly used lidocaine, first made in the 1940s, to numb the mouth and gums. The medicine stopped electrical transmission in nerves, silencing the pain sensors from reaching the brain. At Stanford University in Palo Alto, California, Donald Harrison MD (1934-) and his colleagues recognized the possibility that the drug might also be able to stop the electrical transmission in the heart. They knew of a few case reports from anesthesiologists who had used the drug to suppress extra heartbeats in patients undergoing surgery; however, more testing needed to be done.

Harrison went back to the animal lab and created heart attacks by occluding the heart's main artery. He knew that in these animals that stimulating the heart with a pacemaker wire could easily produce ventricular arrhythmias, not a surprise in a heart deprived of blood and oxygen. But when the animals were treated with intravenous infusions of lidocaine, much higher energy electrical pacing was needed to induce the malignant arrhythmias. It was time to use lidocaine in patients with heart attacks. The Stanford team studied lidocaine in twenty-nine people after heart attacks. In nineteen of twenty-nine, there was a greater than fifty percent reduction in the number of extrasystoles when the drug was given continuously. There were twenty episodes of ventricular tachycardia in five patients, and in all of these cases, another injection of intravenous lidocaine corrected the problem.

The CCU world welcomed this good news, and lidocaine quickly became the go-to drug to treat arrhythmias once they appeared. This advancement begged a new question: Why wait for "warning arrhythmias" to appear on the monitors before giving lidocaine? A group of cardiologists in Holland, led by Heins Wellens MD (1935-), had a bold proposition: what if all heart attack patients received lidocaine *at the time of diagnosis?* The Dutch doctors devised a rigorous scientific experiment to find out. The 105 patients in the control group received standard care and did *not* receive "prophylactic" lidocaine when they entered the CCU. The 107 experimental patients did. The results were astonishing. The untreated group had nine (8.6 percent) cases of ventricular fibrillation. The treated group had *none.* Lidocaine prevented the cause of sudden death in heart attack patients even before there was a warning, and almost overnight, the worldwide standard of care changed. The use of lidocaine for the prevention of malignant arrhythmias lasted for almost twenty years.[74]

---

74   Over those two decades, the incidence of ventricular fibrillation at the time of an acute heart attack dropped to less than one percent due to drugs and treatments used to decrease the extent of heart muscle damage.

HEART PRESSURES IN REAL TIME: NEW TOOLS IN THE CCU

In the early 1970s, trying to assess the effects of a heart attack on the physiology of the heart and the circulation still caused great frustration. How bad was the damage? If the blood pressure was low, did the patient need more fluid? If the pressure in the heart was high, would diuretics remove the excess lung water? What drug combinations led to a better outcome? Precise management in the first few hours or days after the cardiac event was crucial in improving outcomes.

The combination of CCUs and catheters showed promise, but there were challenges, too. The catheterization procedure did uncover the true effect of a blocked coronary artery on heart function; the "hemodynamic" data recorded the measurement of pressure inside of the left ventricle, the chamber damaged by severe heart attacks. But these data could only be obtained in the cath lab, not in the CCU, and this had major drawbacks. In addition, catheterizations were expensive and required a full staff to complete. Sometimes arteries got damaged. Also, the data gave pressure measurements for only one point in time because the catheter could not remain inside the left side of the heart without forming blood clots on the outside of the plastic tube. These clots could break loose and travel to the brain and cause a massive stroke. Doctors needed a safer, simpler, and less expensive way to follow the patient's data and response to medications over time.

Cardiologists grudgingly accepted that they still had no way to prevent heart attacks but continually sought more information. Inspired by the work of Eugene Braunwald and others who were studying the ways that the heart could survive a myocardial infarction, perhaps they could prevent the victims from succumbing to the damage. While not a cure, maybe the new ideas could palliate the consequences. In the 1970s, cardiac research was in high gear. The

National Institute of Health provided funding for unique scientific centers, Myocardial Research Units, that gathered data on patients with heart attacks in the CCUs around the US. They were looking for the missing piece: how to safely obtain reliable, frequent data about the pressures inside the heart after a myocardial infarction.

H.J.C. "Jeremy" Swan MD PhD (1922-2005) thought he had a way to solve this. Born and educated in Ireland, he moved to the US in the late 1940s and began his academic career at the Mayo Clinic in Rochester, Minnesota. He was obsessed with his idea: instead of using a leg artery, he wanted to place a catheter in an arm or neck vein to measure the important pressure value in the left ventricle after a heart attack. *If* it worked, the procedure could be safely done right in the CCU, at any time, and without a full staff. The big if was learning how to measure pressure in the left side of the heart from a vein because a vein took blood back to the right side of the heart, not the left. The pressure on the right side was just not that important most of the time, but the data on the left was gold.

There was a significant problem to this approach. The lungs separate the right and left side of the heart, and when blood leaves the right ventricle, it enters the pulmonary artery and then is carried into smaller and smaller blood vessels called capillaries, where the oxygen enters from the lungs. Any catheter pushed far into the pulmonary artery would stop when it reached the tiny capillaries, a physical obstruction that could have read "Road Closed."

Swan realized this problem with his idea, but he also knew something else from his cath lab training: if he pushed a needle on a catheter through the pulmonary artery and "wedged" it into the lung, he could record a pressure. What was the meaning of this "wedge pressure"? Did it reflect pressure from the right side or the left side of the heart or something in between? Earl Wood MD (1912-2009), Swan's boss at the Mayo Clinic, showed that this wedge pressure was very close or equal to the pressure in the left atrium. With the right tools, it was possible to measure the left side of the heart from the right side. Even so, using a needle to puncture a hole in the pulmonary artery of a sick heart attack patient didn't seem like a safe idea.

Swan considered another approach and would soon meet someone who would help him bring it to fruition. What about placing a flimsy catheter into a vein, floating it through the bloodstream, and allowing the cath lab doctor to push the tube into a wedge position while watching it under the fluoroscopy screen? When Swan became the Chief of Cardiology at the Cedars of Lebanon Hospital[75] in 1968, he was determined to pursue this project, and there he met his new collaborator. William Ganz MD (1919-2009) was a Holocaust survivor. Born in Slovakia, Ganz survived a Nazi labor camp and was then sent to Auschwitz, where he miraculously escaped. He was living in Communist Czechoslovakia in the 1950s when he gained permission to take his family on a vacation to Italy. Instead, the Ganz family went to Vienna, Austria, applied for visas, and escaped to the United States, joining up with a relative living in Los Angeles.

Swan and Ganz' first catheters were a disaster. The flimsy plastic tubes curled up in the right atrium, never coming close to the "wedge" position. Then one day, while Swan sat on the Santa Monica beach in Los Angeles, watching sailboats tack and jibe, twisting and turning their sails in the wind, he got an idea. What if he attached an inflatable balloon onto the end of the catheter? Maybe then the forward flow of blood from the beating of the right ventricle would just push the catheter along out to the end of the lung circulation. The catheter would get stuck out there, enabling it to record a pressure without having to puncture an artery in the lung.

Swan and Ganz' colleagues at Cedars were not impressed with this notion, but the two pushed forward anyway. One of their fellow cardiologists said that he envisioned the balloon catheter "wafting through the circulatory system like Mary Poppins' umbrella." The two immigrants disagreed with their critics. Working with the plastic engineers on new balloon designs, and persistently practicing with

---

75 Now known as Cedars-Sinai Medical Center.

their catheter, they succeeded. Their new diagnostic tool collected vast amounts of minute-to-minute information about the heart chamber pressures, allowing doctors to determine the best treatments for the patient and buying some time so the heart could heal. The CCUs had a new weapon against the Widowmaker—the Swan-Ganz[76] or "right heart catheter." Werner Forssmann would have been amazed.

Jullian and Day believed a specialized heart attack unit could save lives, and they were right. Future numbers would tell the story.[77] The coronary care units married the continuous heart rhythm monitoring, the bedside defibrillator, specifically trained nurses, the Swan-Ganz balloon catheter, and later pharmacology. Together, these techniques transformed the care of the heart attack patient, blunting the work of the Widowmaker.

In spite of all of these great advances, a huge problem remained. Too often patients came for their care too late, hours after the heart attack began, and heart muscle cells had already died. Survival rates are usually calculated as survival for one month after a heart attack. But in the long term, there were still too many people left with major scars to their hearts, the pathology that leads to congestive heart failure and Sudden Cardiac Death.

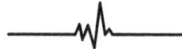

LESSON LEARNED

... Though the patient had seemed fine only seconds ago, as I was preparing to enter the room, a nurse tore by me and raced to the bedside. Cautiously, I approached the bed, still clueless.

---

76 The Swan-Ganz catheter was widely used for many years, but over the last two decades, its use has decreased significantly over concerns about the risk of infection from indwelling catheters. In many situations, prompt cardiac catheterization and angioplasty has limited the extent of heart muscle damage and the complications previously seen.

77 The mortality rate from a myocardial infarction dropped from about forty percent in the early 1960s to twenty percent in 1980, and to less than ten percent by the mid-1990s.

The nurse, with many more years of experience and training than me, threw the patient's newspaper on the floor, removed the reading glasses, and ripped open her hospital gown. In a calm, steady voice, she said to me, "Look at the monitor." Kindly, she didn't follow that with "you idiot." Instead, she asked, "I'm charging the defibrillator. Do you think you can push the button when it's ready?" The patient's heart rhythm was now ventricular tachycardia, the fast heart rate that often changes to ventricular fibrillation followed quickly by death.

She grabbed the two defibrillator paddles and smeared them with electrode gel then leaned hard on them as she placed the round discs on the patient's chest. I heard the defibrillator machine whine, the signal indicating that the device was fully charged. The nurse glanced at me, gave a slight head nod, and as a safety precaution said, "Clear." I pushed the button to deliver the shock. The poor woman clutched her chest. The nurse and I stared at the monitor. It worked! Miraculously, her heart rhythm was normal again.

I continued to do as the nurse instructed and wrote in the doctor's orders that we were starting the woman on an infusion of lidocaine, the antiarrhythmic drug to suppress the extrasystoles and prevent a recurrence of her ventricular tachycardia. An hour later, my patient was reading the newspaper again. I gave her some mild medication to ease the pain on her chest wall from the shock procedure, and the next two days of her stay were uneventful. As her heart muscle healed, we expected her arrhythmias to disappear.

She went from the CCU to a regular hospital bed and then went home in a few days. She had a good prognosis. The right location, the right equipment, and a properly trained and experienced nurse saved her life. A young medical resident learned to keep his eye on the heart monitors and the true meaning of Sudden Cardiac Death. The CCU was an enormous advance, but it was not the final solution. Prevention was still untouched.

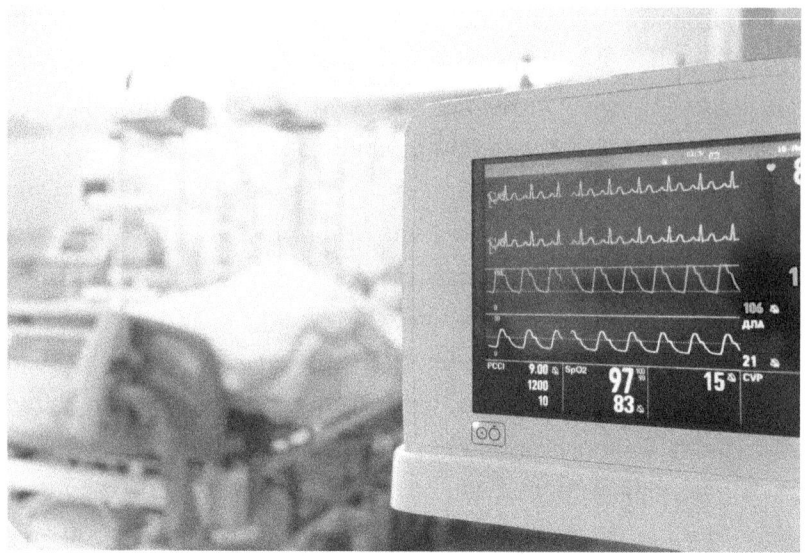

Figure 17. Typical monitors of cardiac rhythm, heart rate, oxygen saturation, blood pressure, and intracardiac pressures in a modern Coronary Care Unit. (Copyright Shutterstock)

CHAPTER 15

SLOW DOWN, YOU MOVE TOO FAST: HARNESSING THE POWER OF BETA-BLOCKERS

Time has always been on my side the way the heart races to compensate for its slow destruction but in the end cannot catch up.

Are scientists using the fable of such a race, to harness the power of opposites?

THE BALLROOM DANCER AND HIS HEADACHE

"Why are you here to see me?" I asked the man in my exam room in the 1980s. His answer to my routine question was prompt, almost taunting: "I'm not sure, doc, but when I dance with my wife, my head hurts and I need to stop dancing. And I love my wife, and I love to dance." For months, after seeing other doctors, he was certain his problem was just a profound, unsolvable medical mystery.

Mr. D had good reason to question why he was seeing a cardiologist. Although he was in his early sixties, he had never had any heart problems. When the head pain started, he went to his family doctor, who referred him to a neurologist, logically assuming that the symptoms were some type of headache. The neurologist concurred, but several types of headache pain medicine did nothing for the problem.

After those failures, his brother-in-law, who I had cared for years ago when he had a heart attack, convinced him that I was the best diagnostician in the world and advised, "Why don't you see Dr. Meshkov? He's a smart guy, and maybe he can figure this out for you." But when I saw him a few days later, I also didn't know what the problem was, and where heart problems are involved, I can usually tell after five minutes of observation and some pointed questions whether or not the symptoms are really due to heart disease and could be serious. He answered no to all of my basic questions about chest pain, shortness of breath, dizziness, palpitations, and passing out. A negative response to these five symptoms usually dramatically lowers the chance of active heart disease.

I asked him to focus on the headache. It only happened after he and his wife were dancing their ballroom style and only after they'd been dancing for about ten minutes. He did admit that he felt his heart beat faster as the pain began and then had this throbbing pain in the top of his head only. He was forced to stop dancing and sit down, and within five minutes, the rapid heartbeat and headache were gone. That was the limit of the problem.

Mr. D was in my office to find out the answer to one key question: Could this throbbing headache be angina pectoris due to coronary artery atherosclerosis? I wanted to keep an open mind, but I had never seen the disease present this way. Usually, the pain is a heaviness in the center or left side of the chest, often extending into the left arm. Sometimes the pain can be in the neck, the jaw, the back, on the right side of the chest, and even only in the teeth. The pain is almost always in the same spot over and over again; it doesn't happen one day in the jaw and the next day in the back. There were many variations, but no one ever said angina pectoris could cause headaches. Still, as a cardiologist, I could not ignore the striking relationship of his pain to physical activity, so I ordered an exercise stress test . . .

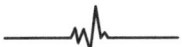

STOPPING ADRENALINE:
THE BETA-BLOCKER REVOLUTION

When you're young, the trauma of watching a parent suffer can scar for a lifetime. But ironically, the experience may also inspire you. When his father got anxious or angry or tried to exercise, James saw the life drain from the man's face. Angina pectoris was already well known to the young future doctor and his family.

James Whyte Black MD (1924-2010) was convinced he wanted to become a doctor, so he went to medical school in Scotland and received his degree in 1946. But his education left him conflicted about the path of his life's work.[78] He thought that "the way patients were treated was unacceptably insensitive." Too often he saw people regarded as if they were a heart or lungs or kidneys, not entire complex human beings. Though Black desperately wanted to make a great advance in patient care, he preferred the laboratory to the clinic. His passion became physiology, the science of organs and systems, like the circulatory system or the nervous system, and he was soon offered an opportunity to begin a physiology department, not at a medical school, however, but at the Veterinary School of the University of Glasgow, a perfect place to perform experiments in animals. And Black already had a focus in mind.

Based on his father's experience and then his medical education, Black obsessed about only one enemy molecule, the organic compound that he was convinced caused the misery of his father and so many others: adrenaline. Researchers first isolated adrenaline from extracts of the adrenal glands in the late 1890s and naturally

---

78 He suspected that his quest for greatness would be long and tedious, with no certainty of success. The splendid final drama might need to wait many years. There would be no one "Aha!" moment.

named it *adren*aline.[79] Adrenaline is one of the molecules known as hormones[80] and has remarkable properties: it increases both heart rate and blood pressure and is crucial for exercise. It also relaxes the muscle of the airways and can effectively alleviate asthma attacks. But adrenaline is a "dual-edged sword," life-saving many times but a danger if one has coronary artery atherosclerosis.[81] The three causes of his father's angina, mental stress, anger, and physical exertion, had a common denominator in Black's mind—high levels of adrenaline.

James Black had no formal PhD-type training in organic chemistry and pharmacology, but he had an exquisitely clear hypothesis that he was out to prove and enough skills to embark on a scientific journey. If he could stop the effect of adrenaline on the heart with a drug, that medication would reduce the heart's use of oxygen by slowing the heart rate, and in this way, he could control or eliminate the chest pain of angina. How to do this was a daunting task without first fully understanding not just adrenaline, but the function of the body's system of hormones.

Years later, when Sir James Black was a Nobel Laureate, he described the essential criteria for a good drug research project: first, identify a clinical problem with a known basis in physiology; secondly, define a "chemical starting" point. Black's project met both criteria: the clinical problem was angina and the molecule of adrenaline was his starting point. But he needed to understand the fundamentals first, and those fundamentals were few.

---

79 At the time, no one had the faintest idea what these two small lumps of tissue, the adrenal glands, were doing lying on top of each kidney; their average size is only about 1.2 inches wide, 2.0 inches long, and less than half an inch thick. But there was an Englishman, Thomas Wharton MD (1614-1673), who noticed the proximity of the adrenal glands to the nerve "plexuses" the gathering places of nerves from multiple locations. The future would confirm his belief that the adrenal glands had a great deal to do with the nervous system, the heart, and angina pectoris.
80 From the Greek word *horman*—to set in motion.
81 In the 1930s, doctors used adrenaline injections as a diagnostic test for angina. The molecule caused chest pain in many patients, but the test had questionable reliability and was pursued by only a few doctors.

A SURPRISING FAMILY EXPERIMENT: THE HEART HORMONE SURFACES

George Oliver MD (1841-1915) could have been accused of child abuse and attempted murder. The good doctor practiced in Yorkshire, a city in the north-central portion of England on the North Sea. Its latitude is just short of fifty-four degrees North, further north than Labrador, Canada, and for sure the winters are long, cold, and dreary. Dr. Oliver had his practice of course but not too much else to occupy his time, especially during the winter. But he was a very curious man—why not conduct a few medical experiments on a family member? Times were different in the late nineteenth century. And he had an unexplored area to research: the adrenal glands and their completely mysterious reason for existing in the first place.

Oliver wanted to test the effects of pulverized cow adrenal glands (acquired from the local butcher), which he mixed with water, alcohol, or glycerine, as he thought the solutions could affect the circulation, the blood pressure, and the heart rate. Checking the pulse was no problem, and blood pressure measuring devices were already available. But Oliver was also an inventor, and he wanted to attempt to document not just the pressure in an artery but how large or small it became; so he created a new device that measured the width of the radial artery in the hand. The wider the artery became, the more blood was flowing into the hand; if the artery narrowed, there was less flow.

With his invention perfected, Oliver needed a human subject to try out his experiment, and he had someone who was easily available. The legend, told by Sir Henry Dale PhD (1875-1968), the Nobel Prize–winning English pharmacologist, is that *Oliver injected a small amount of his adrenal gland solution into one of the arm veins of his only son, a young man in his twenties.* Then good fortune smiled on George Oliver. His son's radial artery blood flow shut down dramatically—the blood vessel constricted, but fortunately for Oliver and his son, the blood flow to his hand returned to normal in a few minutes. There was something very potent in that solution of adrenal glands. Oliver needed help to explain this power he had discovered. He knew where he wanted to go next and who to talk to. He headed south to London.

Oliver met with Edward Albert Sharpey-Schafer PhD (1850-1935), a physiology professor who was an expert on the circulation. He was as startled as Oliver was when he saw the effects of the cow adrenal glands on blood pressure, and soon the duo began doing experiments on dogs using Oliver's concoction. In 1894, they presented their findings at the Physiological Society of London: Dr. Oliver's potion repeatedly caused marked increases in blood pressure and seemingly paradoxically a slowing, not an increase in the heart rate. This finding would become a key clue to the true nature and complexity of the body's nervous system, its role in the circulation, and its relationship to heart disease. An entirely new field of "endocrinology," the study of "internal secretions," the hormones, was opening up. But what was in those cow glands creating such remarkable effects in such a short time and then disappeared almost as quickly as they began?

In the next few years, the organic chemists got to work with their magic. In 1899, the American John Jacob Abel MD (1851-1938) and then in 1901 the Japanese chemist Jokichi Takamin PhD (1854-1922) both isolated a molecule that Takamin named "adrenaline." Abel chose to name the same molecule differently; he called it "epinephrine," "depi" meaning in the Greek "upon, near to," and "nephrine," related to the kidneys.[82] Then Friedrich Stolz PhD (1860-1936) and Henry Drysdale Dakin PhD (1880-1952) synthesized adrenaline from the molecular "spare parts" of a six-carbon structure known as a benzene ring, some oxygen and hydrogen atoms, and finally nitrogen combinations known as "amines." Stolz, Dakin, and other chemists produced a new group of biologically important molecules that could be synthesized in laboratories, a collection of "catechols," carbon, hydrogen, and oxygen atoms, with amines—the "catecholamines." Adrenaline was just the first of many more to come.

---

82 To this day, the terms adrenaline and epinephrine are used interchangeably.

Over the next fifty years of research, it became clear that the catecholamines were crucial "transmitters" of powerful signals affecting the brain, the heart, and the blood vessels. They also affected the muscle in the airways, those "smooth muscles" that can't be controlled by the conscious brain and become constricted in patients with an asthma attack. For many years, an injection of adrenaline was the most important medication used to stop an acute asthma attack. The question of how doctors could use this knowledge to treat many other conditions, especially coronary artery disease, with its clear relationship of symptoms to fast heart rates, was still obscure.

THE NERVOUS SYSTEM'S YIN AND YANG: MAKING SENSE OF THE CONFUSION

If James Black was going to manufacture or discover a drug that arrested angina, sorting out how the whole system of the catecholamines worked was the key to unlocking the ability to produce medications that were useful in patients with coronary artery disease. Discovering new catecholamines that were natural products of the body and making new one in the organic chemistry laboratories was wonderfully exciting to the researchers. But understanding how each one of these molecules affected the circulation, the heart, and the nervous system was a mental quagmire.

Some of the catecholamines caused the blood vessels to contract, and others made them relax. Some increased the heart rate, and others slowed it down. Sometimes there was only a bit of constriction or dilatation. To make matters more perplexing, scientists discovered other types of transmitters, not catecholamines, in particular a compound called acetylcholine, a substance that in many ways has directly opposing effects from molecules like adrenaline. But there was a much more important "black hole" of understanding.

Physiology, how organs act individually and collectively, explains how systems work, not cells or organs alone. In the specific case of the circulatory system, how do blood vessels constrict when we go into the cold, and how do they dilate when the temperature rises or we need to walk faster? What happens to the circulatory system when there is heart disease? Can a drug "block" the effects of molecules like adrenaline and acetylcholine? By the 1940s, there was acceptance of the idea that these molecules worked by attaching themselves to other very specific molecules on the surfaces of the cells of all the organs— "receptor molecules." But the unanswered questions were endless.

James Black's quest for a new drug for angina needed major new scientific help, and he had a particular focus in mind. He had his sights on a specific part of the nervous system, not the part that allows us to read and speak and move our arms and legs, but the part our conscious brains do not control but is crucial for life, the "autonomic" nervous system. This is the part that keeps us breathing when we fall asleep and make us salivate when we smell something good to eat. It also controls the blood pressure and heart rate, as we can't "will" our blood pressure or heart rate to rise or fall, no matter how hard we try.[83]

Even more precisely, Black's first interest was in the "sympathetic" part of the autonomic nervous system. The name originates from the Greek idea of *pathos*, the root of the word sympathy. The premise was that this organization of nerves, the brain, and the adrenal glands can respond to perceived danger, "the fight or flight reaction." Black was convinced it was this system that was responsible for angina by releasing adrenaline and increasing the heart's demand for blood and oxygen. But the sympathetic system, releasing substances that speed up metabolism, blood pressure, and heart rate, should require a counterbalance to tone down possible excess of catecholamines. This second part of the autonomic nervous system is called the "parasympathetic" nervous system. Confusion ruled the day about how to understand how these two distinct parts of the autonomic nervous system worked together.

---

83 Unless you are a very dedicated yoga swami, few have been able to make those changes with their meditation practices.

When James Black graduated medical school in 1946, no one knew that a pharmacologist in Georgia was doggedly trying to make sense of the neurotransmitter confusion. Raymond Perry Ahlquist PhD (1914-1983) was the son of Swedish immigrants in Montana. In 1940, he accepted a faculty position at the Medical College of Georgia in Augusta and became obsessed with transmitter molecules. Ahlquist extensively studied their effect, concluding that there were only two types of receptor molecules that controlled constriction and dilation of blood vessels, and named them alpha receptors and beta receptors. His work in the late 1940s would serve as scientific fundamentals for Black just a few years later.

Ahlquist's research delved into the mystery of the sympathetic part of the autonomic nervous system, finally making sense of the myriad effects of the transmitter molecules traveling endlessly throughout the circulation. Black was thrilled by Ahlquist's finding of a fundamental property of the beta-receptors on heart cells; when adrenaline landed on them, the heart muscle started to beat stronger and faster and use more oxygen.

Black now had his most important target for a drug: in patients with coronary artery disease, adrenaline caused angina by binding with the beta-receptor molecules on the surface of heart muscle cells. His idea of blocking adrenaline was correct; now he needed to find that blocker drug. Black could see a path forward but knew that the trek would continue to be tedious and treacherous. Ahlquist's discovery was the key.

MAKING THE BEST DRUG

Black needed to find a place with more resources than his veterinary school to pursue his antidote to adrenaline. He chose the right company in the drug industry. In 1958, Black went to work for Imperial Chemical Industries (ICI) in England. Since 1948, ICI had been vigorously looking for new drugs to treat high blood pressure and produced a group of drugs that decreased the catecholamine molecule production of nerves called ganglia. These "ganglionic blockers" did lower blood pressure but with frequent intolerable side effects. These medications did not transform the treatment of high blood pressure.

Upon arriving at ICI, Black's laboratory had only one catecholamine molecule other than the ganglionic blockers to work with—isoprenaline, a "close relative" of adrenaline. Dedicating themselves to tedious work without any glamor, Black and his colleagues tried many organic chemistry tricks to add or subtract different atoms and molecules to the basic molecular structure of isoprenaline but were unable to find a new compound that effectively shut down the normal beta-receptor response to adrenaline of increasing the heart rate and blood pressure in the animal heart models. In hopes of finding a valuable chemical trick to try, Black began researching what other researchers were finding.

As it turned out, in 1958, two other pharmacologists, Neil C Moran PhD (1924-1997) and Marjorie E. Perkins PhD of Emory University, found that a molecule they named DCI, dichloroisoprenaline (developed by the Eli Lilly Corporation) "annulled" the cardiac stimulation effects of adrenaline on the heart. Moran and Perkins had shown that organic chemistry could manufacture a brand-new molecule that also latched on the beta-receptor molecule on heart cells even more tightly than adrenaline and swept the catecholamine past the heart and back into the circulation and metabolic destruction. The fast heart rate and the angina might disappear. Moran and Perkins coined the now-logical term "beta-blocker."

However, Black knew he needed to find an even more potent beta-blocker and continued doing extensive research on variations of adrenaline on guinea pig hearts until he struck gold. ICI Compound 38 174 caused great celebration in Black's lab. The molecule they named pronethanol was a pure antagonist of the effect of isoprenaline on heart rate and blood pressure. It created just the effects Black was looking for in the hearts of animals. But what about human beings, especially those with angina and coronary artery disease?

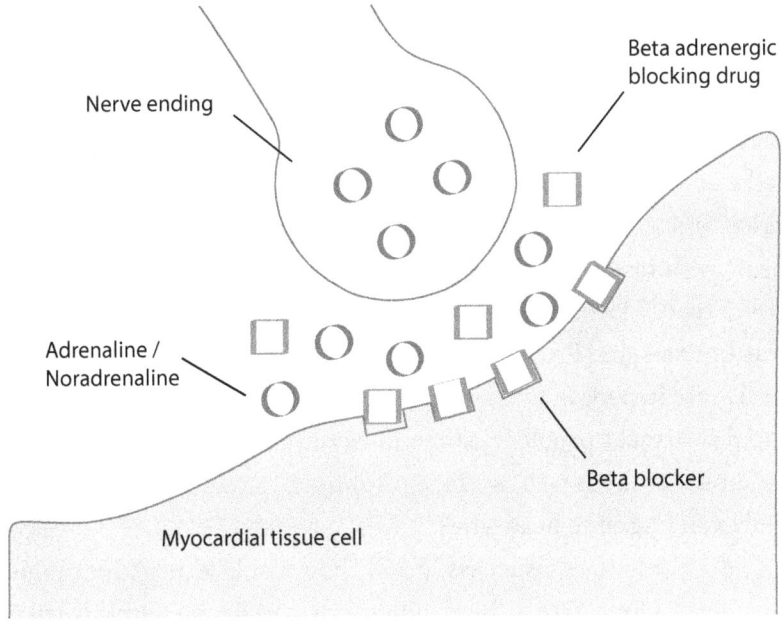

Figure 18. Mechanism of action of beta-blocker drugs such as propranolol on heart muscle cells by blocking entrance of adrenaline and noradrenaline through beta receptors on the cell surface. (Courtesy of Meredith Dawson Designs, LLC)

Though their next trials using dogs looked promising, in order to cross the finish line, Black and ICI had to do tests on humans and were ready to try using pronethanol in patients with angina. Starting out with small doses the studies did confirm that some patients did have fewer episodes of angina and less use of nitroglycerin tablets. However, a high number of the patients reported gastrointestinal and neurologic side effects. So the search continued for a safer compound. Black hadn't yet found his prize drug and kept working. Then Black's lab came up with ICI 45520. This new compound was what Black was searching for, a medication that was safe, stable, and had few side effects from slowing of the heart rate. Black named his creation propranolol.[84]

With the help of others, James Black had done it.[85] Propranolol became the standard of care for thousands of patients with angina, often allowing them to lead normal lives with excellent levels of activity. In describing propranolol's effect in his Nobel Lecture, he wrote, "There were telltale signs that the cardiac reserve was reduced, but I persuaded myself at the time that this was a reasonable price to pay for the possibility of increasing the work capacity of a heart with restricted blood flow." His idea of twenty years prior had come true. Black had his best beta-blocker, and its use in angina was only a start. Propranolol proved to be effective in slowing the heart rate in people suffering from cardiac arrhythmias, a variety of rapid heartbeat problems sometimes unrelated to coronary artery atherosclerosis, as well as effective for the treatment of hypertension and even migraine headaches.

With this major success at ICI, one would expect that James Black had a long career there. But after six years, he abruptly left to take a position at Smith, Kline and French (SKF), a major American pharmaceutical company.[86] He was described as charming and genial outside of his lab but also as an "irascible maverick" with "prickly independence" and an "antipathy to big institutions." But one thing is certain: James Black's ideas about drugs and receptors changed pharmacologic research from "molecular roulette" into logical science. The beta-blocker era in cardiology that he began flourished exponentially from its first use for angina patients in the mid-1960s.

---

84 ICI sold it as Inderal.
85 Many more patients and studies were conducted through the 1960s and into the 1970s with great results in most patients.
86 In 1975, only one year after being at SKF, Black and his colleagues released the drug cimetidine, trade name Tagamet, the drug that revolutionized the care of millions of patients with ulcers of the stomach and the esophagus. Tagamet became the first drug to yield sales of over $1 billion a year, topping the sales of Inderal.

While modern medicine would improve on his discoveries,[87] Black's propranolol revolutionized the care of patients with coronary artery disease, providing long acting medication that markedly decreased the fearful physical and mental burden of angina pectoris. A problem for clinicians was taken into the science lab arena and then back to the doctor and the patient—"translational research" had triumphed. Though James Black never personally took care of patients with coronary artery disease, he gave cardiologists one of the major tools to help people suffering from the work of the Widowmaker.

TURNING DOWN THE HEART'S REQUEST

... The stress test was abnormal. The changes in his electrocardiogram told me that the exercise jeopardized his heart's blood supply— which for unknown reasons caused his headache! And sure enough, as predicted, the headache went away after he rested for just a few minutes. When I shared these details with Mr. D, he was startled but optimistic that perhaps this cardiologist had stumbled upon the correct diagnosis and, more importantly, could treat the condition.

The work of the heart was the explanation for Mr. D's exclusive form of angina pectoris. When he danced, his heart received signals from his nervous system that told his heart to step up its output of blood. His heart could only respond in two ways: it could increase the speed that it contracted and pushed blood out into the circulation, or it could increase the volume of blood pumped out with each heartbeat. The fuel to drive these two responses were those two transmitter molecules, adrenaline and noradrenaline. The faster he danced, the stronger the signal came from the nerve cells located on his muscles. The alarm activated Mr. D's brain, other nerves, and the two adrenal glands in the abdomen. And adrenaline and

---

[87] There are now many types of beta-blockers even better than propranolol, used to treat not only high blood pressure and cardiac arrhythmias but migraine headaches and congestive heart failure. They are also useful in blunting "performance anxiety" in those who develop a fast heartbeat, dread, and sweating before speaking in public. Beta-blockers are among the most commonly prescribed medications worldwide.

noradrenaline streamed out into his blood vessels and queued the heart muscle to spring into action.

But Mr. D's heart blood supply was compromised. The atherosclerosis in his coronary arteries blunted the amount of oxygen and blood his heart could supply to its own cells as they tried to beat faster and stronger. Mr. D's heart couldn't keep up with the demand. The metabolism of his heart cells ground to a halt, sending a signal to the brain that they were struggling—his headache. When he stopped dancing and his heart rate slowed down, the headache was gone, as if nothing had happened.

I hoped I had the cure. I prescribed a powerful medication to take several times a day—a beta-blocker. I asked him to take the medication for three or four days and then try to return to his ballroom dancing. I was anxious for Mr. D's next office visit, and I hustled into the exam room as soon as he came in. I didn't even wait for my assistant to take his blood pressure and electrocardiogram. I had a one-word question. "Well?"

"Dancing better than ever, doc."

"No headache?"

"Not a bit."

The magical medication, the beta-blocker propranolol, solved his difficult-to-diagnose problem. Before treatment, his heart rate probably jumped from seventy beats a minute at rest to 120 with exercise. With propranolol the rate likely increased to only eighty-five beats a minute. The lower rate didn't stress his heart beyond its limits; it could produce enough output of blood to meet the demand of his muscles, but now his heart muscle cells could function with less oxygen, and he didn't develop the headache. His rare form of angina was gone.

Mr. D remained my patient for years, and he never did need a heart catheterization, angioplasty, or bypass surgery. Like the majority of people with stable coronary artery disease, he took his beta-blocker to control his angina, aspirin to reduce his risk of a heart attack, and a statin drug to lower his cholesterol. He returned to his normal life. Modern treatment blunted the relentless progression of his coronary artery disease, so common in decades gone by.

I have seen thousands of patients with angina over my career, but he was the only one with an exercise-related headache from coronary artery disease. I have no idea why his unique symptoms of angina showed up this way, but it was his body's way of telling him, "Slow down, you move too fast." The development of propranolol was the first new treatment for angina since the discovery of nitroglycerin almost ninety years prior. Perhaps there was also a way for cardiac surgeons to enter the treatment arena.

CHAPTER 16

THE DRESSMAKER'S SON AND THE GIFT OF THE CABG

Favaloro may be a name you have never heard of, but it is one that haunts me still. For my work has always depended on the eventual obstruction
of the finite channels to the heart.

But what if they were not so finite after all?
Would all my methodical work be in vain?

MY FRIEND THE PATIENT—2009

"Are you here trying to break my treadmill machine again?" Bill Van Decker MD said kiddingly to his patient Ed. Ed is my very good friend, and when he came to me for advice, I explained why I could not see him and instead referred him to Bill. I knew that having a close friend as a patient is not a good idea because it's nearly impossible to be objective. But this was not Ed's first time on Van Decker's machine.

In his mid-sixties and at the peak of his legal career, Ed felt great and didn't have any major risk factors for coronary artery atherosclerosis, but a few months earlier, he began to have shortness of breath and some pain in his left shoulder. The pain was unpredictable; it happened at rest and not often with exercise.

When I had referred Ed to Van Decker, Bill suspected coronary artery disease was Ed's problem and ordered a stress test. But the exercise test using nuclear images of the heart showed just a small degree of lack of blood supply to one part of the heart muscle, a result that usually means you can treat the problem with medication only. Given that Ed himself was convinced that the pain in the shoulder was not due to his heart but some kind of muscular pain, and his busy life went on.

However, just a few weeks later, as Ed was walking up steps into the courthouse, he broke out in a cold sweat that he described as much more alarming than a sweat caused by overheating or overexertion. Frightened, he sat down on a bench, and in a few minutes the sweating stopped. Still in denial, he continued with his day in court. Ed called me at the end of the day, and I insisted that he come in to see Bill the next day, and despite his previously benign stress test, I was worried enough to want another one and suspected Bill would agree.

This time the test was very different: Bill saw the electrocardiogram go from normal to abnormal after only a few minutes of exercise and abruptly stopped the test. The nuclear image pictures looked much worse than on the test performed just a few weeks earlier, but at least now there was an answer to the cause of Ed's problem. His atherosclerosis was becoming more severe, now depriving his heart muscle of blood even with only mild exercise. Something needed to be done right away . . .

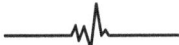

ANOTHER IMMIGRANT'S STORY: THE BIRTH OF CORONARY ARTERY BYPASS GRAFT SURGERY

It was now or never, he thought. René Favaloro MD (1923-2000) was thirty-nine years old when he flew from Argentina to Cleveland, Ohio, in 1962. He had been dreaming of one specific goal since he graduated from medical school thirteen years earlier—becoming a trained lung surgeon. He really had no interest in heart disease. He knew he could learn and excel at the manual skills of surgery. His mother was a dressmaker and his father a furniture craftsman. Working with his hands carefully and with great skill was second nature to him. But the English language was not. Favaloro's arrival in the United States was unnoticed by almost everyone at the Cleveland Clinic, the institution leading the way in the progress of cardiac and lung surgery. But Favaloro's young life, as well as the thirteen years since he had graduated from medical school, had taught him something about perseverance.

At a young age, Favaloro was driven by a passion for helping others and, despite his situation,[88] planned to have a medical career. As a youngster, Favaloro was inspired by reading a book about the life of Louis Pasteur (1822-1895), the great scientist of immunology and vaccines, and by his uncle who was a family doctor. He enrolled in medical school in Buenos Aires and was certain that he would have a career as a surgeon after his graduation in 1949. But Argentina at the time was a country ruled by a dictator, and in order to gain acceptance at a prestigious institution for graduate training in surgery, all medical students needed to sign a document pledging their allegiance to the National System, the political party of Juan Perón (1895-1974). Favaloro refused,[89] giving up the opportunity to become a trained surgeon. He could still practice medicine, but his options were few; he only had the skills and training of a general practitioner.

In response to this turmoil, Favaloro fled the big city of Buenos Aires and began medical practice in a town of two thousand inhabitants, Jacinto Aráuz, located in the Argentinian La Pampa Province. He could not have chosen a more remote spot in his large country, but fortunately his younger brother agreed to join him in practice after his own graduation. The Favaloro brothers practiced in a town without

---

88   By his own description, his family was "low middle class," living in La Plata, a town fifty miles south of Buenos Aires.
89   This would begin Favaloro's many problems with the government of Argentina.

a hospital or an emergency room, so they scrimped and saved every fee they received, built a medical center for the town, and then added operating rooms. Between 1950 and 1962, the pair performed over eleven thousand surgeries in spite of their lack of formal training in surgery. The local people couldn't travel to a major city for specialized care and the town loved the two dedicated brothers.

But Favaloro had never forgotten his dream of becoming a lung surgeon, and despite being an almost forty-year-old, Spanish-speaking family doctor, Favaloro secured a training position at the Cleveland Clinic[90] through family contacts and his old professors from his medical school days. With his limited English-language skills, Favaloro was very unsure that he would survive any training program in America, but after only a few weeks, he realized that he landed in a place that believed in teamwork, with a rare spirit of collegiality. In a stroke of unbelievable luck, he met Mason Sones, already a major star in the cardiology firmament, and Sones asked him to help with his analysis of images of coronary artery atherosclerosis. The task had nothing to do with lung surgery, but René Favaloro was in no position to turn down a request for help from Dr. Sones. He wisely agreed.

This decision would immerse Favaloro into a new and previously unimaginable world. Coronary artery angiograms, the technique that Dr. Sones had stumbled upon by accident only four years prior, were stunning to Favaloro. The doctor had never seen such images before, nor had many others at the time, and hadn't known that these pictures were even possible. He had never really been interested in the heart, but now he was mesmerized. In addition, the Chief of Cardiothoracic Surgery, Donald Effler MD (1915-2004), and his colleagues at the Clinic were performing remarkable new surgeries for patients with heart valve and congenital defects. He and Mason

---

90 The Cleveland Clinic was founded in 1921 by three surgeons who had worked together in the US Army in World War I and has been regarded by many as the top hospital in the world for cardiac care for decades.

Sones, however, had a new frontier of surgery in mind: they were interested in surgery for patients with angina and coronary artery disease. They took their surgical ideas from articles published over a decade earlier by a surgeon from Montreal, Canada, Arthur Vineberg MD (1903-1988).

NEW BLOOD: SURGERY TO TREAT CORONARY ARTERY DISEASE

In the early 1960s, Sones and Effler were fascinated by the brave efforts of Dr. Vineberg. Vineberg was born in Montreal, Canada, and received his education at McGill University in his hometown. His own life had been affected by coronary artery disease in a profound way as his father had died of this very condition. The idea that surgery could help, if not cure, patients with angina pectoris from coronary artery atherosclerosis had had a brief moment of notoriety in the early twentieth century. Surgery to cut the nerves of the sympathetic nervous system in the neck, those that controlled the perception of pain in the chest, had very limited success and was quickly abandoned. But working as a general surgeon at the Royal Victoria Hospital, Vineberg came up with a novel method—a way to supply new blood to a heart deprived of its own blood supply by blocked arteries.

Vineberg's idea did not spring out of nowhere. The anatomists had shown that the heart had a very complex network of arteries and veins, not just the two major arteries, the left and right coronary arteries that originated from the aorta as it attaches to the top of the left ventricle. At the smaller blood vessel level, there were elaborate and numerous connections between the veins, called the "sinusoids," and the tiny "capillaries" of the arteries. At the microscopic level of the heart muscle, blood and oxygen were shared between the much smaller arteries and veins.

Knowing these anatomic facts, Vineberg reasoned that if he could surgically plug the end of another large artery into the heart muscle, he could flood the tissue with much more oxygenated blood and diminish the chest pain of angina. He thought his technique might work like burying a large water hose into a garden to allow water to percolate through the soil to the plants. Vineberg's idea, if it worked, would supply a large volume of blood to spread into the heart tissue, and the oxygen in the blood would be sucked up by the tiny capillaries in the heart muscle. There would then be a new source of oxygen for the tissue starved of blood because of atherosclerosis in its normal pipeline of the coronary arteries, the left and the right coronary arteries. Vineberg needed a "third coronary artery" to attempt his experiments as this artery was going to "bypass" the normal path for blood into the heart muscle.

As a trained and experienced surgeon, Vineberg thought carefully about where he could find a new blood supply for the heart. The artery to use needed to be very close to the heart so that Vineberg could dissect it out, clean it up, cut one end open, and then sew the open end into the rich vascular bed of heart muscle. He needed a large artery but one that would not cause the tissue supplied by that artery to die from lack of blood supply if a surgeon diverted its blood flow. There needed to be other arteries in the area that would pick up the burden. Where would he find such an artery?

The breastbone, the sternum, lay right over the heart and had some ideal qualities for Vineberg's purposes.[91] The sternum, like every organ or bone, has its own blood supply. Traveling along the underside of both sides of the sternum are two large arteries that are branches of the thoracic aorta, the large conduit that takes blood from the left ventricle of the heart and carries it throughout the chest via smaller vessels to supply the lungs, the spine, the skin and breasts, and the bones of the chest wall. These arteries are called the "internal thoracic arteries," or the "internal mammary arteries." Fortunately for Vineberg, the thoracic

---

91   At surgery, it is stunning how close this plate of bone is to the heart and how carefully cardiac surgeons must be when opening the sternum to not nick the heart muscle and cause rapid bleeding.

arteries are not the only blood supply to the sternum. He thought that diverting one of them from the chest bone into the heart would not result in problems with the sternum's oxygenation and viability.

In 1946, Vineberg began his animal experiments using one of the internal thoracic arteries of dogs, peeling it away from the sternum and sewing it directly into heart muscle. Vineberg's surgical skills for this unique procedure were inadequate at first; only one out of thirteen dogs survived the surgery. But practice paid off, and within four years, his success rate was up to seventy-five percent short-term survival in his animals. Vineberg was ready to try his operation in patients with debilitating angina, as for these unfortunates there were no other options, either from surgery or medication.

In April 1950, Vineberg performed his first human surgery using the "third coronary artery." The patient survived but only for sixty-two hours. His second patient did much better and lived another ten years! Vineberg concluded that for the first time he created a surgical treatment for coronary artery disease, an operation based on knowledge of how the heart's own blood supply worked. His operation demonstrated "proof of concept"—more blood to the heart could overcome the shortfall in oxygen supply caused by atherosclerosis. A simple idea was proven and hope for millions was perhaps on the horizon.

Vineberg continued his practice, and in 1958, he published his results and others were soon eager to build on his work. He documented that in fifty-seven patients, sixty-seven percent were now free of angina. Vineberg had data to show that clearly it was possible to perform surgery and re-supply the heart muscle with blood, have patients survive, and in many, eliminate their chest pain. The Cleveland Clinic team of cardiac surgeons and cardiologists pushed first to duplicate and then improve on Vineberg's procedure. Because Mason Sones showed that he could image the blood supply of the heart in the cath lab, Effler and his colleagues had a technique that could document what happened to the heart's circulation after the surgery.

Sones knew how to take advantage of Vineberg's work to expand the knowledge and hopefully improve on his results. Knowing the location of the internal thoracic artery as it sprung from the aorta, Sones was able to place his dye-filled catheter into its origin, inject the contrast material, and produce a stunning picture of the blood flow through the internal thoracic artery into the heart muscle. The dye saturated the tiny mixed up mass of arteries and veins, creating a "blush" of white easily seen on the fluoroscopy of the heart in the cath lab. Throughout the early and mid-1960s, the Clinic's operating room was busy performing "Vineberg's" and in 1968 reported that ninety-two percent of the time, the re-positioned internal thoracic artery had excellent blood flow shortly after the surgery.

The combination of these skills and discoveries was monumental. The Cleveland Clinic team now had very useful tools to look at atherosclerotic plaque and distortions of the heart's blood supply; cardiac catheterization with angiograms of the coronary arteries had changed everything. Now they were looking into projects to alleviate symptoms, restore some of the damage from the Widowmaker, and perhaps prevent heart attacks using surgery.

But there was more to come. After scrubbing in on Vineberg procedures, Favaloro began to mull over a new idea. He was deeply confident in his surgical skills, hand-eye coordination he learned from his mother, the dressmaker. But Favaloro realized that as spectacular as he thought his surgical talent was, dissecting out the thoracic artery firmly secured under the breastbone would be a challenge. So he invented a special surgical instrument, called a "retainer," that made the job easier. By 1966, he and Effler were performing surgery using not one but both internal thoracic arteries from the underside of the sternum, a "double" Vineberg operation.

However, disappointing information came to light: the cath images showed that the internal thoracic arteries only created visible communications with the patient's own coronary arteries about fifty percent of the time. These data raised two major concerns. First, was some of the improvement in the patient's symptom a placebo effect?[92] Secondly, even though there was a large flow of blood through the internal thoracic artery right after the surgery, was the artery closing off due to blood clots over time? Perhaps the new blood supply lasted only months.

The Argentinian knew that the Vineberg advance was just a start and knew what should come next. He thought there must be a better way than just plugging an artery into the heart muscle and hoping that new connections would evolve between the internal thoracic arteries and the patient's own coronary arteries. His idea crystallized, and it was bold: he was sure that he could directly sew a mammary artery into the heart's own arteries, not the muscle, connecting it beyond the point of an atherosclerotic blockage in the native artery. This new artery would propel new blood right into a coronary artery, not just spray it out through the tiny veins and arteries of the heart muscle. And he knew it could be done.

FAVALORO WAS NOT ALONE

As it turned out, the idea of revascularizing a patient's own coronary artery with a direct connection from an artery under the breastbone did not originate with Favaloro. In 1960, an American surgeon, Robert Goetz MD (1910-2000), a German immigrant who fled antisemitism in 1929, was confronted with a desperate man. A thirty-eight-year-old cab driver from the Bronx, New York, had such severe angina that he was using seventy to ninety nitroglycerin tablets a day. Goetz thought about what he might be able to do to help the man. He knew he had the surgical speed and talent to perform an arterial bypass operation, without using a heart-lung machine. But Goetz remembered the days of the late 1940s, when a few surgeons like Dwight Harken tried to perform surgery on a beating heart, usually with a high mortality rate.

---

92 Placebo from Latin meaning "I shall be pleasing." Placebo effect is a beneficial effect produced by a treatment not attributed to the properties of the treatment and must be due to the patient's belief in the treatment.

Nonetheless, given free rein,[93] Goetz performed the surgery, and his confidence in his skills was confirmed. The operation went well, and the patient survived. Reportedly, his patient remained without angina for at least one year. Details of his long-term course are obscure, but it is likely after a year the bypass grafts developed blood clots or recurrent atherosclerosis. Regardless, Goetz' surgery was a successful short-term treatment for horrible angina.

Despite the fact that Goetz was hindered from performing more coronary bypass surgeries, his achievement had a lasting impact on the history of heart disease. Years later, he wrote that other than the cardiologist who referred the man to him for surgery "our medical colleagues were violently against the procedure. We even came in for severe criticism from some of our surgical colleagues."[94] But throughout the history of medicine, skepticism about new ideas arises over and over again, doubt often driven by the inertia of old concepts but also the need for verification before acceptance. Although Goetz did not have the determination to proceed further Favaloro would take his one successful surgery as additional proof of concept. He was ready to "push the envelope" on his own.

There were others in the world, again hidden from the West by the Cold War, who also were performing revolutionary bypass operations for coronary artery disease. No one outside of Russia, and certainly not Favaloro, was aware of the work of a brave surgeon named Vasilii I. Koselov MD (1904-1992). He was the son of rural peasant farmers who used his ambition and intelligence to gain him a medical degree in St. Petersburg and whose gumption would soon be put to the test.

In the early years of his career as a surgeon, he, like millions of other Russians, was faced with a profound challenge by the Second World War. Koselov was living and working in St. Petersburg when the Nazi

---

93 Goetz's plan really needed to be presented to an ethics committee at his hospital before he proceeded. But not in 1960.
94 It is likely that the criticism focused on Goetz' failure to at least use the heart-lung machine rather than depend on his quick hands to save a sick beating heart.

invasion reached the city in September 1941. Koselov somehow was able to care for patients and perform surgery in the most unimaginable deprived conditions, he himself suffering from a lack of nutrition and barely surviving bouts of dysentery. This must have been an incredibly distressing time and place to be a doctor, as during the siege of over two years, 640,000 people in St. Petersburg died from malnutrition alone.

After the war, Koselov returned to his position as an academic surgeon in St. Petersburg, and it is here that he would have a lasting impact on the fight against heart disease. His boss, Vladimir Demikhov MD (1916-1998), was also intrigued by the idea of using arteries to bypass blocked coronary arteries. In 1953, Demikhov performed internal thoracic bypass procedures in dogs, four of whom survived for the next two years without any heart problems. The technique of revascularization of the heart became Koselov's obsession. Over several years, he invented surgical instruments that allowed him to carefully tease open the wall of the coronary artery, maintain blood flow, and do his suturing of the mammary artery into the native artery. In dogs, his technique worked beautifully, usually without using a heart-lung machine!

Koselov was now ready to try his operation in humans. On February 25, 1964, he replicated the surgery done by Robert Goetz a few years earlier. The patient survived, and Koselov was off and running to perform many more arterial bypass procedures. Eighty percent of the time, his heart surgeries were done without the use of the heart-lung machine, instead using two new aids to Koselov's work—magnifying glasses and specially designed scissors.

In the late 1960s, just at the time Favaloro was generating and beginning to act on his new ideas in Cleveland, Koselov published excellent results in his patients in the Soviet medical literature, showing markedly reduced or completely eliminated angina. But his data had a serious flaw; very few of the patients had undergone a cardiac catheterization either prior to or after the procedure, meaning the precise anatomy of Koselov's patients' coronary arteries was not known. That would be like a surgeon saying that their new technique to remove an appendix was a terrific advance, without showing the pathology reports saying that a diseased appendix was taken out. Who in the West was going to trust the work of a Soviet surgeon at the height of the Cold War, especially without these key data?

His data also left other big gaps. Given the complexity of the coronary artery circulation, especially in blood vessels with cholesterol blockages, how could one be sure that the bypass graft was used to treat the most important blocked artery, the one supplying the largest amount of heart muscle? How could one be certain that the graft was open long-term, even if the patient's chest pain was gone? Scientists knew that the heart develops detour routes around blocked arteries over time; perhaps it was these collateral arteries and their additional blood supply that was abating the angina.

The skepticism about Kolesov's work was profound. When he published his first paper in English, a forward to the text read, "The opinions expressed concerning the management and surgical therapy of angina pectoris as expressed in this paper by Professor V. I. Kolesov are at variance with concepts of many surgeons in the United States." Koselov's doubters were even more strident in his own country. After presenting his data at a conference in 1967, the Cardiology Society of Leningrad issued the following resolution: "The surgical treatment of coronary artery disease is impossible and has no prospects for the future." Koselov's doubters had concerns about his results because of the lack of information about the coronary anatomy before and then after the surgery, rather than the idea of revascularization of heart muscle. Favaloro and his Cleveland Clinic colleagues were about to start down an uncertain path of cardiac surgical experimentation.

ON THE BRINK OF BREAKTHROUGHS

By the mid-1960s, Effler and the Cleveland Clinic team made their decision—they were going to go far beyond Vineberg's operation for severe angina patients. Instead of tying the internal thoracic artery into the heart muscle, they were going to follow the lead of Goetz, Koselov, and their brand-new South American trainee, René Favaloro. Ironically, when Favaloro first arrived at the Clinic, he did not have a license to even assist on surgeries, and one of his first jobs was to simply clean the heart-lung machine after surgery. Just a few months later, after completing the paperwork for his medical license, he was going to be one the leaders of a breakthrough surgery.

The team began suturing the internal thoracic artery directly into the heart's most important artery, the left anterior descending, the favorite location of the work of the Widowmaker, when there was a major plaque buildup to bypass. But the surgical technique remained challenging. If the patient had more than one or two arteries that had severe blockages, the surgeons were limited to using only one or two thoracic arteries. What if the patient needed four or five different bypasses in order to really revascularize that heart? There had to be a better technique to use for those people.

Favaloro quickly brought his brand-new idea to Dr. Effler: what about using pieces of vein from the leg to serve as the bypass conduits? There were long veins in the legs that could be easily "harvested" just prior to the surgery, trimmed up neatly, and then cut into pieces for use. The surgeon might have many potential veins to use and do as many bypasses as necessary. Again, the idea did not arise without any previous knowledge and experience. Favaloro knew that vascular surgeons at the Clinic had success using pieces of veins to reconstruct damaged arteries in the legs and the kidneys; but would the veins (much thinner than arteries) hold up to the increased pressure a heart can exert?

By early 1967, Favaloro was ready to try out his ideas. He started modestly; he used a piece of vein to bypass a blockage in just one artery on the right side of the heart, sewing the upper end of the vein above the blockage point identified by cath images obtained prior to surgery and then attaching the other end of vein again into the artery but below the blockage.

Sones anxiously waited for the time that he could again perform a cath on a patient that Favaloro had operated on. He got his first chance in May 1967 when Favaloro completed a bypass of the right coronary artery in a fifty-one-year-old woman. The cardiac cath showed that the bypass was open three months later! Still, Favaloro was concerned about the long-term blood flow using a short piece of vein; he wanted to use a longer piece and get more blood flow through it. His next idea was the real breakthrough: he was going to sew the upper end of the vein bypass graft into the aorta, just about the top of the left ventricle, a location from which the vein could receive much more blood flow.

Within a year, Favaloro and the clinic surgeons transformed the world of cardiac surgery, showing that pieces of vein, usually from the saphenous vein of the leg, could serve as successful conduits for blood and oxygen to enter the myocardium beyond ("distal") to where the Widowmaker's plaque blocked blood flow. Cardiac surgery at the Cleveland Clinic exploded, and their surgeons began using coronary artery bypass graft surgery, the "CABG," in patients not just with angina but combining the procedure with heart valve replacements, removal of dead heart muscle tissue called aneurysms and even in patients with an imminent or definite myocardial infarction.

By January 1, 1970, Favaloro and his colleagues had the information to answer so many previously unanswered questions. They had data on 224 patients who had undergone CABG surgery at their hospital, including those who had bypasses performed using leg veins as well as the internal thoracic arteries. The cardiology world held its breath—did the CABG operation work? Did the patient's angina disappear? Was it a safe procedure? Did it prevent heart attacks?

Favaloro first presented his data to the medical community at the World Congress of Cardiology in London, England, that year. Interviewed in 1997, Favaloro remembered the day well: "The room was jammed with people when we began the debate and the doors were closed, but the doctors in the foyer began pushing to get in, and after four to five minutes, they broke the handles off the doors[95] and crowded the room." The frenzy proved well-founded as Favaloro's results were spectacular. Nearly every time the surgery resolved the angina, sick patients returned to normal lives, and the heart-lung machine and skillful technique led to a very low mortality rate of four to five percent, remarkable for cardiac surgery at that time. If others could replicate his data, Favaloro's work would be revolutionary, the first successful surgery for a disease that had plagued mankind for thousands of years.[96]

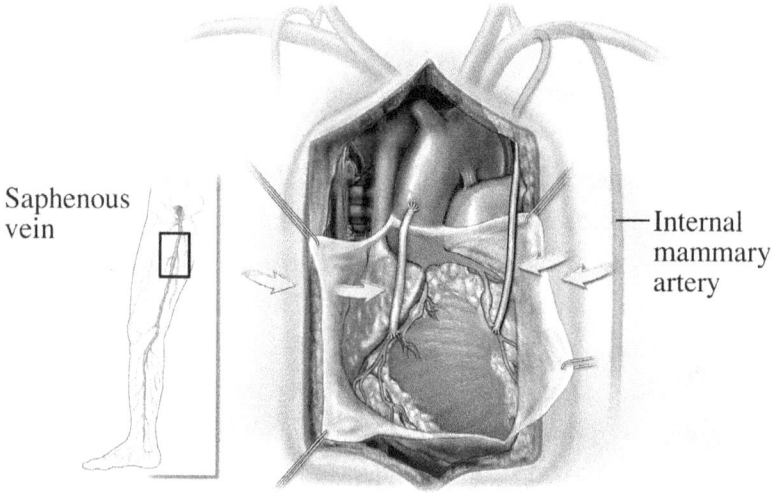

Figure 19. Two methods of performing coronary artery bypass surgery, using a piece of vein from the arm or leg, or the internal mammary artery under the breastbone (sternum) as a bypass conduit.
(Copyright Shutterstock)

---

95   Perhaps the doctors who broke down the doors to hear him speak took their inspiration from some of the enormous music festivals of the late 1960s. René Favaloro was indeed the first "rock star" of coronary artery bypass graft surgery.
96   About a decade later, analyzing their data over eleven years and several thousand patients, from 1967 to 1978, the Clinic team, now including other luminaries of cardiac surgery such as Floyd Loop MD, Delos Cosgrove MD, and Bruce Lytle MD, reported that the chance of surviving the operation was an astounding ninety-nine percent.

Sones and his cath team also had data, the kind that the Russian Koselov had not provided. They showed that twenty-one months after surgery, seventy-five to eighty-five percent of the grafts remained open, and the five-year patient survival rate of the patients ranged from ninety to ninety-three percent. Sixty-five to seventy percent of the patients no longer experienced angina. Now there was documentation that indeed "re-vascularization" could eliminate angina, that most of the bypasses functioned properly over time, and that the surgery could be done safely.

In spite of his success at the Cleveland Clinic, René Favaloro pined for his native country. He made the difficult decision to return to Argentina in 1971. His goal was to establish a medical foundation based on the Cleveland Clinic model. By 1975, he had put together a group, and they opened the Fundación Favaloro in Buenos Aires. He and his new partners performed thousands of cardiac surgeries, operating on patients regardless of their ability to pay. They counseled patients about disease prevention and hygiene and offered a smoking cessation course. Favaloro did the first successful heart transplants in South America. Favaloro's foundation also established a research laboratory in 1980, and by the year 2000, he had helped prepare 450 young surgeons who had come to the Fundación,[97] just like the Cleveland Clinic had trained him.

But the effect of Argentina's chronic political and economic turmoil on Favaloro's personal life was intense. He railed against corruption and the abduction and murder of political dissidents. Finally, his angst brought him to a breaking point. On July 29, 2000, he committed suicide, shooting himself in the chest and heart with a pistol. Favaloro left a note explaining his decision to end his life—he was worn out from being a "beggar in his own country." His death was a national tragedy for Argentina, the untimely death of a man who had placed Argentinian medicine on the world stage. His absence slowed the progress of cardiac care in South America.

---

97 The Favaloro Fundación became a national treasure in Argentina and the Universidad Favaloro was founded in 1998.

René Favaloro's legacy holds a profound place in the history of medicine and cardiology. Taking inspiration from the few others who had attempted resupplying a heart muscle with a fresh blood supply to relieve the chronic ischemia caused by coronary atherosclerosis, he settled on a new technical idea about how to achieve the goal of revascularization. In addition, the success of his idea of using veins to bypass atherosclerotic coronary arteries created a new reality in technique that improved the outcomes of surgery that was thought to be impossible. He was passionate about training others in the technique and welcomed the entire nascent world of coronary artery surgery to follow his lead. Within a few years of his famous London presentation, almost every major medical center in the United States and Europe had established CABG surgery programs.[98]

Dr. Favaloro helped millions. Although his character and beliefs often were those of a "Don Quixote," Favaloro wasn't seeing imaginary windmills and foes; he was effectively dealing with the Widowmaker. He had guts, backed up by a faith in his own skill, and the science behind his ideas. His name may only be recognizable by a select few,[99] but the impact he made was universal.

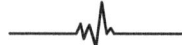

A GREAT OPERATION

. . . Putting him quickly into a hospital bed, Bill arranged for a cardiac catheterization for Ed the next day. To no one's surprise,

---

[98] In 2000, the number of CABG surgeries in the United States peaked at slightly more than 500,000. This accrual of massive amounts of data allowed the cardiologists and cardiac surgeons to better assess which treatment—surgery, medications, or angioplasty—would benefit their patients most. As a result, the number of CABG procedures decreased over the years. Nevertheless, the operation continues to save thousands of lives each year.

[99] The world-dominating website Google many times posts a cartoon of someone their staff feels is important to honor on their homepage; they call it a "Google Doodle." On July 12, 2019, there it was: a drawing of René Favaloro in his surgical cap and scrubs, in honor of what would have been his ninety-sixth birthday. In the twenty-first century, that honor might rival a Nobel Prize. Certainly, more people will know about it.

there were severe blockages of atherosclerosis in three coronary arteries. Bill arranged for our colleague, James McClurken MD, a top cardiothoracic surgeon, to evaluate Ed as soon as possible. Ed, of course, had never met Jim and was very concerned not only about the surgery but also the person to whom he was entrusting his heart and his life. But Bill and I knew Jim was the right person for Ed on many levels. The patient and heart surgeon met, and Ed felt he had made a human connection with Jim almost immediately.

Within a day or so, Ed underwent the surgery, an arterial bypass placed to his left anterior descending coronary artery, and the two other major arteries as well. After we resolved a few complications post-surgery, Ed went home, never to return to the hospital for any cardiac problems in over a decade. Instead, he re-engaged in a full and normal life after his bypass surgery, a technique deemed impossible until just over fifty years ago. I suspect without the surgery, his life would have been very different, punctuated by many more heart problems and possibly serious myocardial infarctions that would have threatened his life.

Atherosclerosis had caused significant damage to the coronary arteries of my friend Ed, but the Widowmaker's end result was thwarted by a procedure first developed by an unlikely person—René Favaloro, the son of a dressmaker from Argentina. For the first time, there was an effective surgical treatment for coronary artery disease. There was still no valid means of prevention, however. For that, the lab scientists would need to lead the way.

CHAPTER 17

METABOLISM MEN: UNLOCKING THE CHOLESTEROL CODE

Who could blame doctors for wanting to ride in on a white horse at the last moment and save the day? They are valiant defenders and it makes the game all the more unpredictable.

Not so with this new team of chemists. They are ready to play dirty by creating an offense that will thwart my most trusted moves. If they perfect this strategy, it would certainly tip the odds.

ELIMINATING THE DRAMA: QUIET PREVENTION

Joan's problem started slowly in 1999. It was just a "rub," an odd feeling in her chest. She liked to walk after dinner, and that feeling would happen but then go away when she slowed down. Sometimes when she was walking more quickly, the sensation was more like a "burning."

The symptoms were not a terrible surprise to her, but the timing was. Her parents and her uncle had all died from heart disease, but they had a bad diet, full of "Polish food." So given her moderate lifestyle, she perhaps anticipated heart problems as she got much older, but not when she was only fifty-three. Women didn't get heart disease this young, did they?

Her physician recommended a stress test, one during which she would first exercise and then images of her blood supply would be taken using a radioactive tracer; it was going to "light up her heart" she was told. The test was abnormal. She needed to see a cardiologist, and she told her husband Joe, "We'll fix it."

In my office ten days later, I had the stress test results and immediately told her she would need a cardiac catheterization and medications for angina pectoris. There was only one problem—Joan's son's wedding was just a few days away, and she wasn't going to miss it. Besides, she said, "The dress is in the closet."

Just a few days later, while shopping for the earrings in cold weather, she could barely walk before the symptoms began. For the first time, Joan was scared . . .

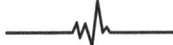

THE GENIUSES OF CHEMISTRY: RECEPTOR MOLECULES AND MAGIC BULLETS

Firemen love to fight fires; they are incredibly brave and risk their lives to save people and buildings, and along the way they get an adrenaline rush from what they do. Though not risking their own lives, cardiologists and cardiac surgeons aren't that different. By the late 1960s, CCUs and CABG surgery provided new fire for their adrenaline surge. But prevention of heart attacks—while those who treated heart disease wished there was something they could do, that task seemed relatively boring. But the heart attacks just kept coming and coming. More victims of the Widowmaker were surviving, but there wasn't any way to "flatten the curve" of the epidemic.

It is important to note that by the mid-nineteenth century, the organic chemists proved that all of the chemical elements and molecules of the body were in motion. They were going in and out of cells, like oxygen being absorbed through the cells of the lung from the atmosphere. But how did this happen? What means of transportation did these crucial substances rely upon to reach their correct destination? What was occurring at the level of the individual cell of, say, the intestine that allowed food into the body to be used to supply energy and build and repair cells? A young scientist from southwestern Germany, and his keen eyes, helped provide the answer.

Paul Ehrlich MD (1854-1915) was entranced by the small, odd-looking black instrument that his older cousin, a medical student, gave him as a teenager. Probably like most youngsters, he might have looked at pond water to observe the tiny creatures and plants living there, or the wings of dead insects. Then something else caught his attention. Ehrlich's family owned and operated a successful textile business, and Paul wondered what the fibers of cloth looked like under the microscope, especially after they were exposed to dyes. He knew that cotton, linen, and wool were organic materials; his cousin told him they were made out of cells and have cell walls surrounding them. But why did some dyes stain the cell walls better than others? Ehrlich realized that there must be something in the cell wall that grabbed on to some dyes tightly and others not.

Before he was twenty years old, Ehrlich had an insight that hadn't dawned on generations of older scientists. The cell walls of the cloth fibers must have specific *"receptor molecules"* that were able to latch onto specific molecules and shepherd them into the cells, like a key fitting into a lock. How else were only some dyes able to enter the cell wall or the various organelles of the cell and others not?

Paul Ehrlich saw the future of his life in science and medicine. He followed his cousin into medical school, already with a microscope at his side. But now he was interested in the cell walls of another mysterious form of life seen only under the microscope. The science of microbiology was in its "salad days" in the late nineteenth century in France and Germany, after the discovery by Louis Pasteur that the dreaded fatal disease of rabies was caused by bacteria.

Inspired by Pasteur's work, Ehrlich took his ideas even further. Ehrlich and others discovered that a wide variety of dyes, called "stains," could reliably create a specific color on not just the cell walls but also the organelles, the internal components, of cells of not just bacteria but human cells as well.[100] But Ehrlich did not stop there. He carried these concepts into treatment. He reasoned that there might be certain compounds that could grab on to the cell walls of bacteria, get into the cell, and the right molecule could alter the metabolism of the bacterial cell and kill it. With incredible diligence, Ehrlich studied thousands of compounds to attempt to find ones that killed bacteria. The world became a believer in Paul Ehrlich's "magic bullets" when, in 1909, he discovered the first drug effective in treating syphilis, a horrible incurable disease prior to his work. Ehrlich's drug named Salvarsen was used extensively until penicillin was invented in the 1940s.

Ehrlich's legacy of the receptor molecule has lived on and changed the world. Just like Newton's ideas about gravity, his brilliance emerged from a "thought experiment," allowing him to envision a molecule he could not see. Ehrlich's work was foundational for modern immunology and pharmacology. He received the Nobel Prize in Medicine in 1908, and his life was celebrated in the 1940 film *Dr. Ehrlich's Magic Bullets*. In 1915, at the age of sixty-one, one of the great scientific geniuses of the last millennium succumbed to the work of the Widowmaker—he died of a heart attack. But his life's work would help others come closer to catching this elusive foe.

THE NOBEL PRIZE DUO: UNLOCKING THE MYSTERY OF CHOLESTEROL

Michael S. Brown MD (1941-) and his close friend Joseph L. Goldstein MD (1940-) were just embryos in their academic careers in 1968. Two years earlier, Brown, from suburban Philadelphia and the University of

---

100 This is the science of Histology, the identification of cells and bacteria under the microscope by their appearance and response to dye stains.

Pennsylvania, and Goldstein, a small-town boy from South Carolina and the University of Texas Southwestern in Dallas, were thrown together as interns in internal medicine at the Massachusetts General Hospital in Boston. They became friends within days, both having an intense interest in clinical medicine but also in medical research. They liked taking care of patients, but it was basic laboratory research that they sought, and now they were studying genetics and biochemistry together at the National Institute of Health in Bethesda, Maryland. The two were unified by a common fascination with metabolism, the processes that all living beings use to produce the molecules that drive life, such as insulin and its ability to allow sugar to enter the cells for energy.

Despite their research focus, for a few hours a week, Brown and Goldstein did see patients in a clinic, usually people with very unusual problems of metabolism that could not be understood or treated by their local doctors. Often, they and their families came to Bethesda in desperation for any kind of help. Sure enough, one day Dr. Goldstein was assigned to care for two desperately ill children, ages six and eight. Both children had suffered from multiple myocardial infarctions—heart attacks in children? Why? The two children Brown and Goldstein saw were suffering from a very rare disease that was first noticed in the 1920s and 1930s. A Norwegian, Carl Müller MD (1886-1983), discovered this malady. These unfortunates had extremely high levels of cholesterol in their blood. In addition to forming cholesterol blockages in their coronary arteries, they often had deposits of cholesterol in the tendons of the body, lesions called "xanthomas." There was just so much cholesterol in their bodies; it had to gather somewhere.

By looking at the patients' family histories, Müller concluded that this disease was genetic, not due to diet or some other factor. He knew these people must have a major problem with how they metabolized cholesterol. He called this an "inborn error of metabolism" and named this disorder Familial Hypercholesterolemia (FH). What made these genes function so poorly? Müller didn't have a clue.

In 1968, no treatment or medication could reduce cholesterol levels and the risk of more heart attacks; Joe Goldstein was frustrated that he could do nothing for his sick children patients, and he shared his chagrin with his friend Dr. Brown. Brown and Goldstein became obsessed with trying to figure out what was the cause of this horrible disease. They knew that the answer would come in the biochemistry lab; without a clear understanding of the fine details, no rational treatment would ever be possible. Their hope was greater than explaining and helping the one in a million patients with Familial Hyperlipidemia. Often extreme forms of a disease can serve as a model for a problem that occurs in many others to a lesser degree. Brown and Goldstein dreamed that their work could unlock the causes and possible treatments for atherosclerosis, the handiwork of the Widowmaker.

This medical duo knew the fundamentals of the metabolism of cholesterol. Cholesterol comes into the body from the diet, where once absorbed through the intestine, it is coated with protein molecules to form the lipoproteins, the molecules that John Gofman found in the late 1940s. But the lipoproteins from food are not the only source of cholesterol; the liver, the major "metabolic factory" of the body, is also involved. To make matters daunting, there are thirty chemical reactions leading to the final product of cholesterol. But Brown and Goldstein realized that only one of the steps was likely the most important step in the entire process.

Each of them understood the kinetics, the all-important speed of biochemical reactions, and that in all series of reactions there is one step, the slowest one, that determines the overall rate of the process and controls the amount of a molecule produced. This is the "rate-limiting" step. The human liver controls cholesterol metabolism. Cholesterol chemistry's slowest step is driven by one specific protein-enzyme with the tongue-twisting name of 3-hydroxy-3-methyl-glutaryl-coenzyme A reductase (its only slightly shorter name is HMG CoA reductase). A malfunction of this key enzyme looked like the best target to look at to understand the problem of elevated cholesterol levels.

Another characteristic of cholesterol was particularly significant to those who studied its metabolism trying to understand its relationship to atherosclerosis: exactly how does cholesterol get inside of cells? All cells of living things need to control their internal environment and their interaction with the outside world, be it the bloodstream or the atmosphere. Many atoms and molecules don't have free access to the inside of cells; they can only enter through channels in the cell walls containing specific molecules, those Paul Ehrlich receptors, unique ports of entry, similar to the need for a cargo ship moving west across the northern Atlantic Ocean to enter the United States through New York and not the beaches of the east coast of New Jersey. In these special "harbors" on the cell membrane, the receptors are waiting, like the large mechanical cranes you see on docks that unload cargo from ships. But the bulk of the cell membranes is made up of cholesterol, which doesn't like water—it's a "hydrophobic" molecule. The cell membrane is a barrier to the molecules and elements in the blood vessels and only lets in those molecules it needs through specific channels and receptors imbedded in the cell wall.[101]

Brown and Goldstein knew that cholesterol metabolism has four steps:

Step One: cholesterol gets into the body from our food and enters the intestine; in response to the presence of food, hormone molecules in the gut signal the liver to secrete bile, which forms an emulsion, a combination of proteins, fat, and cholesterol, that envelopes the cholesterol with a "hydrophilic" coat. Only then can the cholesterol cross from the inside of the intestine and into the water-welcoming channels in the cells of the intestinal wall. The lipoproteins like water, unlike pure cholesterol. They are the carrier molecules of cholesterol.

---

[101] These properties of molecules are why salad oil, which like cholesterol is hydrophobic, doesn't mix with vinegar, which is acetic acid and highly hydrophilic. Just another example of the power of organic chemistry to explain the world.

Step Two: from the small intestine cells, the cholesterol is repackaged by other gut protein enzymes into new particles, shipped into the circulation, and then grabbed up by the liver cells.

Step Three: the liver changes the cholesterol again, using not just the cholesterol from the diet but also the cholesterol made by the liver itself.

Finally, *Step Four:* cholesterol is shipped out to the cells again where it is used to form a major part of the backbone of the wall of the cells, those hydrophobic barriers. Cholesterol didn't like water when we ate it, the body created a new form of it so it could cross through the intestine and get to the liver, and then it goes back out to form cell walls, and still not like water!

FINDING A TARGET

Brown and Goldstein were trying to make some sense of the mental entanglement of cholesterol metabolism. If they were going to solve the cause of the disease in the two sick children with heart attacks, they needed to find an initial target in the metabolic sequence to focus on, a molecule, preferably an enzyme, that made some sense. They knew very well another equally crucial and fundamental concept in metabolism: the body needs to control the production of its molecules. That is to say, the body needs to make enough cholesterol to supply its own needs, but when the level rises, there must be a biochemical signal that tells the liver cells that enough is enough and to slow down or even shutdown the production of more cholesterol. This process is called "feedback regulation" —what goes up must come down, the Yin and Yang of metabolism.

The pair thought that perhaps the problem might be with the most obvious molecule, malfunction of the HMG CoA reductase molecule, the rate-limiting step enzyme that determined the entire overall speed of cholesterol metabolism. If that enzyme was malfunctioning, the answer might be easy to uncover. Perhaps the failure of the HMG CoA reductase to respond to the signal from the blood that too much cholesterol was present was why the Familial Hyperlipidemia patients' liver cells continued to make cholesterol that was not needed. That would cause a profound failure of the feedback regulation of cholesterol in the people with FH. The enzyme just kept producing cholesterol out of control.

But first the team had a practical hurdle to overcome. The liver manufactures the body's cholesterol, but how can you study liver cells outside of a living person? Yes, a patient can undergo a liver biopsy and the liver cells can grow in a dish of nutrients, but this procedure carries considerable risk of bleeding and liver damage. Was there a safer choice of human cells to study that could be easily accessed with less risk and also manufacture cholesterol? With the breakthrough discoveries about DNA, there was the realization that every single cell of the body contains all of the DNA for the entire body. So there was a chance that just about any cell you choose might express an enzyme or protein abnormality, particularly in rare genetic diseases. Brown and Goldstein needed to find the right cells to test. They thought that the fibroblast cells of the skin would be perfect.[102] The fibroblast cells had all of the enzymes needed to produce cholesterol.

After their NIH experience, Brown and Goldstein both moved to Dallas and took junior faculty positions at the medical school of the University of Texas Southwestern and picked up where they had left off. Jumping into their experiments, they developed a specific assay, a chemical test that allowed them to measure the concentration of HMG CoA reductase in their experiments. Next, they wanted to be sure that the fibroblasts cooperated with "feedback regulation." They added various types of lipoproteins to the tissue cultures. The fibroblasts of normal volunteers did decrease the activity of HMG CoA reductase after exposure to only one type of lipoprotein—low-

---

[102] Fibroblasts live in the dermis of the skin just below the skin's top layer, the epidermis, are easy and safe to biopsy, and grow well in tissue culture dishes in a laboratory.

density lipoproteins, LDL. But what about the cells of the two sick children? In these patients' cells *the level of HMG CoA reductase was fifty to one hundred times the level in normals, clearly explaining their extraordinary levels of blood cholesterol!* These cells were working overtime producing LDL cholesterol particles. The HMG CoA reductase enzymes were running amok with no controls to stop them—they were in violation of the fundamental law of metabolism, feedback regulation.[103] But why exactly was this happening?

So here was the dilemma confronted. Brown and Goldstein knew that there were two ways that molecules got into cells—the receptors, often grabbing onto hydrophobic molecules like LDL cholesterol and shepherding them into the cells, and another way, direct entrance into cells through specific molecular channels in the cell wall, locations where many common hydrophilic molecules can enter very quickly. They were sure that there was a Paul Ehrlich–type receptor molecule on the fibroblasts' cell walls, and they were going to try to bypass it and fast track LDL into the cell through channels, not the receptor. To achieve this, they synthesized a hydrophilic form of cholesterol by mixing it with alcohol and a protein called albumin then added it to their fibroblast cell cultures. If the water-friendly LDL, getting directly into the cell without interacting with any receptor molecule on the cell wall, also did not affect the cholesterol production, the question was settled—there had to be a problem with the HMG CoA reductase molecule. But what if the new hydrophilic LDL particle suppressed the enzyme and slowed down the cholesterol factory, consistent with normal feedback regulation? Then there was a very different explanation for the problem in the FH people.

The results were stunning. The hydrophilic cholesterol concoction went right through the cell wall membrane and *did suppress* the production of HMG CoA reductase, both in normal cells as well as the patients with FH! The HMG enzyme was subject to feedback

---

103 These cells in the FH people were similar to cancer cells, which also grow and grow incessantly.

regulation—if it was exposed to a water-friendly form of cholesterol. Thus, the FH patients' genetic defect was *not* due to a problem with HMG CoA reductase function; it had to be due to something else. It must be in the process by which LDL, the normal hydrophobic particle, got into the cell. Could this malfunction involve a receptor molecule on the surface of the cell? Was the receptor thwarting the entry of the normal hydrophobic lipoprotein containing cholesterol the cause of the problem?

The receptor for the LDL particle then became the focal point of Brown and Goldstein's research. There is a term for the process by which molecules are grabbed by receptors as they approach the cell wall, endocytosis,[104] and they thought this process might be the key to the whole mystery. First, they had to prove that there was an LDL receptor on the surface of the fibroblast cells. LDL was isolated easily from blood by using a high-speed centrifuge. Brown and Goldstein then labeled the LDL particles with radioactive iodine and added them to their cell culture of fibroblasts of people with normal cholesterol levels and the patients with FH. Next, they took some pictures—radioactive iodine emits particles that collide with a crystal in a device called a nuclear camera, a detector of radioactivity. Then these collisions create an electrical signal; if they had used a Geiger counter, they would have heard a crackling sound from the radioactive energy bombardment. In this case, the detector created an image—dark spots on a film that they could easily examine.

Looking at the film, the results were clear. Normal cells grabbed onto the radioactive LDL particles zealously; lots of spots were seen on the film attached to the crystal on the detector. But in the FH patients, there was almost no uptake of the radioactive LDL particles. These people had very few LDL receptor molecules or their receptors

---

104 By the 1960s, electron microscope images of cells documented how they can envelope molecules by pushing out a portion of the cell wall, just like a long tongue, grab onto the molecules and ingest them, taking them out of the external environment and into the cell to be used for particular functions. The microscopists might have thought that they were looking at very tiny Venus Fly Traps.

were defective (or both problems!), a metabolic disease due to their DNA, not their diet. The LDL had no way to enter the cells and interact with the proteins that control cholesterol metabolism. If LDL didn't get into the cells of FH people, the HMG CoA reductase enzyme was not receiving a metabolic signal to slow down making cholesterol; there was no feedback regulation.

Brown and Goldstein's discovery resulted from their commitment to the Scientific Method of always questioning a first assumption. The HMG CoA reductase enzyme, their first suspect for the problem, was innocent. The LDL receptor defect was the guilty party and explained the disease of Familial Hyperlipidemia, a disorder that allowed huge numbers of LDL molecules to circulate through the blood and find their way into the walls of arteries and cause heart attacks, even in young children.

But even more discoveries emerged. The LDL receptors in the normals were most efficient when they were clustered together in specific areas of the cell wall. The receptors were not randomly distributed on the cell wall; they had specific locations of concentration. They really were molecular harbors for LDL. These harbors are named "coated pits." Brown and Goldstein also investigated the life cycle of the LDL receptors; they are produced in the endoplasmic reticulum, another of the cell's organelles. They carry the cholesterol from the cell surface into the cell in about ten minutes, making several hundred round trips during their lifetimes. They function well for about twenty hours until they are degraded by enzymes.

But how could Brown and Goldstein be sure that all of this work in a dish of fibroblast cells was also relevant in intact animals and humans, what is known as "in vivo"[105] rather than "in vitro"?[106] Additional studies resolved the doubt; LDL receptors were found on lymphocyte white blood cells and then on the cells of the adrenal glands and most importantly the liver. Further research by Brown

---
105 In vivo: inside a living organism.
106 In vitro: cells growing outside the body in a tissue culture medium of nutrients.

and Goldstein identified the actual structure of the LDL receptor, a chain of 839 amino acids creating a folded protein. They were even able to determine the location of the gene that creates the molecule.

By the late 1970s, the two Texas professors had fully worked out the scheme for how cholesterol and LDL particles entered cells. The first step was binding by the LDL receptors in organs (especially the liver), followed by internalization of the particles by endocytosis, transportation into the cell for splitting into cholesterol-containing lipoproteins, and movement to other cells through the circulation. Finally, there was entry into other cells to fulfill the role of the production of cell membranes, hormones, and bile acids. In normal cells, the cholesterol and LDL served a regulatory function that kept the LDL levels in the blood stable. This function was gone in the FH patients.

The metabolism of cholesterol helped explain why a diet high in fat, LDL, and cholesterol is so damaging. In the presence of this type of food, the LDL receptors become saturated; each receptor molecule can accommodate only one LDL particle at a time. The latecomers to the cell surface just float around in the blood. To make matters worse, when there is excess cholesterol and LDL in the blood, feedback regulation decreases the production of the LDL receptor. Enough cholesterol and LDL were already in the cells. As far as the liver cells are concerned, that was a normal response, but the result was damaging. So all combined, there were three problems: overworked LDL receptors, not enough of them, and those that were present were sometimes dysfunctional. The defects in metabolism allowed LDL and cholesterol to remain in the bloodstream, with nowhere to end up other than inside of the walls of the arteries of the body, especially those small arteries supplying the heart muscle. The result was atherosclerosis.

IMPLICATIONS FOR THE FUTURE

By the time Michael Brown and Joe Goldstein were awarded the Nobel Prize in Medicine in 1985, research had been going on for a decade, using their elegant explanation of the metabolism of cholesterol and the LDL particle to search for medications that would lower blood cholesterol levels and hopefully reduce the numbers of both old and young people worldwide from succumbing to the work of the Widowmaker. Their work provided the scientific roadmap for this work, offering new avenues of research in many directions.

The model of Familial Hyperlipidemia served as the basis to explore the genetic implications of elevated cholesterol levels in the population as a whole. The patients Brown and Goldstein studied had the rare form of the disease, an incidence of one in a million. These people inherited faulty DNA from both their parents; their form of the disease is called "homozygous." But there were many more people who inherited just one abnormal gene, either from their father or mother. Millions have this partial but still potentially deadly disease. These people, the "heterozygotes," do have LDL receptors but only one half of the normal number. But just like the patients with the severe form of the disease, the risk of atherosclerosis in the heterozygotes is very high. The prevalence of this genetic disorder in people with ischemic heart disease is ten-fold higher than in the general population.

Brown and Goldstein's work led to a much more profound understanding that elevated cholesterol levels were due to a combination of diet and genetics, and the details of the metabolism of lipoproteins. Their work offered the possibility that new medications could attack some of the key components of the system, lowering lipid levels and reducing the risk of heart attacks.

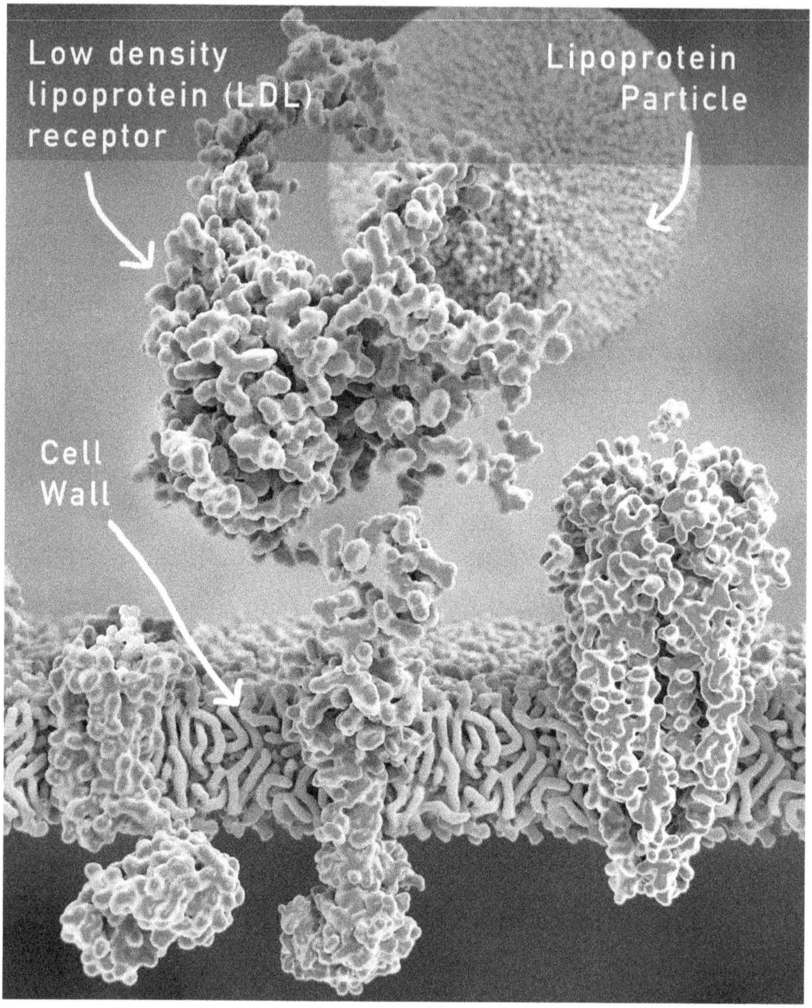

![LDL receptor figure with labels: Low density lipoprotein (LDL) receptor, Lipoprotein Particle, Cell Wall]

Figure 20. The LDL receptor on the cell wall surface, about to grab hold of a lipoprotein molecule. (Copyright Shutterstock)

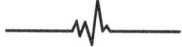

TWENTY YEAR FOLLOW-UP

... Fortunately, my patient Joan made it to her son's wedding, but when one of her relatives asked her to dance a Polka, she had to turn her down; she thought: *She's going to kill me.* Knowing she was "too young to sit in a corner" her whole life, Joan resigned herself to the upcoming hospitalization.

The catheterization found what Joan's symptoms and her stress test predicted; all three major coronary arteries were severely diseased, and triple CABG surgery was needed. I asked my heart surgeon colleague Dr. Furukawa to perform the operation.

While Joan now felt fine—her post-op course was completely benign, and about two months later, out to dinner with Joe, the couple went dancing—I knew the battle was far from over. The task ahead was to stop Joan's coronary arteries from slowly becoming obstructed again. I would need to make use of some miraculous chemical discoveries to achieve that goal. Considering Joan's high cholesterol and her family history, I suspected that she did have the heterozygous form of Familial Hyperlipidemia. I placed her on aspirin to slow down her platelets from clumping together inside of the heart bypasses and medication to reduce her blood cholesterol. For the last twenty years, Joan has led a normal life and never had angina pain again.

Brown and Goldstein had opened the scientific door to help me accomplish my job for Joan.

EPILOGUE: ALWAYS A PHYSICIAN AT HEART

In September 2019, it was a great honor for me to get the chance to speak to Michael Brown. Before we got to his medical and scientific accomplishments, we reminisced about growing up in the same suburb of Philadelphia and attending the same high school—his photograph hangs in the display case of my high school's "Hall of Fame" —as well as the same college and medical school.

Then Dr. Brown told me that he was thrilled by both his career and the fact that after fifty years, he and Dr. Goldstein still maintain an active research lab at the University of Texas Southwestern, continuing their quests to further uncover the secrets of lipid metabolism, and work with and train so many new researchers over the years. He also greatly respects those who practice medicine and cardiology.[107]

It was striking to me that such an accomplished researcher could see how his work on skin cells had helped patients so directly. Dr. Brown told me that his parents, raised in New York City, always wanted him to be a "rich Park Avenue doctor." Although this would have been a wonderful job, the work of Brown and Goldstein helped save many more lives than any clinician in practice could over an entire career.

He also relayed a story that few know. He and Dr. Goldstein had always assumed that the two children they cared for at the NIH, who sparked their interest in cholesterol, had died at a young age from their severe atherosclerosis. But in 2015, Dr. Brown gave a lecture to an endocrinology group and mentioned the two ill children. After his talk, a doctor approached him and told him that the young girl had been his patient for many years and was fifty-seven years old. The woman received treatments called plasmapheresis to clear her blood of cholesterol, had coronary artery bypass surgery at age nineteen, and for many years took medication orally to lower her cholesterol. Her brother unfortunately died at age fourteen just before he also was scheduled to have bypass surgery. Dr. Brown was very gratified that his work had helped at least one of the children to live a pretty good life. He is a physician-scientist at heart.

In the last ten years, Brown and Goldstein's elucidation of the structure and function of the LDL receptor has led to the development of an astounding group of medications that lower cholesterol by allowing the LDL receptor to work more efficiently and live a longer life. These drugs may revolutionize the treatment and prevention of atherosclerosis.

---

107 Dr. Brown's comments resonated with me. I reminded him that I met him once before. He and I were buying sweatshirts in the University of Pennsylvania bookstore after I attended a talk he gave. Gingerly, I walked up to him and introduced myself. After telling him how much I admired his work, he felt obligated to ask me what I did. I said, "I'm a cardiologist seeing patients." He replied, "Oh, you're one of those guys on the frontlines." I have always regarded that as high praise from one of my heroes, a Nobel Prize winner.

By the late 1970s, the discovery of the LDL receptor accelerated the research intensity to find medication that could lower cholesterol levels and the risk of heart attacks. But there was another piece to the puzzle to try to solve: how to identify those with atherosclerosis more accurately than by using EKG stress tests and the judgment of doctors. Was prevention on the horizon?

CHAPTER 18

STOPPING TIME: THE RADIOACTIVE HEART IMAGES

A fractured bone, a twisted spine, these are perfect candidates for the glowing pictures, but my damage is about muscles and blood flow. Thus I am free to continue my work in the shadows.

Yet what if they find a way of easily peering inside; what would stop them from finding the evidence of my approach?

UNCOVERING THE SILENT KILLER

Mr. E's back was really bothering him. He just couldn't walk more than a few feet without the pain shooting down his legs. He had tried medication, physical therapy, and even some injections of steroids and anesthetic medication into his spine, but without any real benefit. He was in his early sixties and just couldn't see himself leading the rest of life so disabled.

The next step was to see an orthopedic surgeon to operate on his lumbar spine to remove the bone spurs that were putting constant pressure on the nerves leaving his spinal cord and traveling to his legs, severe "sciatica." The orthopedic surgeon agreed that surgery would probably help him, but he told Mr. E that he needed to see a cardiologist first to determine if he was a "safe candidate" for surgery. "What's not 'safe' about me? You're worrying me," was Mr. E's response. The surgeon noted that Mr. E had high blood pressure and diabetes and at his age needed to be sure his heart was healthy enough to withstand the stress of the anesthesia and surgery.

Reluctantly, Mr. E saw a cardiologist who asked the usual questions about chest pain and shortness of breath, and while Mr. E pointed out that his back hurt so much he wasn't able to exercise, he had no cardiac or respiratory problems that he knew about. Then Mr. E laid back on the exam table for his electrocardiogram. The technician ran the test and left the room to hand the tracing to the cardiologist, who returned in a few minutes with a strange look on his face. He said in a monotone, "I'm not sure, but Mr. E, you may have had a silent heart attack."

Mr. E appeared as if he didn't believe the doctor. "How in the world could that happen?" He then pulled out a little notebook and started writing.

"Well, sometimes the heart arteries can get blocked up very slowly over years and slow down the blood supply gradually, until the heart muscle dies, and I can see that on your electrocardiogram."

"So now what? Can I have my back surgery?" he asked, his pen poised again.

"Not yet. Sometimes the EKG can be misleading. We need to do a stress test to confirm that the changes I see are in fact due to a heart attack."

Mr. E began to perspire and seemed doubtful. "Doc, I'm not sure I can do any kind of exercise test."

But the cardiologist still needed to uncover the truth about Mr. E's heart . . .

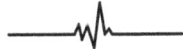

MOMENTS IN TIME: IMAGES OF THE HEART
NEW HAVEN, CONNECTICUT—SUMMER 1979

By the late 1970s, the diagnosis of slowly developing atherosclerosis was still not accurate in many patients, often requiring a cardiac catheterization to determine if their chest pain was due to coronary artery disease or not. Stress tests had helped to be sure, but they had two major drawbacks: the results were often inconclusive, and they could not be used in many patients who had medical or orthopedic problems that didn't allow them to walk safely on a treadmill. A new generation of cardiologists had better ideas.

I was planning to be a member of that modern cadre, and despite my first night on call as a cardiology trainee with numerous phone calls and a two a.m. trip to the ER, I was as determined as ever. As I drove into the Yale-New Haven Hospital parking lot, I noticed through my grogginess a strange color in front of me—the pale purple paint job of a hatchback car, a Gremlin, vintage late 1970s. Not a common sight. But something else was weird; the license plate read "LVEF." After a few seconds, it came to me—I was driving behind my boss's car, Barry Zaret MD. Dr. Zaret had already achieved international recognition for his work as a young star of a new breed of cardiologists: an imager, a picture-taker.

But one with a twist. Zaret was not one whose images were obtained in the cardiac cath lab by injecting dye into the coronary arteries; rather he wanted to capture images in time without "invading" the arteries of the leg and the heart itself. His obsession was not just the blood flow to the heart muscle to look for the work of the Widowmaker, but the blood flow out of it. Dr. Zaret was driven to measure the function of the heart, and in particular, the function of left ventricle, the "business end" of the heart that pumps the blood out to the rest of the body. If successful, these images would dramatically change the ability of all cardiologists worldwide to diagnose the presence and extent of coronary artery disease, methods far more accurate than the EKG and stress tests that had been used since the 1940s.

The "LVEF" on Dr. Zaret's license plate stood for the left ventricular ejection fraction, the percentage of blood pumped with each heartbeat, a percentage keenly observed by every cardiologist. The heart fills up prior to each beat but does not empty completely; only about half of the blood gets pushed through the aorta into the arteries. That's the ejection fraction; normal is fifty to sixty percent, and in people who have had major heart attacks and scar tissue instead of normal muscle in the front wall of the left ventricle, that number is much lower, often fifteen to thirty-five percent. The LVEF has a direct bearing on their prognosis. That's not too surprising—the greater the damage, the worse the prognosis.

Dr. Zaret was leading the charge to determine this number using radioisotope imaging, a way to determine this crucial parameter without the need for a cardiac catheterization. He wanted to see what the Widowmaker was up to before it was too late. He was going to teach many others and me how to do that. He was depending on decades of research as the foundation of his work.

CAN YOU STOP TIME? IMAGES

The desire to create images is an innate human desire; painting and sculpture are the hallmarks of any culture, going back thousands of years. But all art is only a vision of reality, not the reality itself. Yet over a hundred years ago, the ability to create real images of the human body at a particular moment in time would change the world. For this reason, every history of medicine must tell the story of Wilhelm Roentgen PhD (1845-1923).

Roentgen was a German physicist, and in November 1895, he discovered that a device called a Crookes tube generated invisible energy that created dark spots on a photographic plate; he called them "x-rays." Within weeks, Roentgen also proved that the x-rays created an exact image of the bones of his hand and his wife when he exposed them to the mysterious energy that hurdled unseen through the air. Roentgen would win the first Nobel Prize in Physics in 1901, and the use of x-rays, then called "Roentgenography," would rapidly revolutionize the care of patients. Doctors could determine the extent of fractures in trauma patients, decide if surgery was needed, and then see the results of their work. Chronic diseases affecting the lungs and the bones, like tuberculosis and arthritis, could be accurately diagnosed.

The budding specialty of cardiology also looked to these images as tools into the structure and function of the heart and blood vessels. Now doctors could determine the size of the heart by looking at images of the chest and see the effects of all forms of heart disease; an "enlarged heart" became an important determinant of prognosis. A clinician could see if fluid had built up in the lungs as an explanation for a patient's shortness of breath. The x-ray of the chest could often distinguish if a person's breathing difficulty was from a heart disease or a lung disorder. Often that heart disease was the heart attack. X-rays were only a start at looking at the heart and the effects of coronary artery disease.

But x-ray pictures of the heart too often only showed the end of a process—the heart enlargement that occurred only after a massive myocardial infarction. By that time, the patient's fate was usually sealed. Heart attack victims with an enlarged heart developed shortness of breath and fluid in the lungs, congestive heart failure, and there was little doctors of the early twentieth century could do. They were still too often only able to predict the future for their patients, and it was usually a grim one.

The pioneer cardiologists dreamed of learning much more about the blood supply of the heart; if they could somehow create accurate images of the flow out of the heart itself and into the coronary arteries and the heart muscle before a heart attack happened, then perhaps treatment would follow. They might be able to tell that atherosclerosis was slowly but surely blocking up the tiny coronary arteries of the heart. At that time, cardiac catheterization and coronary angiograms were decades away. The top echelon of pure scientists might offer a clue to creating better images of the human heart and prevent heart attacks—the physicists like Roentgen.

Antoine Henri Becquerel PhD (1852-1908) was the perfect physicist for his time. Born in Paris, he was the fourth generation of his family to become physicists. By 1895, he was Chairman of the Physics Department at École Polytechnique in Paris. When he discovered that there were elements of nature that emitted invisible particles that flew through the air just like x-rays, there was a possibility that these elements, referred to as being radioactive, might be of use in medicine sometime in the distant future. But how could these fascinating natural elements ever be used to track down the Widowmaker?

RADIOACTIVE HEARTS

In the first half of the twentieth century, two medical adventurers, Hermann Blumgart MD (1895-1977) and Myron Prinzmetal MD (1908-1987), undertook some unique experiments. Just by trying a fanciful idea, they discovered that some radioactive elements could stick to red blood cells, and they used these elements to measure the flow of blood through the lungs and the circulation. Their work was regarded as a curiosity. Although using the radioisotopes to "label" certain organs, like the bone and the thyroid gland, were attempted, there was no meaningful advance in medicine in using radioactive element isotopes (radioisotopes),[108] until an electrical engineer from Denver, Colorado, began working on imaging scanners in the Donner Laboratory at the Lawrence Research Institute in Berkeley, California.

---

108 Radioisotopes are forms of an element with a different number of protons and electrons than the basic element but are radioactive; they emit particles. For example, the element carbon usually has twelve protons and neutrons, but there is a rare form that has fourteen protons and twelve neutrons and is radioactive. Carbon 14 is used to "date" ancient artifacts and documents.

Hal Oscar Anger (1920-2005) loved science all of his life. Anger thought he could build a better machine than the primitive radioisotope scanner his lab was working on, and by 1952, he was ready. He introduced imaging using the first "gamma" camera, one using photomultiplier tubes that could record accurately both the intensity and position of radioactive gamma electromagnetic energy (similar to x-rays) released by the decay of the nuclei of specific radioisotopes.

Anger learned how to target particular areas of the body such as the thyroid gland, the bones, and the liver, but the moving beating heart was proving challenging to image, and researchers would again need to turn to physics for the answer. By the 1950s, the "atom-busters" in Berkeley were busy using their cyclotrons[109] to bash electrons and other subatomic particles into many normal elements to see what would happen. In one of their experiments, they were able to convert the element molybdenum into a radioactive form called technetium 99m, the m indicating the atomic weight of the new element. Other radioactive elements were also created, and these survivors of the cyclotron opened the door to radioactive imaging of the heart.

Alexander Gottschalk MD (1932-2010) was a radiologist who went to California in 1962 to work with Hal Anger and used technetium 99m to create improved images of many organs, but that's not all. He also discovered that the technetium would stick to so many red blood cells that the Anger camera could detect and produce images of the "blood pool," an outline of the volume of blood passing from the veins into the heart and back out again, black and white anatomy imaging in a living person.

Gottschalk's early heart images didn't attract much attention for almost a decade, likely because the computer technology was so primitive that there was no way to use Gottschalk's images to accurately assess the heart's blood flow or overall function. Better ideas about how

---

[109] A cyclotron is a large machine used by physicists to accelerate subatomic particles in a circular path using powerful magnets. It was invented in the 1930s by Ernest Lawrence PhD and M. Stanley Livingston PhD.

to image the heart and discover the work of the Widowmaker needed to come from another generation of heart specialists.

STALKING THE WIDOWMAKER

Barry Zaret MD was born in Far Rockaway, New York, in 1941, the son of a kosher butcher who fled pogroms[110] to come to America. His interest in chemistry led him to medicine after college. He received his MD from New York University, found his interest in cardiology, and began specialty training at Johns Hopkins University in Baltimore. There he would foster a connection that would greatly advance the progress of cardiology.

One of Zaret's close friends, William Strauss MD, had gone to Hopkins a year before him. Under the tutelage of Bertram Pitt MD of the Hopkins faculty, the two young trainees began projects in cardiac imaging[111]; this work was an attempt at a "quantum leap" in cardiac diagnosis and treatment decisions. Determined to find a way to understand and deal with the work of the Widowmaker, they planned a two-pronged attack: to image the heart muscle blood supply and then to measure accurately the "holy grail" of the LVEF, the ejection fraction number that had such important implications of treatment and prognosis of coronary artery disease.

The Hopkins team had a big idea; if they could inject the radioactive material directly into the coronary arteries of dogs, the images would reveal much more detail about the flow of blood in and out of the myocardium. If their idea worked, the radioisotope would penetrate all of the small arteries and then the veins of the heart and create a much broader picture of the heart's blood supply than had

---

110 Pogroms were organized massacres, usually of Russian and Eastern Europeans Jews in the nineteenth century, a major factor leading to mass emigration of Jews to the United States.
111 Zaret, Strauss, and Pitt were not the first to use radioactivity to image the heart muscle itself. In the late 1960s, PJ Cannon injected a radioactive element called xenon into the heart muscle of dogs and produced images of the "washout" of the radioactive blood as it circulated through the heart's arteries and veins, even in a heart that was still beating.

ever been done. Working late into the night after their clinical duties during the day, Zaret and Strauss became expert catheter doctors for dog hearts and found that the radioactive tracer did yield images that could be interpreted much more clearly. The pictures were "grainy" for sure, but the locations of where specifically the heart's blood was going within the heart muscle was specific. Their Anger gamma camera was working well.

For the first time, accurate images depicting the flow of blood through all of the areas of the heart muscle were created. The "labeling" of red blood cells by a radioactive element and injecting them into the heart's largest arteries was followed by capturing the imprint of the invisible radiation particles as they left the heart blood vessels. They flew through the air at the speed of light and crashed into a thin sheet of crystal sodium iodide in the Anger camera. The result was an electric current that was converted into an image on a photographic paper. Physics of the early twentieth century had led to heart images that could help people.

Measuring the LVEF involved some mathematics. The idea was pretty straightforward but getting it done, not so much. For example, if a balloon is filled with water and some of it is pushed out, how much is left? If 100 cc of fluid were put in first and 50 cc are left after a push, then fifty percent of the water was ejected; then the "ejection fraction" of that balloon would be fifty percent. Though the left ventricle isn't really shaped like a balloon (it's more like a football), the idea of the LVEF is the same as the balloon example. But how can you measure that in a human body?

For sure, the radioactive labeled red blood cells swirling around in the left ventricle were the answer, but then came the key assumption: the number of times the gamma rays coming from the radioactive cells struck the Anger camera should be related to how much blood was present. More "counts" of radioactivity meant more blood; less counts, less blood. When the ventricle beat a few hundred times, if a computer could keep track of all of the counts, then there would be enough data to estimate how much blood was in the left ventricle.

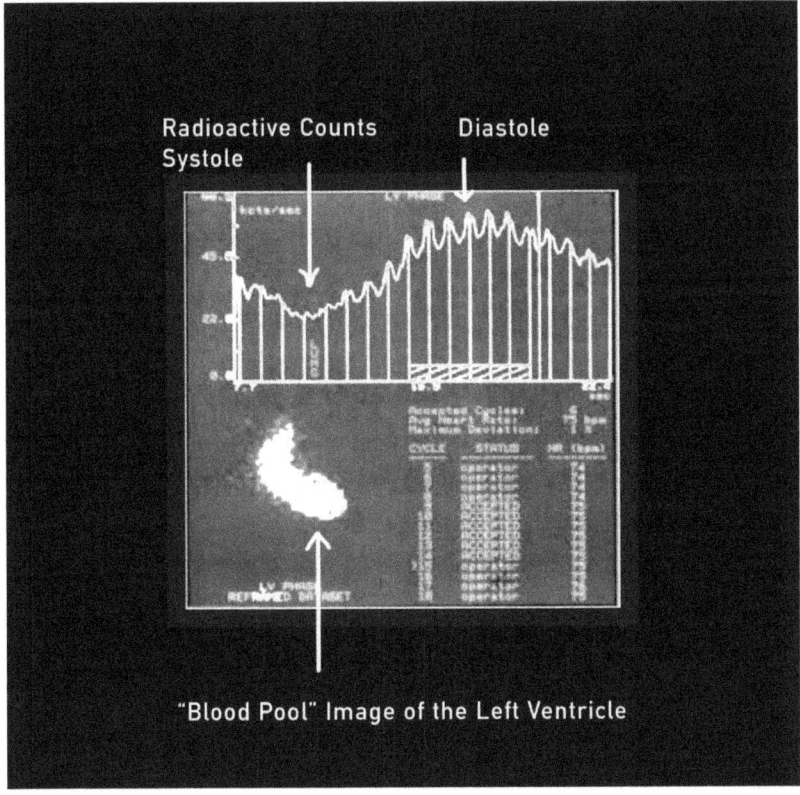

Figure 21. Example of "first pass" technology showing the left ventricle during systole and diastole, numbers allowing calculation of the Ejection Fraction (percent of blood pumped with each heartbeat; normal fifty-five to sixty percent). (Courtesy of J of Nucl Med Nicholas K, et al., 1994, Hindawi Publishing.)

When they compared the results to the ejection fraction the team had gotten from doing traditional measurements using contrast dye injected in the left ventricle in the cath lab, the correlation was remarkable; but the final goal was the most ambitious. Could Zaret and his colleagues image "ischemia," lack of blood supply from atherosclerosis? Considering that a heart muscle with normal blood vessels would emit gamma rays, if the blood supply to one area was blocked up, no gamma rays would emanate from that area of the heart muscle. Could the gamma camera images show a "cold" area of no blood and "hot" areas with normal blood supply? In effect, could the images stop time and show if an area of heart muscle had been damaged by a heart attack or was in danger of damage from cholesterol buildup?

Combined with a measurement of LVEF, these pictures depicting normal radioactivity versus no or less radioactivity would open up a brand-new way to diagnose and then decide how to treat coronary artery disease, using a technique that was completely different, safer, and much easier to perform than a cardiac catheterization. If these tests were really as good as the young Hopkins upstarts thought, then thousands, maybe millions of people could be studied to identify atherosclerosis lurking in their heart's arteries before they succumbed to a heart attack. This was an audacious idea, relying on data to make recommendations to patients about medication and heart surgery, without the need for a cardiac catheterization involving the puncture of a large artery and the injection of contrast dye.

A revolution in cardiology was about to begin, a dramatic change in the ability to diagnose the presence and severity of the work of the Widowmaker, and it started with a study of only twenty patients. Using technetium 99m labeled albumen injected into a vein, Zaret and his colleagues were able to show that nine patients without significant coronary artery disease, confirmed by cardiac catheterization, had normal ejection fractions and their images were virtually identical to the left ventricular pictures captured by injection of contrast dye into the heart chamber. However, the remaining eleven patients in the study all had significant coronary artery disease by cardiac catheterization. Every one of their nuclear images of the blood pool in the left ventricle were abnormal, giving visual evidence of a previous myocardial infarction or severe lack of blood supply (ischemia) that slowed down the motion of a portion of the heart muscle wall when it tried to contract during systole.

Even Dr. Zaret was amazed that the results were so good.[112] Here was a test that could dramatically improve the accuracy of the prognosis of patients compared to the electrocardiogram, chest x-ray, and stress test. It involved sophisticated technology but was safe for patients and agreed with the "gold standard" of diagnosis, the cardiac catheterization. Clearly the path was open for much larger studies.

But the events of the outside world created obstacles for Zaret and Strauss, just as they had affected Werner Forssmann and John Gibbon: a war, this time the United States' involvement in Vietnam in the 1960s and 1970s. Both Zaret and Strauss joined the military and worked at Travis Air Force Base in California. They were lucky to have a boss who encouraged them to continue their nuclear cardiology studies there, and military retirees on the base, many with heart disease, received their care. However, the work that emerged from Travis took a different tack from the previous studies. Zaret and Strauss were convinced that *exercising patients* with significant coronary artery blockages would induce the ischemia caused by the extra workload on the heart and that their nuclear technique could detect the lack of blood flow, yielding information about the area of the heart that was in trouble from atherosclerosis.

Using radioactive potassium, the two "nuclear cardiologists" collected forty-three patients and performed seventy-eight studies, forty-seven at rest and thirty-one with exercise. The radioactive potassium was injected just at the end of the exercise session and the patients imaged within five minutes. The group included twelve normals, and in those patients, the radioactive tracer spread throughout the myocardium in a smooth uniform pattern, easily seen on the images. But in thirteen of the fifteen with a history of previous heart attack, and in sixteen of nineteen of those with a history of angina pectoris, "cold" spots were seen on the image; the radioactive

---

112 The findings were so significant that they caught the attention of the very conservative and often just suspicious editors of the world's most prestigious medical publication, the *New England Journal of Medicine*.

potassium carried in the blood just could not enter that area of muscle of the left ventricle because its path was blocked by atherosclerosis.

Nuclear techniques had now proven that they could be used to detect essential pieces of information about coronary atherosclerosis and answer plaguing questions. Was the cholesterol buildup severe enough to impair blood flow so that permanent heart damage was present? Was the blockage severe enough to create abnormal function and motion of a part of the wall of the left ventricle with exercise, where it had been normal at rest? Was the overall function of the left ventricle, the ejection fraction, normal or not? Diagnosis had reached a new plateau.

After leaving the Air Force, Zaret joined the faculty at Yale University, and over the next three decades, important research studies in nuclear cardiology emerged from Yale on a regular basis.[113] Nuclear cardiac images were used in studies in patients with "false positive" stress tests, showing that the blood supply to the heart in those patients was normal. The images were used to study the heart's blood flow in those who had undergone coronary artery bypass surgery to assess the long-term success of the bypass grafts. Zaret and others also did very important work about the effect of chemotherapy drugs on the heart (especially in patients with breast cancer) and the effect of heart valve disorders on the ejection fraction with important implications for the timing of heart valve replacement surgery.

In 1975, Zaret chaired the first session on nuclear cardiology at a major cardiology meeting and became editor of the first journal on the use of nuclear imaging of the heart. A radical change in the accuracy of diagnosis was achieved, and I was fortunate to be in the right place at the right time to be on the cusp of that emerging knowledge. It is difficult now to imagine practicing cardiology without those tools and its modern variants. Barry Zaret's license plate matched the man's goals well.

---

113 Dr. Zaret became the Chief of Cardiology at Yale after only five years on the faculty, a remarkable achievement in academic medicine. He maintained that position for the next twenty-six years.

The world of nuclear cardiology exploded exponentially in the 1970s. New radioactive elements that provided more accurate images were discovered, and new techniques to measure ejection fraction sprung from computer technology. In 1977, James Ritchie MD and his colleagues at the University of Washington reported on seventy-six patients with coronary artery disease confirmed by coronary artery imaging in the cath lab. Fifty-eight of them (seventy-six percent) had a defect, a "cold spot," an area of little or no blood flow, on the images either with exercise or before the exercise portion of the test. Sixty-nine of the seventy-six (ninety-one percent) had either an abnormal stress EKG or a thallium defect. Many other investigators were able to report similar results, using superior radioisotope techniques to sort out the difficulties in identifying the atherosclerotic lesions of the Widowmaker.

Although nuclear stress testing took off as the major diagnostic test to look for coronary artery disease, what about people who couldn't exercise because of severe shortness of breath with exertion or orthopedic problems, like Mr. E? A major advance in the portfolio of nuclear cardiology techniques was the use of medication injected intravenously that increased the size of the coronary arteries, shifting more blood flow through arteries free of atherosclerosis and starving cholesterol-blocked ones of blood. This difference could be easily seen after then injecting radioactive thallium or technetium, and accurate nuclear stress tests could be performed in patients who could not exercise.

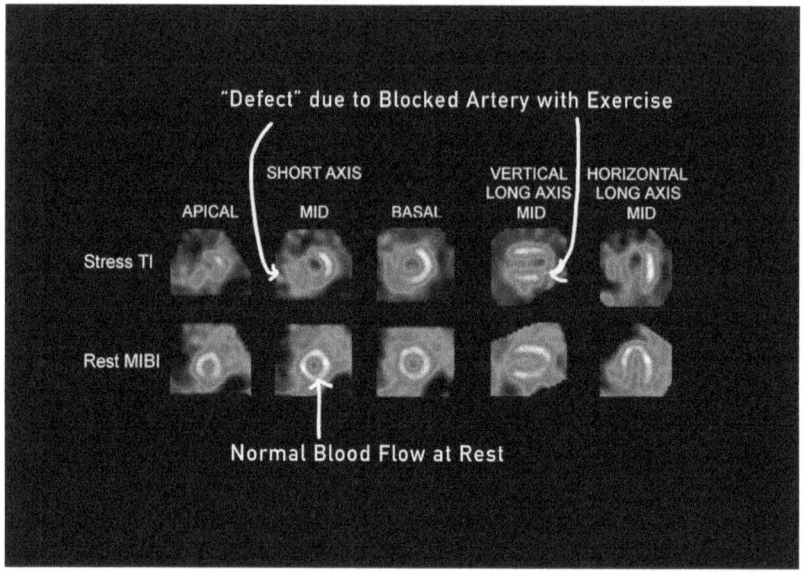

Figure 22. Example of normal myocardial blood flow at rest, and lack of blood supply with exercise ("Stress TL" images) using radioactive tracer imaging. (Courtesy of Alan Maurer MD)

Though the future would bring about debate on their efficacy,[114] these tests confirmed important scientific assumptions about the effect of atherosclerosis of the coronary arteries on the heart—that the ejection fraction is a good measure of how much damage has been caused by a heart attack and its effect on long-term prognosis; that the normal response to exercise is for the ejection fraction to increase; and that blockage of certain arteries caused the motion of that portion of the heart muscle dependent on the flow of blood through that artery to falter and then improve with rest, showing that those heart cells were not permanently damaged.

---

114 Controversy has existed for many years now, asking the question of how many of these tests are really medically necessary. There has been significant pushback from health insurance companies and Medicare in the United States over this issue, not only because of the inevitable "false positive" tests but also the cost. For these reasons, stress testing of any kind, with or without nuclear imaging, is not recommended in people without possible cardiac symptoms and a normal electrocardiogram.

Improvement on these tests,[115] as well as better treatment and prevention, were on the horizon. Using radioactivity, sophisticated cameras, and computers, the medical scientists had indeed "stopped time." Not everyone needed a cardiac catheterization to see if they have coronary artery atherosclerosis. An army of young cardiologists, trained by Dr. Zaret and others, had a new tool to use in their efforts to make a diagnosis and then a prognosis. But treatment and prevention had much further to go in the 1970s and early 1980s. More revolutions were needed.

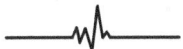

CONFIRMATION OF A SUSPICION—THEN THE PLAN

. . . Mr. E's cardiologist had an answer for his concerns about the prospect of having to do an exercise stress test. "I understand how you feel. The good news is we have a stress test we can do where you don't need to exercise. It's called a 'chemical' or 'pharmacologic' stress test, and it's used commonly in this kind of situation where someone can't exercise on a treadmill. First, we put an intravenous line in your arm and then inject a very tiny amount of a radioactive element that gets into the heart muscle. Then we give you a medicine by vein that makes the heart's arteries get bigger, just like what would happen during exercise. If the blood flow to the heart muscle is normal, the picture of the radioactivity we see looks like a doughnut. If there is a blocked artery, the picture looks like someone took a bite out of the doughnut."

Realizing he wasn't going to have his back surgery unless he had the cardiologist's blessing, Mr. E agreed to the test for the next week.

---

115 Over the forty years since these breakthrough techniques of cardiac imaging were developed, other advances in nuclear cardiac imaging have occurred using computed tomography (CT scans), in which multiple "slices" of images are obtained, yielding much more accurate results. The advances in stress testing using radioisotopes have pushed the accuracy of stress testing to eighty to eighty-five percent when compared to cardiac cath as the "gold standard." This is still not one hundred percent but is far better than using the EKG and stress testing alone. Millions of nuclear cardiology tests are performed worldwide.

His test's ability to image his heart's blood supply and the function of his left ventricle, that most important chamber of the heart, was the result of over one hundred years of research into how to "stop time" and create powerful information about the state of the heart that guided his treatment.

On the day of the test, an intravenous line was inserted in Mr. E's arm and a small amount of the radioactive element injected. He was lying under a big round camera, and the technologist told him that the radioactivity was going to create a picture of the blood supply to his heart. That was part one of the test. Mr. E sure didn't like the idea of being "radioactive" for a while but was assured that it would last for only a few hours and that he wouldn't "glow in the dark."

In about twenty minutes, he was ready for part two. The technician told him that he was going to receive a medicine that was going to "open up" all of the blood vessels to his heart, that he would get another small shot of the radioactive liquid, and then another set of pictures of his heart would be made. The medicine made him feel "weird" and gave him a headache, but it passed in just a few minutes, and then the technician said, "You're done. The doctor will look at the pictures and call you with the results." Having had no problems with the test, Mr. E didn't lose any sleep that night. He recounted his day in his notebook.

Mr. E was surprised that the call from the cardiologist came so early in the morning. "Mr. E, there's a real problem here. The blood supply to the front wall and sidewall of your heart is likely pretty badly blocked up, and the front wall of the heart doesn't move normally. The EKG was right."

"Can we go over that again? I am going to write it down."

"Sure, take your time. But there's no doubt there's something wrong with your coronary arteries; they're full of cholesterol blockages. You need another test now."

Not surprisingly, the catheterization showed that Mr. E did have two very severe blockages, one a complete blockage in the left anterior descending coronary artery, the heart's largest and most important artery. He needed a bypass operation. The surgery went smoothly, and Mr. E went home about a week after.

Mr. E's life-threatening heart problem, his "silent heart attack," was discovered by using a radioactive element emitting invisible particles called gamma rays. The big round machine lying over Mr. E's chest captured an image of the heart and its blood supply, stopping time, creating a picture of the reality of his heart's circulation on that day. He had never had angina.

Mr. E became my patient some years later, to follow up on the success of his surgery. When he sees me, Mr. E still writes everything down in his spiral notebook, but he never did have that back operation. The technology that saved his life began in the early 1970s, and the surgery that restored his heart supply began a few years earlier. Yet another revolution in the treatment of atherosclerosis was on the horizon in the late 1970s.

CHAPTER 19

THE GERMAN ICARUS: ANDREAS GRÜNTZIG AND THE ANGIOPLASTY REVOLUTION

Now they can hear and see my path and I feel them,
like never before, nipping at my heels. Still their only cure
for the damage I am threatening is to sharpen their knives
before I arrive and cut my victims open.

Thus it will stay, if no one dares to dream higher.

THWARTING THE WIDOWMAKER—WINTER 2018

There was no warning. The chest pressure started abruptly as he was sitting at his computer about ten a.m. My physician friend shook off his disbelief and knew exactly what was happening. He and his wife had just gotten off an airplane a few hours earlier, returning from a delightful trip to a beach town in Mexico, away from the winter gloom of Philadelphia. The chest pain worsened. In spite of being active, in good health in his sixties, able to practice medicine, exercise, and travel when and where he wanted to, Harold was having a heart attack.

He told his wife and instructed her to drive him to the hospital, a trip of about ten minutes. "No," she said emphatically, "I'm calling 911."

When the EMTs arrived, Harold's instincts as a doctor kicked in, and he told them, "You need to activate the cath lab." Harold knew he was having a heart attack and that he needed an urgent angiogram.

After arriving in the emergency room, the electrocardiogram confirmed Harold and the ER doctor's suspicion; he was indeed having a major heart attack, with the EKG changes strongly suggesting there was a blood clot in the left anterior descending coronary artery, a clot that had likely formed only in the last few hours just before he began to have chest pain. A classic "Widowmaker" heart attack was evolving minute by minute, heart muscle cells starving for blood and oxygen, about to die if quick action was not taken . . .

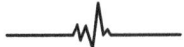

FLYING HIGH

We know the Greek legend of Daedalus and Icarus and how it ends: a father built wings for his son to fly like the birds, but his work ended in disaster for his son, who refused to heed his father's warnings about flying too high. It is a tale of both the glory and hubris of humans that has resonated through the ages. Andreas Grüntzig MD's (1939-1985) journey to become an innovator in the arena of heart disease is a testimony to his determination, his brilliance, and the openness of free societies to those with new ideas. The heights he reached were limited, however, by his ego and the resulting jealousy of others. For this modern Icarus, his path in life started in the desperation of a world war.

Andreas and his brother Johannes Grüntzig were born in Dresden, Germany, in 1939, just months before the start of World War II. After much turmoil during which their father, a Nazi soldier, disappeared, at the end of the war their mother Charlotta realized that her sons had no future in the "communist block" of the Cold War. It is difficult to imagine the emotional turmoil of teenagers thinking about leaving their home and widowed mother behind, but Andreas and Johannes knew it was the right thing to do, and they escaped to West Germany. Andreas knew he was a good student, studied hard, and in 1958 gained acceptance at medical school in Heidelberg, West Germany, graduating in 1964. There he explored internal medicine, vascular surgery, and epidemiology, searching for a passion.

A CAPTIVATING IDEA

In 1969, Grüntzig happened to attend a lecture on "dottering." Charles Dotter MD (1920-1985), a radiologist from Oregon, and previously unknown to Grüntzig, was using catheters to unblock leg arteries without surgery. Physicians had recognized the symptoms of atherosclerosis of the arteries of the legs for centuries and called this disease "claudication."[116] The ambitious "interventionalist" radiologist Grüntzig was listening to, Charles Dotter, was performing previously unimagined procedures at the University of Oregon. His ambition was to conquer atherosclerosis of the legs with catheters that could do the job of "wedging, just as you would put a nail through a piece of cheese," improving the blood flow through these diseased arteries and relieving claudication. He thought this would become a far superior and safer procedure than major vascular bypass surgery, the only other treatment available at the time.

At the age of thirty-two, the free-thinking Dotter became the youngest person to become the chairman of a major academic radiology department in the United States. His colleagues called him "Crazy Charlie." One of his staff radiologists said Dotter "had thirty brilliant ideas a day. It took the rest of us to figure out which one was really worthwhile." Dotter created a new field of treatment—interventional radiology, the use of catheters and other clever tools to clear up blockages in arteries all over the body. He was convinced that "if a plumber can do it, we can do it in blood vessels." His love of

---

116 The name claudication comes from the history of the Roman Emperor Claudius (10 BCE-54 CE), who could only walk a short distance, needed to stop, and only after a few minutes of rest could return to walking. The Latin word "claudicare" means to limp.

things mechanical was exemplified by his custom trademark on his personal documents—a crossed pipe and wrench. And while Dotter was working with his catheters on animals into the early 1960s, he wanted to be doing work on humans. His frustration increased, as he continued performing angiograms on patients with atherosclerosis of the legs to provide the surgeons with a road map for their bypass operations. Dotter yearned to not just be involved with the diagnosis but the actual treatment of patients.

Dotter's opportunity to use his new invention, a combination of telescoping catheters that would fit on top of each other to allow a smooth and gradual opening up of a blocked artery, on a human patient came in January 1964. An eighty-three-year-old woman had such severe disease of the blood vessels in her legs that her toes were dying from gangrene, and her vascular surgeon told her that the only option was an amputation. Urged by the patient to find another option, the surgeon agreed to have Charles Dotter see what he could do. Dotter performed the angiogram and found a localized blockage in a major artery to the leg, a perfect target lesion for a brand-new procedure: an angioplasty. Dotter's catheters were put into the artery of the woman's leg in the groin area and then snaked down to the area of the atherosclerosis of the blood vessels around her knee. In a matter of minutes, Dotter's catheters did their job: they physically pushed the cholesterol plaque into the wall of her arteries, clearing a path for new blood flow. In a few days, the woman's foot became warm again from the return of blood flow, her gangrene healed, and she was able to walk again.

In that lecture hall in 1969, Andreas Grüntzig reveled in Charles Dotter's[117] work, seeing the potential of "dottering," and soon angioplasty became Grüntzig's passion.

---

117   Charles Dotter died in 1985 at age sixty-five, the "father of interventional radiology."

THE PURSUIT OF A LIFETIME BEGINS

In the early 1970s, Grüntzig began working at the University Hospital in Zurich on the tedious task of trying to make special catheters to use in the peripheral arteries of the legs but all the while with a much bolder idea in mind: to make catheters to perform angioplasty in the small coronary arteries of the heart. Grüntzig's new idea began to take form. The telescoping catheters would become obsolete if he could manufacture a plastic *inflatable balloon,* one that could be wrapped on the outside of a small diameter catheter and then be inflated and push aside the debris of atherosclerosis. Drs. Swan and Ganz in California had manufactured catheters with inflatable balloons to use with their special catheters they placed into the right side of the heart, so the balloon idea, while not his own, could be useful. The concept of dilating arteries with a balloon was simple; the engineering task was not. Grüntzig's balloon catheter needed to be much sturdier than the one of Swan and Ganz; it needed to not just expand inside of a blood vessel but physically push plaque into the wall of an artery. He needed help.

Gruntzig needed a dedicated and tireless team to persevere through the trial and error and found one in his wife Michaela and another assistant, Maria Schlumpf. Night after night in the Grüntzig's apartment in Zurich, on the kitchen table, the trio of novice plastic engineers tried a "rat's nest of materials" to create a stable balloon catheter. They tried old catheters, different kinds of plastic molds, and used knives, thread, and glue to try to place rubber on the tip of the catheters to form a balloon. But when inflated, the rubber balloons leaked air, and the catheters were pathetic when they were opened against some resistance; they just got bloated at the ends and didn't push back against the blockage. The team got so desperate they even tried a drill, which was obviously too traumatic to even consider using in a human artery.

The breakthrough came when Grüntzig consulted a plastics expert, a retired professor named Heinrich Hopff PhD (1896-1977).

Hopff suggested that Grüntzig try using the same plastic used in Coca-Cola bottles—polyvinyl chloride (PVC). This remarkable substance was very strong and once molded preserved its shape. Sheets of the stuff were pretty easy to slice and mold into the shape of a sausage and maintain that shape when subjected to external pressure. PVC could withstand five to eight atmospheres of pressure; a PVC balloon would work. Grüntzig was sure of it. After Grüntzig and his team figured out how to mount balloons onto the tips of their catheters, he began using his PVC balloon catheter to treat patients with claudication in 1974. His success rate rose to eighty percent, a marked improvement from the era of using the stiff telescoping Dotter catheters.

Grüntzig was on fire, and it didn't take him long to achieve his next goal of creating a catheter with two channels, one for the balloon that would be inflated using a foot pump to drive it open with compressed air, and a second corridor to inject contrast dye so he could visualize the artery accurately. In January 1975, Andreas Grüntzig used his new two-channel device to open up a blocked leg artery. He was elated but not surprised. At age thirty-seven, he was becoming world famous, and many believed that his ultimate target for angioplasty was the heart and its arteries, not just the legs. The coronary arteries were "where the money was," and the future would prove that this was true in two ways, not just one.

At the American Heart Association convention in 1976, he described his great results in 220 cases of claudication, and few missed the hint of where he was headed. The responses to his work and its potential application to other parts of the body were extreme. Richard Myler MD (1936-2013) of San Francisco saw the enormous promise in the work, and many others could see where Grüntzig was headed with angioplasty—to the arteries of the heart. However, Spencer B. King III MD, the head of the cardiac catheterization laboratory at Emory University in Atlanta, Georgia, was convinced that "This will never work." His opinion would change in a few short years.

When Grüntzig presented his data at Stanford University in California, John Simpson MD thought, *This guy's either going to revolutionize the treatment of coronary artery disease or he's going to jail.* Undaunted, Andreas Grüntzig continued his work; the arteries of the human heart were in his sights.

THE DAY OF DAYS

On September 16, 1977, Andreas Grüntzig was poised to reach for the sky and revolutionize cardiology. His partner would be Dolf Hartmann, a thirty-eight-year-old German insurance salesman with a big heart problem.

Hartmann came to Zurich to see what he could do about his debilitating angina pain. A cardiac catheterization done a few days prior showed a major plaque of atherosclerosis in the middle part of his left anterior descending coronary artery. Hartmann had not had a heart attack; there had been no damage to his heart muscle, but the constant angina indicated he was at risk for major damage from the Widowmaker in the near future. The doctors in Zurich told Mr. Hartmann that coronary artery bypass surgery was his best option, in which they would take a piece of vein from his leg and use it to bypass blood flow around the blockage. But Dolf was terrified of cardiac surgery. Was there another option? Grüntzig was very eager to provide one.

Undeterred by a challenging first attempt on another patient,[118] Grüntzig believed coronary angioplasty could work for Hartmann. He told Dolf that if successful, the experimental procedure would end his need to take fifteen nitroglycerin tablets each day to get rid of the severe chest pain. On the day of the surgery, Hartmann was strapped on a table in the catheterization laboratory, hoping for the

---

118 A few weeks prior to September 1977, Grüntzig had attempted coronary angioplasty for the first time, but the man had such severe atherosclerosis in the arteries of his legs that he couldn't even pass his balloon catheter anywhere near the heart.

best. About thirty doctors and nurses gathered to watch Grüntzig, the handsome "angiographer" in his surgical cap shaped into a beret, wearing clogs instead of traditional operating room shoes. Surgeons stood by, ready to take the patient for emergency bypass surgery, likely suspecting that when he inflated the balloon and put severe pressure on the wall of the heart artery, Grüntzig's procedure would tear a hole in it.

Hartmann was not completely sedated and could see the small catheter going inside of his own heart on the fluoroscope, as well as witness the many challenges that arose. Once again, coronary angioplasty was off to a bad start. Grüntzig's first two balloon catheters wouldn't even inflate while he was testing them before trying to insert them into Hartmann's leg artery. But trying a third time, the balloon catheter expanded and remained full of air. Grüntzig deflated the balloon and was ready to go. Then after first imaging the left anterior descending coronary artery to confirm the location of the blockage found in the earlier procedure, Grüntzig slid his invention over the guidewire, but there was another problem. The balloon catheter wasn't that flexible. It took Grüntzig about forty-five agonizing minutes to get the balloon catheter in the right spot.

The moment of truth arrived. Would the balloon inflate under the pressure of five atmospheres of compressed air and remain open as it pummeled the atherosclerotic plaque blocking blood flow into the artery wall and expand the diameter of the artery? Or would the balloon collapse under the pressure? Grüntzig was confident, and his faith was soon rewarded. There were many held breaths in the room as the compressed air opened up the hourglass-shaped balloon and it morphed into a full-blown sausage as it pushed the plaque aside. *The blockage disappeared.* A repeat injection of contrast dye showed that blood flow in the previously severely diseased coronary artery was normal!

The groundbreaking procedure could not have been more successful. The entire procedure had lasted about one hour, and

Dolf Hartmann recovered completely, having no more need for nitroglycerin tablets. He had left the hospital in a few days and began leading a normal life; his angina pain was history. Hartmann was so elated that he contacted a local newspaper to report on his doctor's epoch achievement.

Over the next few months, Grüntzig performed a string of successful angioplasties, and the buzz throughout the world of medicine was powerful. Who was this unknown guy and was his procedure really working, or were the stories just rumors? Did his angioplasty really work, restoring blood flow in the heart's most important artery without the need for a coronary artery bypass graft surgery? Grüntzig's fame swelled quickly. A Swiss magazine, *Schweizer Illustrierte*, ran a nine-page article on Hartmann's procedure entitled "Is Death from Heart Attack Vanquished? The Struggle for the Heart," featuring a scantily clad female with a heart logo on her left chest on the cover, and in the article photos of Grüntzig and Hartmann in a swimming pool together a few days after his angioplasty.

Grüntzig traveled to Miami, Florida, in November 1977 to present his cases at the world's premier cardiology meeting, the convention of the American Heart Association. All of the prominent names in the field awaited the presentation. Among those was Mason Sones, the first person to perform a coronary angiogram. The presentation room was packed, waiting for Grüntzig to speak and show his angiograms, images before and after the angioplasty. The pictures were dramatic: severe plaque beforehand then disappearing after the inflation of the balloon catheter. Medical audiences at national meetings are usually quiet and often bored, but this time the crowd broke into spontaneous applause. They knew that they were witnessing medical history. The angioplasty wasn't just a diagnostic test; this was a treatment, a way to obliterate coronary artery disease without surgery. According to Richard Myler, who became an early devotee of Grüntzig's work, Mason Sones began to cry and said, "It's a dream come true."

In August of 1978, thirty-seven cardiologists and radiologists came to watch Grüntzig do something unthinkable, demonstrate angioplasty in a real patient on television. Although over the years these types of live presentations would become common in the world of interventional cardiology, this was not true in 1978. But such was Grüntzig's confidence in both his angioplasty and his own skill. His results were usually awe-inspiring to his audience. Now the cardiology world was able to marvel at the success of his procedure firsthand and think seriously about learning how to perform angioplasty themselves.

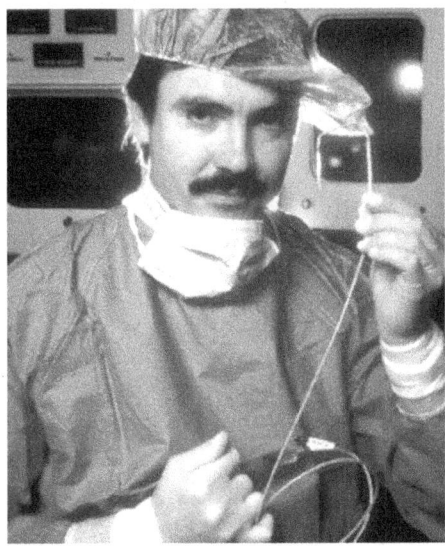

Figure 23. Andreas Grüntzig MD (1939-1985) and his balloon catheter. (Courtesy of cardiacathletes.com)

Grüntzig initially tried to do the responsible thing and gather more information, and by August 1979, he had collected data on 264 cases. There was a sixty percent technical success rate, not as grand as hoped for, and within months, thirty-three percent of the dilated arteries had become blocked with scar tissue—"restenosis." Alarmingly, ten percent of the patients were taken to immediate bypass surgery because the inflation of the balloon severely damaged the inner lining of the coronary artery, creating a "dissection," accompanied by an abrupt cutoff of blood supply to the artery. Clearly angioplasty was going to need to go through a steep learning curve, for Grüntzig as well. But the genie had already left the bottle, and angioplasty spread rapidly throughout the world.

Grüntzig himself was restless, and his fame had not given him the free rein and respect he had anticipated. He thought his status in Switzerland would now be solidified, but his very conservative superiors still did not provide the space, personnel, and technical support he needed to continue and improve the procedure, train others, and help more and more patients. It appeared that his achievements in Zurich had reached a ceiling. Looking elsewhere, he wanted to return to his native Germany as a professor, but the German medical establishment considered him a "plumber," not a real doctor. However, the United States proved much more promising. Harvard, Stanford, and the Cleveland Clinic all pursued Grüntzig, but the most interesting offer came from a charming gentleman from Atlanta, Georgia.

In January 1980, Spencer King, the cardiologist from Emory who saw Grüntzig's presentation on angioplasty of leg arteries four years earlier, met with Grüntzig. King tempted him with the promise of the financial resources of salary and staff, as well as the laboratory space that his hospital could offer, if Grüntzig joined their angioplasty group. The offer was just the acknowledgment Grüntzig needed.

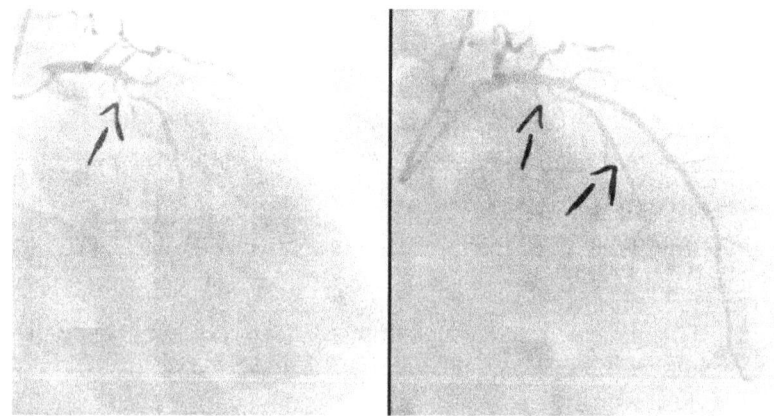

Figure 24. Total occlusion of left anterior descending coronary artery (Widowmaker lesion) and complete restoration of blood flow after angioplasty. (Copyright Shutterstock)

WELCOME TO ATLANTA

Andreas Grüntzig took Emory by storm and was a dynamic celebrity both in and out of the hospital. His flair, boundless optimism, and confidence captivated all that he interacted with, especially the women, what with his handsome looks and gallant kissing of the ladies' hands. One nurse described that time as "a medical Camelot." In addition to his charisma, he lived with an almost manic striving, like there was no upward limit to his life. Symbolically, he had already learned to fly a plane, telling his boss in Zurich, "I like flying because it confirms that I have no fear."

As flamboyant as he was in his personal life, Grüntzig was a cautious careful operator in his laboratory and when choosing his patients. He created meticulous notes and spoke at length to his patients and their families about the risks and benefits of angioplasty. The balloon could tear the artery, causing a sudden complete blockage of blood supply, often requiring emergency heart surgery. For this reason, he needed the support of the surgeons at Emory who were grudgingly willing to just "stand-by" around the cath lab if they were needed. Grüntzig only considered prospective patients who had had a large number of angina episodes each week (sometimes every day) and had *not* had a heart attack. He knew there was no data at the time to tell whether or not angioplasty was safe or effective after a myocardial infarction, when perhaps blood clots were inside of the coronary arteries, and that rapid re-supply of blood after a successful angioplasty might actually damage the heart muscle.

But the rush to learn how to do angioplasty was unstoppable. Grüntzig was invited to speak all over the world as well as inviting others to see his magical workshop in Atlanta. The number of angioplasties done worldwide quadrupled by 1982. Grüntzig and others produced more "steerable" catheters that could slip around the twists and turns of a diseased coronary artery with ease. The medical device companies competed to manufacture the best new catheters, already flush with cash from the sales of their first models.

The effect of Andreas Grüntzig's personal life, which was not just private but public in Atlanta, is difficult to judge in retrospect. He left his wife and married a much younger Emory medical student, Margaret Ann Thornton MD, in 1983 and continued to throw lavish parties, with Grüntzig often entering the party from the upper floor of his luxurious home dressed as an Arab sheik. The alcohol, dancing, and young adoring women were everywhere. There was significant concern from his Emory colleagues, but he still continued his angioplasty work aggressively, training many young trainees in his procedure. Soon others seeking to push the use of angioplasty much further would appear in the limelight.

COMPETITION: MORE PERSONALITIES ON THE WORLD STAGE

In the early 1980s, the technology of angioplasty was running far ahead of the science of atherosclerosis and coronary artery disease. With coronary artery disease still far and away the leading cause of death in the world, and the emergency rooms and doctors' offices full of patients with chest pain, the angioplasty arose as the first cure for coronary artery disease and the prevention of the heart attack. The wave of cardiologists starting to perform angioplasty was like a tsunami.

Grüntzig found himself very concerned that many people just learning angioplasty weren't being careful enough. Did they really understand who was best served by the new technique, when even he himself was uncertain? Coronary artery atherosclerosis can affect so many specific areas of the heart's blood supply. Did every spot of cholesterol plaque require an angioplasty? Millions of people live with atherosclerosis in their heart and die in their nineties of some other disease. There had to be ways to sort out which blockages were really life-threatening and causing angina and which ones could be left alone. Angioplasty was not without risks.

His concerns were well founded at a time when a new sarcastic term entered the cardiology world—the "oculo-stenotic reflex." The phrase meant that if a cardiologist saw any blockage at all in a coronary artery in the cath lab, the balloon procedure was next. He or she would see the blockage and automatically squash the plaque into the artery wall with another balloon catheter. There was just too much power and money tempting some of the new breed of cardiac specialists.[119] Angioplasty, just like coronary artery bypass surgery, was indeed the right procedure but only for the right patient and the right time.

In the midst of this frenzy, another outsized personality joined the publicity fray. Geoffrey Hartzler MD (1946-2012) became known as "the Billy the Kid of heart-probing." Born to a poor family in Goshen, Indiana, Hartzler drove a cement truck in the summers and thought he would become a chemist before he decided he wanted to go to medical school. A bright student who worked hard, Hartzler trained at the Mayo Clinic and joined the faculty in 1977, specializing in electrophysiology, new procedures probing the mystery of the cause and treatment of abnormal heart rhythms. He became very adept at passing wires and catheters into the heart. He loved doing procedures and was so aggressive he claimed, "I was known as the Invader." It's likely his patients did not know his moniker.

After learning of Grüntzig's success in 1977, the Mayo Clinic naturally wanted to pursue its own angioplasty program, but the faculty took Grüntzig's advice and proceeded with caution. They were determined to gain experience first with one hundred angioplasties of the leg arteries before tackling the coronary arteries. A few years later, Hartzler "The Invader" saw a chance to bypass Mayo's careful conservative plan of performing only leg angioplasties. A patient at Mayo with angina heard about angioplasty for the heart and asked

---

[119] In the early 1980s, my hospital hired a new cardiac surgeon to perform bypass operations. After he had been there for several months, I asked the head of our cardiac cath lab what he thought about the new surgeon. He said, "I don't really know; I don't need a surgeon any more—all of my patients have angioplasty."

Hartzler if he would try the procedure on him. Hartzler eagerly agreed, but he wanted to practice at least one coronary angioplasty first, so he experimented on a dog and placed a balloon catheter into the animal's left anterior descending coronary artery. The next day, Hartzler proclaimed to the patient, "We are ready." He did not notify the lawyers in Mayo's risk management department.

That day, Hartzler took advantage of the fact that many of his superiors in the electrophysiology department were away at a conference, and he would have unfettered access to a lab. Hartzler began the procedure, and quickly some of the other Mayo cath doctors drifted into the room. No one stopped Hartzler. Trying over and over again, he just could not get first the guidewire and then the flimsy balloon catheter to obey his command; the plaque buildup in the artery was severe and the path to get beyond it tortuous. Two hours passed and the spectators' under-their-breath comments became more cynical, and some of the faculty members even urged him to stop. But Hartzler persisted. Finally, the guidewire snaked across the atherosclerotic lesion, and Hartzler quickly loaded up the balloon catheter over the guidewire outside the patient and advanced it into his body and into the right spot inside of the coronary artery. He carefully inflated the balloon, and everyone watched on fluoroscopy as the obstruction to blood flow disappeared. No one could have been more relieved than Hartzler. Apparently, he never told the patient that when he inflated the balloon catheter in the artery of the animal he had practiced on the day before, the dog promptly died.

On that day, Hartzler did the first coronary angioplasty done at the Mayo Clinic, but his superiors were horrified by his recklessness, and his employment there was terminated within a few months. Unshakable, Hartzler joined a private practice in Kansas City, Missouri, where he was free to pursue angioplasty as much as he wanted. Within a year, his angioplasty volume rose to eight hundred procedures a year, and he was doing angioplasty on patients with very severe coronary artery disease in multiple locations throughout their coronary circulation. Grüntzig had only done patients with very localized blockages, not diffuse atherosclerosis, and had never done two angioplasties in different locations during the same procedure.

Was Hartzler another Icarus? He was doing angioplasty on patients who had been turned down by other surgeons because of the severe extent of their disease. He was convinced that "the only indication for bypass surgery is failed angioplasty." But too often Hartzler's patient did end up with failed procedures, complications requiring urgent surgery, and even death. He had "pushed the envelope" too far too often.

In 1981, Hartzler took another reckless step that would change cardiology forever, but not until over a decade later.[120] He was so confident in his skills that he was ready to try to destroy another shibboleth, the belief that angioplasty for an acutely blocked artery causing a heart attack was very risky and clearly "uncharted waters." Grüntzig and the others had only done the procedure on people with angina, not acute heart attacks. Standing at the bedside of a patient with an acute myocardial infarction from a blocked right coronary artery, Hartzler decided to act. With consummate confidence in his procedure and his own skill, he whisked the patient off to the cardiac cath lab and quickly opened up the blockage without a problem. The patient left the hospital two days later without chest pain.

But no human is immortal, and after more than a decade of spending hours in the cath lab wearing a heavy lead apron, Geoffrey Hartzler's body succumbed to the burden of gravity. His back gave out, requiring five surgeries. He was forced to give up angioplasty, admitting later that the physical burden was not the only reason he wanted to stop. He was doing so many high-risk patients that death in his lab or shortly afterwards was not uncommon. Nevertheless, Hartzler's work convinced many other cardiologists worldwide that angioplasty could be expertly done outside of the hallowed halls

---

120 Another form of treatment for acute heart attacks was just gaining worldwide traction at time: drugs that broke up blood clots in the coronary arteries, the thrombolytic "clot busters."

of academic medical centers, and the numbers of angioplasties performed worldwide just kept climbing. In spite of his at times unethical behavior, Geoffrey Hartzler had made a major contribution to the advancement of angioplasty technique.

THE END OF ATLANTA CAMELOT

Having reached great heights throughout his professional life, Grüntzig and his wife found a peaceful retreat in a place on one of the barrier islands off the coast of Georgia. He loved that home and flew his plane there on weekends. In late October of 1985, a storm named Juan plowed through the Gulf of Mexico, causing turbulent weather in the southeastern United States and into Georgia. But Grüntzig was determined to spend the weekend on the coast and, not surprisingly, thought he had the skill to avoid the bad weather. He took off with Margaret Ann and their two dogs in his Beechcraft Baron on October 27, 1985. Their plane crashed in rural Georgia.

When the wreckage was finally found a few days later, the airplane contained the bodies of Andreas and Margaret Anne, an unfinished manuscript of Grüntzig's, and some cash. Also found were the bodies of the Grüntzigs' dogs—Gin and Tonic. A modern Icarus had returned to the earth, having lit up the sky.

FAST FORWARD THIRTY-FIVE YEARS

Angioplasty changed the treatment of coronary artery disease forever, but it was not without its problems. The technology continued to improve, with increasing success rates, and the fear of abrupt closure of dilated arteries and the need for emergency coronary bypass surgery virtually disappeared. The restenosis problem, however, became serious; too often an artery that was dilated easily became clogged again, usually with scar tissue, just like any other part of the body responding to an injury.[121] This complication was much more common in women who usually have smaller arteries than men, meaning even mild scar tissue formation could block blood flow. But an even more disturbing problem continued: the tremendous financial incentive for cardiologists, hospitals, and balloon catheter manufacturers to perform more and more procedures.

Too many cardiologists did an angioplasty on mildly blocked coronary arteries, blood vessels supplying only a small amount of heart muscle. These atherosclerotic plaques almost never caused a Widowmaker heart attack. At times, patients who did not have angina or a history of a heart attack but underwent a cardiac catheterization for another reason, like a heart valve problem, were having angioplasty done. Many of the patients who did have angina never received medications like beta-blockers or long-acting nitroglycerin to see if medicine alone could have taken care of their problem.

This overutilization prompted aggressive oversight by Medicare and the major insurance companies and drove a more scientific approach to determine the correct indication for angioplasty. Large studies revealed very surprising results. Although angioplasty was very effective in reducing the frequency of chest pain, there did not appear to be any benefit, at least when looking at many patients, that the risk of heart attack and death was reduced when compared to patients treated with medication for their angina. These results stunned the interventional cardiology world.[122] The findings just didn't seem to make any sense: how could removing a major blocked coronary artery not prevent future heart attacks? As my friend Martin Leon MD, a world leader in interventional cardiology at Columbia-Presbyterian Hospital in New York City, told me years ago, "Angioplasty is the only known cure for coronary artery disease." But Dr. Leon's comment is just a bit tongue in cheek. It is true that if one particular blockage has been

---

121   Pushing plaque into the wall of a small artery is a definite injury. Sometimes angioplasty was called "barotrauma," the result of the expansion of a balloon under high pressure.
122   And still remain a controversy to this day.

dilated and remains open for over a year, it will almost never come back, but coronary artery disease can attack any portion of the coronary circulation and end up creating new blockages in many different areas. It is likely, however, that modern advances[123] have reduced the previously inexorable progression of atherosclerosis, closing the gap between the benefits of angioplasty and medication treatment of coronary artery disease. Regardless of the studies' results, there is no doubt that angioplasty has improved the lives of millions of people suffering from angina and the psychological burden of the fear of chest pain from normal activities of life.

NEW HELP FROM NEW TECHNOLOGY: BEYOND BALLOONS

The restenosis problem was huge. Patients often needed to return to the cath lab several times when one particular diseased artery clogged up again with scar tissue. A thirty-three-year-old radiologist who was in the audience at a presentation by Andreas Grüntzig in 1978, Julio Palmaz MD (1945-), was surprised at how much time Grüntzig spent discussing the pitfalls of angioplasty, especially the restenosis problem. Palmaz had an idea—a scaffold to place inside the artery to retard the scar tissue and also the "recoil" that occurred over time after an artery was stretched open.[124] He wrote up a manuscript about his idea and began to tinker; he wanted to invent a coronary artery scaffold he called a "stent." The stent would be a small tube of metal that could be placed inside the coronary artery after the cardiologist had opened up the artery with the balloon catheter.

Palmaz really had no idea about how to create his stent, but he did not let that stop him. He tried working with pins, pencils, and copper

---

123   Advances such as medications to treat angina, the ability to control blood cholesterol levels and blood pressure, and retard platelet clumps with aspirin and other medications.
124   Recoil is the tendency of the artery tissue to shrink in size after it has been stretched apart by a balloon catheter. Like scar tissue formation, it is part of the body's response to injury.

wire but just couldn't make any progress. But one day he found a piece of metal lathe inadvertently left in his garage by a workman. The metal had a series of staggered openings, and Palmaz was convinced that a "mini-version" of that type of metal would work.[125] Palmaz was on the faculty at the University of Texas Health Center San Antonio at the time and encouraged one of the cardiologists, Richard A. Schatz MD (1950-), to work with him on his stent idea, a product to be used in both the coronary arteries and the leg arteries.

By the mid-1980s, experiments in animals were going well, demonstrating that indeed the Palmaz-Schatz stent kept open balloon-dilated arteries.[126] The new stent device was granted a patent in the United States in 1985, and major clinical studies of the stents began in 1988, culminating in United States Food and Drug Administration approval of the stents for widespread use in 1994. Early on, the medical device companies were drawn to the idea of manufacturing stents by the thousands. Palmaz and Schatz sold their company to Johnson and Johnson in the early 1990s and made J & J the leader in worldwide sales for a few years. But then other companies began their own stent development programs, and the competition was fierce.[127]

It was a few years before the Palmaz-Schatz stent was used in many angioplasties. Many cardiologists felt that by using bigger balloon catheters and higher-pressure during balloon inflation they could reduce the re-stenosis problem. Another unknown was what medication to use to prevent blood clots from forming inside the stent over time. Whenever metal like a stent is put inside of an artery, blood clots will form on top of the metal. It took additional years of trial and error research to discover that it required a combination of

---

125 The stent Palmaz envisioned looks similar to a children's toy called a "Slinky."
126 The two engineers needed an investor to form a development company and convinced Phil Romano, the restaurateur who started Fuddruckers and The Macaroni Grill, to invest $250,000 with them.
127 J & J sued their competitors for patent infringement and after twelve years of litigation resolved the matter with a settlement.

two drugs, aspirin and ticlopidine,[128] to prevent blood platelets from adhering to a stent to combat both the scar tissue and blood clot problem.[129] Finally, the widespread use of many types of stents, not just the Palmaz-Shatz stent, dropped the restenosis rate significantly. But restenosis remained at a stubborn level of fifteen to twenty percent within one year of a coronary angioplasty.

Another innovation was needed, and the most promising option would be from a most unlikely branch of pharmacology—cancer chemotherapy. Scar tissue is made of cells, and cells need to reproduce themselves to form a scar. There is a very potent group of medicines that stop cells from replicating. They treat cancer, the disease of uncontrolled growth of abnormal cells. Cardiologists and engineers figured out a way to imbed just a small amount of cancer medication into a coronary artery stent, molecules that would be seep through the holes in the stent. Maybe the drugs would be powerful enough to stop the scar tissue cells from multiplying and be released in small enough amounts that they would not damage cells in the rest of the body. This audacious idea proved to work magnificently. The "drug-eluting" stents, in combination with the dual antiplatelet regimen, dropped the restenosis rate to only one to two percent after one year, a remarkable decrease from the forty to fifty percent rate seen in the 1980s.

It's crucial to understand that coronary angioplasty in its first fifteen years was used in patients with "chronic stable angina." These were people who developed chest pain with exertion or emotional upset. With rest, the pain would go away, and the result was no permanent heart muscle damage. If this happened once every few months, the use of medication like beta-blockers and the occasional use of nitroglycerin to relieve the chest pain was often sufficient. But if the chest pain got to the point where it was really interfering with someone's life, a person could check in with their favorite local interventional cardiologist and

---

128   A few years later replaced by clopidogrel, trade name Plavix.
129   This combination of two medications is called "Dual Antiplatelet Therapy," usually taken for one year after the placement of a stent in a coronary artery.

improve their life with a successful angioplasty.

But where was the application of this new technology and skill in the most important arena of work of the Widowmaker, the acute heart attack? Only Geoffrey Hartzler had the audacity to use angioplasty to abort a heart attack, and he did so successfully in 1980. One would have thought that Hartzler's bravado would open the door for many other aggressive interventional cardiologists. There was no shortage of them. But just at the time that Hartzler did his heart attack case, another dramatic improvement in heart attack care was just hitting its stride, the use of thrombolytic drugs, the "clot-busters."

By 1984, there were intravenous forms of thrombolytic drugs, medications that could be given quickly and were very effective if given in the early hours after the chest pain of a heart attack began, usually in an emergency room without the need for a heart catheterization.

But within a few years, the warts of thrombolytic therapy were pretty clear. The success rate of opening arteries hovered around eighty percent, there was risk of major bleeding, and there was a one to two percent chance of the thrombolytic drug causing a catastrophic brain hemorrhage. One to two percent doesn't seem like much unless you've given a thrombolytic drug and seen this happen to a patient, as I had the misfortune to see twice in the 1980s. Both times, my patients were alive when I met them and died a few days later, never awakening again because of the pressure on the brain caused by blood leaking inside the skull.

By the mid-1980s, a few interventional cardiologists were thinking about replicating what Hartzler had first done. Even though it was clear that major myocardial infarctions were a combination of both underlying atherosclerosis with a clot on top, why shouldn't a balloon catheter be able to break up a blood clot and push plaque into the wall of the artery at the same time? If this acute angioplasty worked, wouldn't there be another benefit? Successful use of medication to break up a blood clot in the coronary artery was great at aborting the acute problem but did nothing to the underlying plaque. With an angioplasty, that particular very troublesome area of plaque could become a problem of the past.

William O'Neill MD, an interventional cardiologist from Michigan, determined that the time had come to see if acute angioplasty was feasible and safe. He and his colleagues at Beaumont Hospital in Royal Oak, Michigan, organized a team to be available on an emergency basis to try to open up blocked coronary arteries. By 1986, they had data on fifty-six patients and submitted their results to *The New England Journal of Medicine*. In eighty-three percent of the patients, O'Neill's team was able to get the artery open without major problems. Their results in opening arteries was the same as in those patients who got standard thrombolytic medication, but most of those patients (eighty-three percent, to be exact) were left with a large amount of atherosclerosis in the coronary artery that caused the heart attack; in the angioplasty group, the chance of that result was only four percent.

A wave of teams began forming at major medical centers to perform acute angioplasty, but there still needed to be more proof. After all, O'Neill's study only included fifty-six people. O'Neill and his colleague Cindy Grines MD organized a larger study comparing acute angioplasty with thrombolytic drugs at twelve major hospitals. Their report was the lead article in *The New England Journal of Medicine* on March 11, 1993.

The O'Neill/Grines study was more expansive, including almost four hundred patients, "randomized"[130] by a computer to undergo an emergency angioplasty or to receive an infusion of tissue plasminogen activator, the standard thrombolytic drug used worldwide. Their technique had improved since 1986, and an astonishing ninety-seven percent of the time, they were able to open the artery in the angioplasty-treated group. None of the patients required emergency coronary artery bypass surgery.

---

130   Chosen by chance; in this study, one hundred percent of the patients were treated, fifty percent with angioplasty and fifty percent with the thrombolytic drug.

The mortality rate in the angioplasty group was less than half of that in the thrombolytic drug–treated group (2.6 percent vs. 6.5 percent), and the rate of another heart attack or death in the hospital was also much lower. Both groups had excellent preservation of overall heart muscle function. That dreaded complication of brain hemorrhage, however, caused four deaths in the thrombolytic drug treatment group and none in the angioplasty. This finding alone would have been enough to change the standard of medical practice.

Acute angioplasty for major heart attacks is now the standard of care. However, not every hospital, especially ones in rural areas, has the personnel and equipment to deliver that care. Often, they have arrangements for urgent transfer of patients to a regional medical center. The sooner the heart gets what it needs, the less permanent damage.[131]

The idea of Andreas Grüntzig, first developed on a kitchen table by him, his wife Michaela, and Maria Schlumpf, have indeed changed the world of medicine. Grüntzig's accomplishment was not a great breakthrough in the science of atherosclerosis and its treatment but rather a feat of engineering brilliance, a goal first brought to his mind by another innovator, Charles Dotter.

THE DRAMA—AND THEN LIFE GOES ON

... Dr. Cohen, a longtime colleague and friend, came quickly to Harold's bedside and agreed with everyone else's conclusions. The cath lab team was already getting ready, and Harold was given some nitroglycerin and morphine for the chest pain and two drugs to stop more blood platelets from sticking to the blood clot in the now-blocked coronary artery, aspirin and clopidogrel.

---

131   In 2020, the standard of care for acute ST segment elevation (specific changes on the electrocardiogram) heart attacks, those deadly events due to a thrombus inside of a coronary artery, is a "door to balloon time" of ninety minutes or less.

Dr. Cohen was joined by his colleague Dr. Klugherz, and the two doctors and the cath lab team worked quickly and expertly. A catheter was placed in the artery of the right arm and advanced into the aorta and then to the verge of the opening of the left anterior descending coronary artery. The injection of contrast dye into the artery moved swiftly but then came to an abrupt stop in the middle of the artery; there was that blood clot, right where the electrocardiogram said the doctors would find it. The first catheter was removed by exchanging it over a flexible guidewire inserted into its end outside the body and used to propel the treatment, a balloon catheter, ready to be inflated by compressed air and push aside that nasty blockage in the artery.

The angioplasty went smoothly, clearing the way for a return of blood and oxygen into the heart's most important artery. Not only was the acute blood clot smashed apart by inflating the balloon to five times the normal pressure of the earth's atmosphere, the underlying plaque of atherosclerosis was flattened into the wall of the artery. How a small diameter coronary artery can tolerate such trauma without tearing apart is still miraculous.

But the doctors were not done. The next injection of dye revealed another blockage in the left anterior descending artery, further down toward the tip of the heart. A second angioplasty was needed and went as smoothly as the first one. Next the stents, containing a small amount of medication previously used to treat cancer, needed to go in. Once in the correct position, expanding the metal stents with a tiny balloon created a scaffolding inside of the artery.

Within two hours after the onset of chest pain, all of these procedures had been performed on Harold, and his Widowmaker heart attack aborted in its early stages. His chest pain lasted a few more hours but was much improved and subsiding, and his vital signs soon completely stabilized. Later that evening, my friend Harold was able to watch Super Bowl LII[132] on the television.

---

132   An epic heart-stopping victory by my local Philadelphia Eagles over the New England Patriots. Fortunately, my friend Harold is from New York.

Over the decades, like Grüntzig, coronary artery angioplasty achieved great heights in the world of medicine. The procedure has aborted so many heart attacks and saved lives in the short and long term. Grüntzig was a German Icarus and a modern legend. But the angioplasty does not prevent atherosclerosis; it only helps deal with its consequences. Prevention remains the greatest challenge of our time, and there was much more research and treatment to come.

CHAPTER 20

WHO YA GONNA CALL? HERALDING THE AGE OF CLOT BUSTERS

It may be true that I have one trick up my sleeve,
but it is a good one,
and doctors have yet to discover how I do it,
making impediments appear
seemingly out of thin air.

Were they to shift their focus,
much of my magic would dissolve.

IMPOTENCE—SUMMER 1980

Dave poked his head out from behind the curtain of a patient's room, and I could see a worried look on his face. He said, "You better take a look at this guy—I think he's having a big MI." Dave, a nephrology fellow, and I were the "moon-lighters" covering the emergency room at a sleepy community hospital in Stamford, Connecticut, St. Joseph's Medical Center.

A man about fifty years old was in the bed looking very anxious and sweaty. He had finished dinner a few hours earlier and was watching some TV when he started to have very bad pressure in his chest, like an "elephant sitting on me." He had broken out into a sweat and felt short of breath.

Dave showed the man's electrocardiogram to me. We didn't need to say anything to each other; the electrocardiogram gave us the instantaneous answer. Searing the images into our eyes and brains were the typical findings of a major MI due to a blockage of the heart's main artery, the left anterior descending coronary artery. The Widowmaker was hard at work.

The ST segments, that portion of the electrocardiogram signal after the QRS complex, the electrical signal of the contraction of the ventricles, were heading straight up, high above where they were a few hours earlier when this man was just home from work. Dave and I both knew what that meant—we called it the "tombstone sign." This man was in trouble. His blood pressure was low, his heart rate was high, and his lungs were starting to fill up with fluid. His left ventricle, the major pumping chamber, was failing due to a sudden loss of its blood supply.

With the help of the nurses, we went to work. We placed an intravenous catheter in a large vein in his arm and injected a large shot of intravenous morphine to relieve the pain, then gave him oxygen to ease his labored breathing. The man was frightened, his eyes wide open, and beads of sweat formed all over his face and chest. I wanted to give nitroglycerin under his tongue to help with the chest pain, but I hesitated. Nitroglycerin can quickly lower the blood pressure, and his pressure was low already.

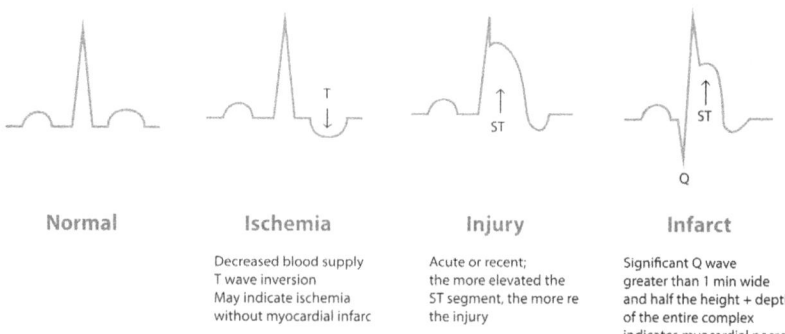

Figure 25. Sequential changes in the EKG signal from Normal to Ischemia to Injury ("tombstone sign") of ST segment elevation to Q wave of completed myocardial infarction and permanent tissue damage. (Copyright Shutterstock)

After several tests and decisions were made, the man was placed in the CCU, and for hours, I struggled to keep him alive as Dave covered the emergency room. But whatever I tried (medication to raise his blood pressure, oxygen, and diuretics to get rid of the lung fluid) only seemed a temporary fix. At about four a.m., his heart stopped. It just slowed down and stopped. I tried more medications to restart it, but I knew the effort was futile. The damage from the blocked artery was just overwhelming. I had given the man "state of the art" care for 1980.

Trudging back to the ER, I was physically and mentally exhausted. Dave told me to grab two hours of sleep before we needed to head back to New Haven. On the ride back, I was obsessed with why I couldn't have done more. What were we missing about heart attacks? We know the arteries were filled with cholesterol plaque, but that took years to build up. Why on this night, at that particular time, had that heart attack happened in this man? What was going on inside of that diseased artery? Because of our ignorance, once the heart attack occurred, how much damage would occur was out of our control. Heart muscle melted slowly but steadily like a snowman in bright sunshine. As a young cardiologist, I felt frustrated and impotent that night.

There had to be something more we could do. I remembered something I heard two years prior when I was an internal medicine resident at Temple University School of Medicine in Philadelphia. Sol Sherry MD (1916-1993) was the chairman of the department and a world-renowned hematologist. Each morning, the residents would present the new cases to Dr. Sherry, and one morning one of my colleagues was describing a patient just like the one I had tried to save that night, a young man with a massive heart attack. Dr. Sherry, I am sure, had heard so many of these cases presented over the years, and he was bored that morning, staring at the floor. But suddenly he picked up his head and said to the group of us, "You know, all of you who are going into cardiology, let me tell you something. Acute myocardial infarction is a hematologic disease." I thought heart attacks were all about cholesterol and atherosclerosis. What did blood have to do with them? Dr. Sherry was back staring at the floor. His words would ring true within just a few years.

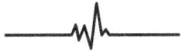

BLOOD CLOTS: THE FINAL ACT OF THE WIDOWMAKER

In the summer of 1980, the cardiology world was unaware that the editors of *The New England Journal of Medicine* were readying to publish a new research study about heart attacks that would finally prove the identity of the most potent weapon of the Widowmaker.

Marcus Dewood MD was practicing cardiology near his birthplace in Spokane, Washington, and was also struggling with how much was still unknown. Dewood learned his cardiology skills well at Cedars-Sinai in Los Angeles, studying with Swan, Ganz, and other luminaries in the world of academic cardiology. But like most cardiologists, Dewood still didn't understand what really caused an acute heart attack. After all, atherosclerosis is a chronic disease.

Trying to get a good handle on why this often-devastating illness happened when it happened in the 1960s and 1970s was like trying to predict when a dam would burst.

Pathologists doing their autopsies had seen blood clots stuck inside of the cholesterol plaque clogging up the coronary arteries for a century. Sometimes the clots looked like they had been there for a long time, and others looked as if they had just formed before the person had died. Sometimes they found no clots, just the cholesterol plaque. Sometimes clots were in one part of the artery and not in others. It just didn't make sense. Pathologists were always viewed with some skepticism by doctors taking care of living patients, but in this case, they themselves just shrugged their shoulders and had no definite opinions about the significance of the clots they found. After all, didn't all kinds of strange things happen to the body and the blood after people died?

Despite the many advances made in the arena of heart disease, some very crucial questions and misconceptions remained. Were the blood clots the crucial culprits, abruptly completely shutting down a partially blocked artery's blood flow, or were they just scavengers, like buzzards hovering over a dead animal's body? The idea of "coronary thrombosis" arose as long ago as the early twentieth century. It was a common expression used to describe what had happened to a patient suffering a heart attack, but it was disingenuous—no one was certain of the significance of the blood clots. The cause of a myocardial infarction by the 1970s had retreated to the idea of the "rusty pipe," the coronary arteries gradually filled up with cholesterol, the flow of blood slowed down, and maybe, or maybe not, a blood clot formed.

But it was believed that the gradual decreased flow of the blood, the "ischemia," did the damage to the heart muscle cells, and on that note, Dewood knew that more had to be done to help patients with heart attacks. He and everyone in cardiology agreed that the longer the time that the heart muscle was deprived of blood, whatever the cause, the worse the outcome would be. Coronary artery bypass graft surgery in the late 1970s was common but was not being used often enough, he felt. Major hospitals had heart bypass surgery programs, and a cadre of young heart surgeons had the skill to perform the operation with great results, but bypass surgery performed quickly after a heart attack was almost never done. The patient had to survive the heart attack first and then undergo a cardiac catheterization and coronary angiography days later. Only then, if the blockages were in a good place along the course of the artery, was bypass graft surgery recommended.

Dewood had an idea, however, that could help with this situation and dramatically speed up the time frame for bypass surgery. He wondered what would happen if a cardiac catheterization was done just after the patient came to the hospital and the definite diagnosis of a major heart attack was established. The cath would show beautiful pictures of where the blockage or blockages were located, and then the surgeons could perform the bypass surgery within hours. The speed of the procedure would save more heart muscle than waiting for several days. Years of research studies in animals all showed that heart muscle cells start to die within minutes after their main heart artery is closed off artificially with a suture and that the sooner the strangling suture is released, the more heart muscle cells recover.

The idea, and especially the way Dewood wanted it done, was not easy to sell. Performing a cardiac catheterization in a patient during the very first hours after a heart attack was risky business. Injection of contrast dye into a diseased coronary artery could decrease blood flow even more, and the dye made heart muscle function worse. The "old heads" of cardiology were convinced that an urgent cardiac cath was not wise and maybe even reckless. But Marcus was going to ask even more from his surgical friends. Bypass surgery was not like removing an appendix, not discounting the skill required to perform that surgery. To perform the bypass using the patient's leg vein, the surgeon needed to open up the patient's own coronary artery that was going to be bypassed. Once the incision was made in the coronary artery and before the vein was sewn into the incision to create the bypass, Dewood wanted his colleagues to do something else.

Dewood had the audacity to ask the surgeons to place a special device into the patient's coronary artery—a Fogarty catheter. This skinny catheter had been used for years to remove blood clots from arteries in other parts of the body. Named after its inventor, Thomas Fogarty MD (1934-), the device is a hollow tube with an inflatable balloon at its tip. When the catheter is pushed into a blood clot and the balloon inflated, the operator can pull the catheter back and extract a blood clot. Marcus wanted the surgeons to use the Fogarty to try to "fish out" a blood clot from the coronary artery even though he wasn't sure what they would find.

Despite these challenges, Dewood's ambitious project was set in motion at his hospital and began working well. The cath lab was used day and night for the heart attack patients, and they were studied very quickly. From 1971 to 1979, Dewood accumulated 322 cases, and 126 of them (39.1 percent) went to the cath lab within four hours after the chest pain started and another eighty-two (25.4 percent) within six hours. Stunningly, when Dewood and his colleagues injected dye into the coronary artery, usually the left anterior descending running right down the center of the heart, *they found a complete blockage in 87.3 percent of those studied in the first four hours.*

This impressive data meant only one thing to Dewood: the images he saw represented a clot, a "thrombus," completely stopping the flow of blood. In another 10.3 percent of the patients studied quickly, he saw a "subtotal" occlusion, a partial thrombus, not one that cut off all blood flow through the artery. The patients who got into the cath lab later, after six hours, had fewer blood clots, but even in those people, blood clots were very common. There was only one logical conclusion: heart attacks started when a clot formed, but then over time the body's system of molecules that break down clots began to work. The longer after the attack began, the less likely that Dewood would find the image of a clot in the artery.

Dewood still needed proof from the surgeons. In the operating room, the confirmation of the nature of the cath findings became clear. The surgeons were able to retrieve a clot from the blocked artery almost all of the time! It was now crystal-clear to Dewood and his colleagues that major acute heart attacks, the ones that killed and disabled people by damaging the heart muscle from the inside surface to the outside of the muscle wall, were caused by thrombus forming inside of the artery.[133]

So it took two separate processes, one long-term and the other acute, to cause a major heart attack. The artery had to first become partially filled up with cholesterol plaque, a process that takes years caused by diet and genetics. But the sudden and unpredictable feature of the heart attack was the complete cut off of the blood flow through a large coronary artery, within minutes or a few hours. A blood clot on top of the cholesterol plaque was in fact the final nail of the work of the Widowmaker. A revolution in the care of the heart attack patient was just over the horizon, using a molecule resurrected from the past, discovered not by a cardiologist but by a blood doctor.

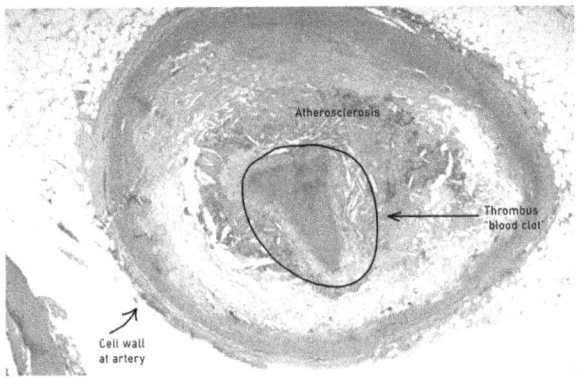

Figure 26. Acute thrombus in the left anterior descending coronary artery similar to findings of Dewood study in *New England Journal of Medicine*, 1980. (Courtesy of Amandeep Aneja MD and Nirg Jhala MD, Temple University School of Medicine and Meredith Dawson Designs LLC)

---

[133] These types of heart attacks are named "transmural," damage through the entire wall of the heart muscle.

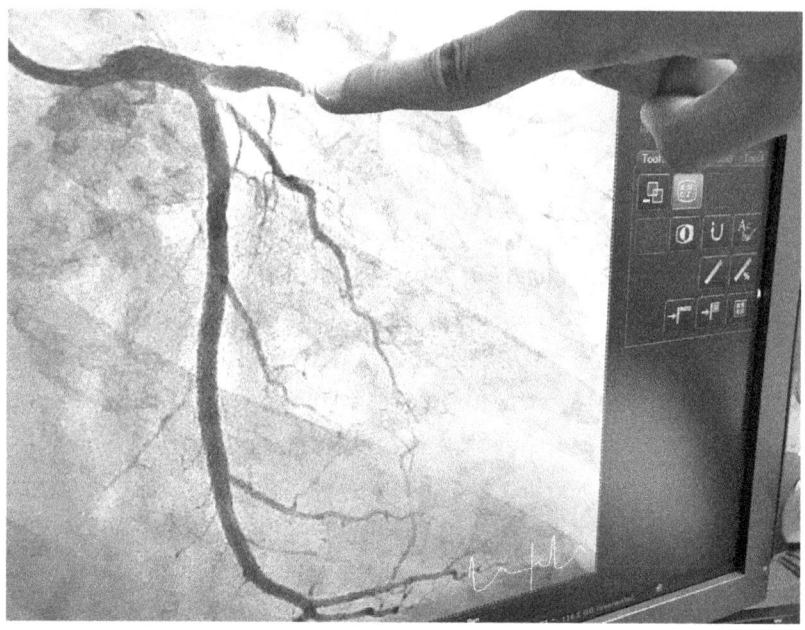

Figure 27. Thrombus seen in a coronary artery partially occluded with chronic atherosclerosis in a microscopic slide. (Copyright Shutterstock)

BACTERIA TO THE RESCUE: BREAKING UP THE CLOTS

Sol Sherry MD (1916-1993) was born in Manhattan and received his MD degree at the NYU School of Medicine in 1939. He then trained in hematology at NYU before serving four years as a flight surgeon during World War II. Sol was fascinated by how blood formed clots and then magically dissolved.

In 1954, Sherry moved to Washington University in St. Louis, Missouri, where he began working with someone who would help hone Sherry's interest in clots. William Tillett MD (1892-1974) was a hematologist like Sherry, but he was studying the bacteria known as the *streptococcus*, the cause of many types of infections, such as those affecting the skin, the heart, and the throat ("the strep throat"). Tillet was fascinated by the microscopic bugs because he discovered that the *streptococci* were making something that broke up the proteins of a blood clot. He isolated the molecule chemically, purified it, and gave it a name—streptokinase.[134]

For over fifteen years, Tillett continued his research into streptokinase and thought that his discovery might be useful in patients but for what conditions was unclear. As someone who was committed to understanding and treating blood clot disorders, Sherry had an idea. He knew well of the controversy of the role of blood clots in myocardial infarctions, but just like everyone else, he was uncertain about their role in this epidemic disease. But now there was a strange molecule made by bacteria that might prove or disprove their importance in causing heart attacks.

In the 1950s, a research project evolved slowly for Sherry. First, he needed to purify streptokinase and make sure that it was safe to use in people; after all, it was made by bacteria that cause human diseases. He didn't even know which heart attack patients had blood clots in their coronary arteries at the time they became ill. The possible problems were many if he was going to treat patients and the answers unknown. Could streptokinase, given by an intravenous infusion, float through the bloodstream into the small holes that opened into the coronary arteries? Could he give enough of the molecules to break up a blood clot that had been forming for several hours, if not longer? How would those patients do after their heart attacks? Would more people survive because less heart muscle was damaged if the streptokinase restored the blood supply? Needless to say, this was a very bold research proposal for the time.

Sherry was determined to try to answer the conundrum of the heart attack and blood clots, and to that end, he and his colleagues recruited twenty-four people for their small study. The patients needed to have had their chest pain for at least six hours and the

---

134 "Kinase" is the last part of the name given to a protein molecule called an enzyme, a molecule that breaks up the chemical bonds on another molecule.

diagnosis confirmed by the electrocardiogram changes typical for a heart attack, along with elevation of specific blood enzymes, protein molecules released from the breaking open of the cell membranes of dead or dying heart muscle cells. Miraculously, of the twenty-four patients, twenty-one survived—*eighty-seven percent*! This was a time when the expected percentage of survival would have been about sixty percent. What's more, in the patients treated within fourteen hours of the onset of symptoms, fifteen of sixteen—*ninety-four percent*—survived. The streptokinase was having a dramatic benefit.

One would have expected that the medical world, as well as drug manufacturers, would have latched on to this remarkable result very quickly and that many larger studies would have been conducted, but this never happened. In fact, Sherry's work remained suspect to most doctors, especially the cardiologists. His study of twenty-four people was so small[135] that the results were regarded with skepticism, and the statisticians, the people who analyzed data, had a major problem with his study. His patients were not "randomized," that is broken up into equal numbers of treated patients and those not given the streptokinase, and he had no "control" group of people who were not treated with streptokinase for comparison. Maybe he was treating a group of people with very mild heart attacks who would have survived just as often without being given streptokinase.

But there were other issues as well. The way the study was set up raised ethical concerns of making patients wait for a definitive diagnosis of a heart attack before having only a chance of getting an experimental drug. And then there were the risks of using streptokinase, including inducing fever and bleeding, especially into the brain. These concerns were significant since a doctor always needs to be sure that the benefit is worth the risk to any individual patient, especially in a research trial. Is a forty percent reduction in the overall mortality rate worth the one

---

135 Getting people to sign up for a study is a hard sell under the best of circumstances, let alone talking someone into it who has chest pain, shortness of breath, and a fear of an acute heart attack.

percent risk of a fatal brain hemorrhage? Something doesn't happen to one person forty percent or one percent of the time; it happens to an individual one hundred percent.

Sherry's data was ignored for decades. Research continued to try to find other medications that might decrease the amount of heart damage done by heart attacks. Candidates were many, including beta-blockers to slow the heart rate, nitroglycerin and other "vasodilators" to increase blood flood, and anti-inflammatory drugs like ibuprofen.[136] Even stranger potions were tried, including glucose, insulin, and potassium combinations, and cobra venom, which does contain a powerful anticoagulant. And of course when all else failed, doctors tried corticosteroids. Nothing tried was able to significantly decrease heart muscle damage once the heart attack process began.

The final "stake in the heart" to thrombolytic treatment of heart attacks in the 1960s came with the establishment of the special care units for patients with heart attacks, the CCUs. These units became the focus of research in the cardiology world, efforts to care for patients after their heart attack, not to try to prevent the heart muscle damage but rather to deal with its complications. Streptokinase use for heart attacks remained dormant.[137]

THE 1980S
BACK TO THE PAST: STREPTOKINASE RESURFACES

Throughout the 1960s and 1970s, the lingering confusion about the cause of a heart attack and the frustration of how to limit heart muscle damage continued. But there were still a few intrigued by the idea of breaking up clots even before Marcus Dewood's results about the prevalence of clots were widely known.

---

136 Trade name Motrin.
137 Dr. Sherry's work with streptokinase in another disease, pulmonary emboli, was much more productive. The results of his studies showing a dramatic decrease in death from blood clots in the lungs earned him international fame. His data were clear that streptokinase is a potent drug for breaking up blood clots.

In the late 1970s, a young cardiologist from Gottingen, Germany, K. Peter Rentrop MD, came up with a new idea. He knew how powerful streptokinase was but thought that the side effects of the drug could be eliminated if they could deliver the clot-buster in a high concentration right into the coronary artery and avoid contact with the circulation as a whole. Cardiac catheterization was fully developed, and if one could infuse contrast dye directly into the artery, why not a drug like streptokinase? Placing catheters into coronary arteries was routine by then. All you needed to do was load the medication into a syringe, place the catheter into the coronary artery, and begin the infusion.

The idea was pretty straightforward: just like Dewood was doing, get the patients into the cath lab as soon as possible and get the blood supply to the heart muscle restored. But the risks were unknown. Some skeptics were concerned that breaking up a clot in a coronary artery and resupplying damaged heart muscle with blood too quickly might make the damage worse. But Rentrop and his colleagues went ahead and, by 1979, had used intracoronary streptokinase in a few patients. Then in 1980, the Dewood report came out confirming that blood clots were the main perpetrators precipitating heart attacks. His study added fuel and inspiration to those studying "clot busting."

Streptokinase continued to step out of the shadows, and a year later, the Rentrop group reported their results in twenty-nine patients. In twenty-two (seventy-six percent), the streptokinase opened up the blocked artery within minutes! Not only did the drug work, but the patient's chest pain went away in fourteen of fifteen patients who were still having pain prior to beginning infusion of the streptokinase. There was more very good news. The pressure inside of the left ventricle, a value that usually rises during a heart attack, dropped—a remarkable finding. This meant that the pumping action of the ventricle improved as the blood clot dissolved and more blood entered the heart muscle. Finally, *only one of the twenty-nine patients died* on the first day after the infusion procedure. These results were absolutely stunning and proof that the horrible damage of the Widowmaker could be aborted and lives saved by restoring blood flow as soon as possible.

A revolution had begun. This time, more than twenty years after Sol Sherry and his group reported great results with using streptokinase by intravenous infusion, the revolt quickly gathered momentum around the world. Rentrop was recruited to the United States and took a position at The Mt. Sinai Hospital in New York City. He and many others began aggressive trials in much larger numbers of patients to determine if streptokinase would really live up to its initial success rates. Worldwide studies were organized, embraced fully by the crème-de-le-crème of academic cardiologists.

Streptokinase lived up to its initial billing, but it was not without difficulties. The commitment on the part of the cardiologists and hospitals doing these procedures was a major strain on the healthcare system. A team of people, not just the cardiologist, needed to be available 24/7. Heart attacks didn't occur on a schedule. In addition, as more patients were given the drug, it was clear that it didn't work in everyone. Using the electrocardiogram, cardiologists realized that the drug was very effective if given within one to two hours after the onset of the chest pain in those people who showed the kind of EKG changes with transmural heart attacks—those with the ST segment elevation, the "tombstone" sign, but not with those who showed inversion (a downward deflection) of the T waves. These people did not benefit from the streptokinase, and in fact, it caused harm in some.

Fortunately, a group of German cardiologists embraced the intravenous streptokinase idea. Rolf Schröder MD of the Frei Universitat in Berlin began giving intravenous streptokinase to acute heart attack patients, mimicking the Sherry study of some many years earlier. Initially, their patients went to the catheterization laboratory first to document an occluded coronary artery. When these studies went well, the Berlin group decided not to wait until the catheterization was done; they would start the intravenous infusion as soon as they were sure of the diagnosis based on the patient's symptoms and the electrocardiogram abnormalities. They reasoned the sooner the drug got to where it needed to go, the better the results. In eleven out of twenty-one patients (fifty-two percent), the blocked artery was opened up within ninety minutes. Their results were not as good as the intracoronary method but were promising.

More cardiologists started using the streptokinase in their communities, and the results were often startling. Cardiologists were used to coming into the hospital at all hours, but now the demand was even more urgent. There could be no more long delays in trying to figure out if the patient was having a major heart attack or not. The entire pace of the process picked up. What's the history? When did the pain start? What does the EKG look like? The EKG again gave the answer. The "frontline" cardiologists were running the show again.

Even the emergency room protocol changed to make the use of streptokinase more effective. As people were rushed into the ER, the patient with chest pain went to the front of the queue—no waiting for triage. Having chest pain? Right this way to a bed and let us hook up the EKG machine. But doctors had to be careful and be sure this was an "ST segment elevation" heart attack. There are other things that can cause acute severe chest pain, like a collapsed lung, which can happen with trauma; like a pulmonary embolism; like severe gastritis or an acute attack of reflux esophagitis; or a dissection of the aorta. But when it was indicated and worked, the effects of streptokinase were dramatic and marvelous. The chest pain disappeared, the sweating and shortness of breath went away, and color came back to the person's face within an hour. It was as if the heart muscle was breathing a sigh of relief, like your arm muscles feel after the doctor releases the blood pressure cuff. Blood was back, oxygen was back, and the heart muscle cells were happy again.

This amazing medication changed the course of people's lives. An hour before, just before starting the streptokinase, a heart attack patient thought the end was near. But when streptokinase worked, in a few hours, patients would often ask the cardiologist when he or she could go home. Real progress was made, and there was more to come. The molecular biologists were poised to help the cardiologists on the frontlines.

BETTER DRUGS FOR HEART ATTACKS: EXPANSION OF IDEAS AND DNA BREAKTHROUGHS

The path that the science of the laboratory, the "basic science," takes until it impacts the way that doctors take care of patients is often a long one. This delay was very true for the field of genetics, a field began by the study of pea pods and fruit flies over one hundred years ago, finally leading to the discovery of genes and their structure by James Watson PhD (1928-) and Francis Crick PhD (1916-2004) in 1952. In the early 1970s, two Californians, Herbert Boyer PhD (1937-) of the University of California at San Francisco and Stanley Cohen PhD (1935-) of Stanford University, experimented with something both bold and shocking. They were going to manipulate genes.

Their idea was groundbreaking and would prove to have wide appeal. They reasoned that if they could insert the genetic code sequence of a protein into the DNA of a virus or a bacteria, then the virus or bacteria would begin producing the alien protein instructed by the newly inserted DNA. Now there was a "factory" that could make any protein you wanted in enormous quantities. Industry was very interested in the idea. What if you could genetically manufacture insulin? The implications for medicine were immense, not to mention the financial return. What was needed was an entrepreneur, and Robert Swanson (1947-1999) stepped forward.

After college on the East Coast, he moved to California, where he found himself unemployed at age twenty-eight. Hoping to find someone interested in working with him to produce something useful, Swanson "cold-called" scientists. One of his calls was to Herbert Boyer. After meeting with Boyer for hours, they decided that they had ideas that might work. Placing $500 each into an account to pay legal fees, the businessman and the molecular geneticist formed a corporation named Genentech. Within two years, their company used the DNA of the bacterium *Escherichia coli* (*E. coli*), to manufacture large amounts of somatostatin, the chemical name of growth hormone produced by the pituitary gland. Quickly thereafter, they had a great triumph; they used bacteria to create an endless supply of pure insulin.

Genentech was on a roll. Dollars poured into the company, and the duo continued to drive the production line hard. Swenson and Boyer knew that they could find the DNA sequence of a molecule that was attracting attention in the cardiology world. The hematologists discovered that streptokinase, made by bacteria, had a cousin in the human body, one of the many molecular members of the coagulation system. It's an enzyme that converts another coagulation system molecule called plasminogen into plasmin. Plasmin is one of the most important molecules that break apart blood clots. Plasmin is just like streptokinase, but before plasmin can work, it needs to be "activated" by another molecule called "tissue plasminogen activator."

The Genentech scientists used their DNA technology to create the powerful molecule in their laboratory in large amounts. In 1982, the company released its commercial version of tissue plasminogen activator, "TPA."[138] Now streptokinase had a strong competitor, one that was a pure substance, without the risk of allergic reactions and with reliable dosing. But it was much more expensive than streptokinase. Which clot-buster was better?

To the cardiologist at the bedside in the emergency room, the victor of the battle between streptokinase and TPA was not clear at all. Both drugs worked most of the time when given very soon after the chest pain began but not all the time. There were still too many patients who continued to have chest pain and EKG abnormalities in spite of

---

138   Genentech has gone onto produce many more incredible products over the years and had sales of over $4 billion in 2017. Tragically, Robert Swanson died of a brain tumor in 1999 at age fifty-two.

receiving one of the two thrombolytic drugs. These people were more likely to end up with a badly damaged heart muscle or die than those in whom a clot-buster worked. Almost all of the articles in the major medical and cardiology journals were about which drug might be better than the other. At national meetings, standing room–only crowds of mostly male cardiologists, dressed in blue blazers, white button-down shirts, striped ties, and gray slacks listened to the royalty of academic cardiology drone on about the differences between the two drugs.

To help answer the controversy about which drugs to use to treat acute heart attacks, not just the thrombolytic drugs, Eugene Braunwald and his Harvard colleagues organized a comprehensive organization to study the new medications that were impacting the acute care of the heart attack patient. Dr. Braunwald hoped the new pharmacologic tools would change the fate of millions and applied the enormous knowledge he and his colleagues had accrued over decades about how the human heart reacts and tries to adapt and survive from the damage of a heart attack.

The Thrombolysis in Myocardial Infarction study group (TIMI), started by Braunwald, began its work in 1984 and within three years published data from a large-scale international trial comparing streptokinase to Genentech's TPA drug. This research study was "double-blind"—neither the patient nor the doctor knew which drug was used. The cardiologist needed to explain everything to the patient and then call an 800 phone number to see which box to use. That way he or she would not be biased in their assessment of how the patient did. The toughest part was convincing the patient and the family that participating in the trial was a good idea for a sick patient. But at least everyone was going to get a clot-buster even if they didn't know which one.

In the end, the large international trials showed that tPA was significantly better in opening up clogged arteries. The report from the TIMI group in 1987 demonstrated that the success rate with tPA was sixty-two percent, versus only thirty-one percent with streptokinase.[139] The streptokinase was much more effective when it was given directly into a coronary artery in a cath lab, but not as potent in its intravenous form. Even so, the molecule first isolated by bacteria in the 1930s had led the way to the widespread use of thrombolytic drugs.

So much valuable awareness and effective action was achieved in the area of treating heart attacks in such a short period of time. The confusion about the acute cause of heart attacks was finally swept away by Dewood and his surgical colleagues pulling fresh blood clots out of the coronary arteries, and by Rentrop showing that a drug from the *streptococcus* bacteria could break up clots in those arteries and save lives. The work of Sol Sherry was confirmed—acute myocardial infarction is a blood disease. Swanson and Boyer were also found to be right that DNA can do marvelous things. Thrombolysis worked in so many cases and dropped the death rate from myocardial infarctions to approximately ten percent from forty percent by the beginning of the 1990s.

The Widowmaker would realize those clot buster drugs were strong work, but researchers still had work to do. What about the unfortunate ten percent? Was there no treatment for them? And significant unanswered questions remained: Why did the clot form and why at that time? Why not two years earlier or two months later? What was going on inside of that coronary artery that we still didn't understand? For the first time, doctors could minimize the death of heart muscle cells from a heart attack, but only if they could get to the patients quickly enough. What about the whole idea of prevention? The monumental task of addressing prevention would get a boost from the world of the microscopic.

---

139   The TIMI group has made so many important contributions to cardiac care for the last thirty-six years. The organization has conducted trials in up to twenty-six thousand patients at a time, involving fifty different countries and five thousand medical centers and clinics. Its work will continue.

CHAPTER 21

THE FUNGUS AMONG US: CULTIVATING THE RISE OF STATINS

Humans believe that an ounce of prevention is worth a pound of cure, but for so long my work has escaped this focus. Thus the chase is only meant to stop me in the nick of time.

Is it possible to find something that would prevent me from ever running my course? And if so, at what price?

MAGIC MEDICATIONS FROM MICROBES

A Family Story

My mother was sixteen years old in the summer of 1945, just as World War II was ending. Spending her weekends away from south Philadelphia at the New Jersey shore with her girlfriends, trying to meet boys, especially the GIs already returning from distant battles, life was grand. Sometime in August, she "caught a cold." Surely not an uncommon problem, usually a short few days of fever, chills, sore throat, stuffy nose, and a cough.

But this "cold" just lingered. After a week of getting worse, with a hacking cough producing nasty-looking phlegm, her aunt took her to the family doctor just a block away in South Philadelphia. (Her mother, my grandmother, had passed away a year earlier.)

Dr. Glick, a family doctor and a legend in his community, listened to her story and then put his stethoscope on her back to listen to the lungs. He told my mother's aunt that her niece had pneumonia, a bacterial infection of the lungs, and that she needed to go to a hospital for some type of treatment, including oxygen to breathe. At that time, the chance of dying from pneumonia was about three out of ten, even for teenagers.

Once my mother was settled in her room, Dr. Glick came to see her and placed a large needle and a plastic catheter into a vein in her forearm. He wanted to give my mother intravenous medication. He said this was much stronger than any pills he could give her to treat her pneumonia. Then every six hours for the next several days, a nurse would enter the room, hang a clear bag of some liquid on the metal pole, and clip a needle into the intravenous line so that gravity would push the unknown elixir down into the catheter in my mother's arm vein, getting that crucial medication into her circulation.

Miraculously, my mother began to feel much better within twenty-four hours, but there was something strange about her care; the nurses insisted that she place all of her urine into a urine basin and not to use the bathroom. She had no idea why the nurses wanted her to do that, but she complied. Dr. Glick came to see her every day, and finally after a few visits, when it was clear that her niece was getting better, my great aunt asked the doctor what the magical medicine that was flowing into her niece's veins every six hours was and why it was necessary for all of her urine to be collected.

Dr. Glick answered quickly, "Haven't you heard about penicillin? It's a miracle drug; it's called an antibiotic, and it kills the germ that causes pneumonia." Although penicillin had been used for several years, by late 1945, it was used almost exclusively to treat and prevent wound infections in injured American and British soldiers fighting the war. Use in the civilian population was very limited because there was no mass production of the drug available at the time. Since penicillin was in such short supply, the excess that made it into the urine had to be saved for reuse, hence the weird protocol at the hospital. Saved by a microscopic life form that we usually regard as a pest, my mother went on with her life, married, and had four sons. Only when I went to medical school did I discover that penicillin came from fungi.

Scientists long ago realized that the natural world, major parts of which are invisible to most of us, can produce substances developed by eons of evolution that give microorganisms like bacteria and fungi a "competitive advantage" in their day-to-day fight for food and survival to reproduce. Over the millennia, healers have occasionally stumbled upon an assortment of these substances that are surprisingly effective in treating human disease. Perhaps someone would find one that would stop atherosclerosis. It would not be easy.

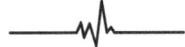

A QUIXOTIC IDEA: A DRUG TO LOWER CHOLESTEROL

Akira Endo PhD (1933-) was a trained scientist and a relentless hunter but not of animals; his passion was the bizarre life forms that have lived on earth for billions of years and are only seen under a microscope. Born into a Japanese farming family, Endo knew by age ten that he wanted to become a scientist. As a teenager, he read about the discoveries of penicillin and then streptomycin, the drug that cured tuberculosis. It always struck him that these remarkable discoveries came from studying microorganisms and the strange substances that they produced for the purposes of their own survival.

After college graduation in 1957, Endo took a job at Sankyo Pharmaceuticals in Tokyo in the microbiology study group, and there he settled on his research interest: cholesterol.

He was fascinated by the role that cholesterol played in the construction of the cell walls of bacteria and all cells. He studied the publications of Konrad Bloch PhD (1912-2000) and Feodor

Lynen PhD (1911-1979), who proved that the rate-limiting step in cholesterol metabolism was controlled by HMG CoA reductase, the enzyme that Brown and Goldstein focused on in their work.[140]

Wanting to come to the United States to further his cholesterol research, Endo found a position with an accomplished cholesterol researcher, Bernard Horecker PhD (1914-2010) at the Albert Einstein College of Medicine in New York City. It was there that Akira Endo developed an idea that drove his research efforts for the next decade. If microorganisms were able to combat their competitors in their fight for survival by producing molecules that were toxic to their neighbors, similar to what the penicillin fungus did, evolution probably had focused their efforts on some key targets in the metabolism of their enemies.

Endo began applying this concept to heart disease and the search for something that could reduce cholesterol. It stood to reason that to destroy their neighbors, a good target for any microorganism would be the rate-limiting step of an important metabolic process. So to destroy cholesterol and shut down the cell wall production of a competitor microbe, Endo knew which enzyme might have a "bull's eye" on it: HMG CoA reductase. Could he find another fungus in nature that stopped cholesterol production in its tracks? Could he find the molecule responsible for this work, make it into a drug that would lower cholesterol levels in people without harming them? The task was daunting. His hunt began.

Akira Endo knew that if he could discover a molecule that stopped cholesterol production, the implications were huge. He reported years later his observation of life in America: " . . . I was very surprised by the large number of elderly and overweight people, and by the rather rich dietary habits of Americans compared to those of the Japanese. In the residential area of the Bronx where I lived,

---

140 Bloch and Lynen won the Nobel Prize in Physiology and Medicine in 1964 for their discovery. At their prize award ceremony, one of the speakers from the committee commented, "Your discoveries may provide us with weapons against some of mankind's gravest maladies, above all in relation to cardiovascular disease."

there were many elderly couples living by themselves and I often saw ambulances going to take an elderly person who had had a heart attack to the hospital." He was a firsthand witness to the epidemic work of the Widowmaker.

A TROUBLED START—THEN PERSISTENCE

Endo was not the first person to look for medication that lowered levels of cholesterol; in the late 1950s, one drug company thought they had produced a breakthrough drug. The Rutherford-Merrell Chemical Company of Cincinnati, Ohio, had a large number of compounds in its supply closets, most of which had no apparent use in human disease. By just trying out all sorts of tests on samples of jars of chemicals gathering dust in dark closets, one of their scientists found one that might help them make a useful drug and make a great deal of money. The compound their employee found inhibited the very last step in cholesterol metabolism; it was not the rate-limiting step, but it did lower blood cholesterol levels in normal volunteers. The company called the new drug Triparanol.

Rutherford-Merrell quickly sent the drug for study to the National Institute of Health. Their researchers confirmed that Triparanol stopped the conversion of the molecule desmosterol into cholesterol, the next to the last step in the metabolism of cholesterol, resulting in lower cholesterol blood levels. But in experimental animals, they still found desmosterol in plaques of atherosclerosis. Ignoring this potential problem, Rutherford-Merrell started clinical trials in humans, supplying doctors with the medication.[141]

At the same time, Merck Sharpe and Dohme, a pharmaceutical giant, also got its hands on Triparanol and began studying it intently, with rising concern. Merck also knew that if Triparanol worked and was safe for people, the economic return on investment could be huge. But the company had found a problem: Triparanol had side

---

141 At the time, the oversight of the Food and Drug Administration was just very lax.

effects, including severely dry skin (ichthyosis), hair loss, and cataract formation in experimental animals. Merck even notified Rutherford-Merrell of its concerns, but the Cincinnati company pretended that it knew nothing about these side effects and kept supplying doctors and patients with Triparanol. Just a few months later, ophthalmologists from the Mayo Clinic reported cases of the same skin, hair, and eye problems in some of their patients taking Triparanol, similar to the animal problems described by Merck. Finally, the Food and Drug Administration got involved and stopped all use of Triparanol. This scandal would result in lengthy and costly lawsuits.

For the decade of the 1960s, both the medical community as well as the public in the United States were understandably suspicious about the development of new drugs to treat anything, but this didn't stop Endo from his work in Japan. He was dogmatic about his idea that nature could provide a substance that lowered blood cholesterol levels safely, and his hunter mentality took over. In 1971, he began many failed attempts to find cultures of microorganisms that interfered with the metabolism of lipids. Clearly a person similar to Thomas Edison, the author of "Genius is 1% inspiration, and 99% perspiration," Endo studied approximately 3,800 strains of fungi in a year. Remarkably, he was able to go to the lab each day without becoming depressed from the tedium and frustration of his quest.

Endo's perseverance finally paid off. In 1972, he was examining a fungus on a rice sample in a grain shop in Kyoto and scooped up another bug to study. This fungus came from the genus *Penicillium citrinum*. Endo was likely particularly interested in this creature because it had similarities to the penicillin found by his hero Alexander Fleming. Perhaps it was just a coincidence that the fungus was from the Penicillin family, but Endo had found his treasure. He took the fungus into his laboratory and went to work with his organic chemistry skills. *Remarkably, the fungus from the rice shop shut down the metabolism of cholesterol in bacteria.* Endo named his prize "citrinin." He actually found three active compounds, and the one he named ML-236B was the most promising to isolate and try to concentrate; he named this special one "compactin."

Endo found that compactin's molecular structure was similar to the HMG CoA reductase enzyme, the perfect shape for a "competitive inhibitor" of the cholesterol metabolic sequence, a molecule that would fool and divert the metabolites in the synthesis cascade into interacting with the imposter, and not the true enzyme on their way to making their final product of cholesterol. Even more promising was that compactin was soluble in water—it was hydrophilic. That meant the molecule could easily get inside of cells and didn't need a specific receptor molecule to gain entry.

But as with most innovative discoveries, there was a major problem: the compactin did not lower cholesterol levels very well when used in the experimental rats. Endo did not let this stop him. In retrospect, he didn't realize that in rats, most cholesterol is not found in the LDL particles like in humans. Undaunted, Endo tried his new fungal compound in other animals, including hens, dogs, and monkeys. In these animals, the compactin was successful in lowering cholesterol and LDL particle levels. Pushing further, Endo studied compactin in human normal cells and in the cells of patients with Familial Hyperlipidemia, the people who inspired the work of Brown and Goldstein. The results were glorious.

All Endo needed now was a collaborator to promote his work. One would have thought that Sankyo would strongly back Endo to pursue using the drug in humans, but Sankyo did not,[142] and Endo left the company in 1979. Not a medical doctor himself, Endo was desperate to continue his work with an MD who was willing to try compactin in humans, and he found Akira Yamamoto MD PhD (1932-2019) at Osaka University Hospital. Dr. Yamamoto agreed to treat an eighteen-year-old girl with Familial Hyperlipidemia with compactin. Her usual blood cholesterol level was about 1,000 mg/dl, at least five times normal. As Brown and Goldstein had proven

---

142 Why Sankyo made this decision was never clear to Endo.

in their patients with the same disease, she had almost no LDL receptors on her liver cells.

The results were a game changer. After two weeks of treatment, the young woman's blood cholesterol level dropped to 700 mg/dl. Treating eight more patients, the two researchers confirmed a thirty percent drop in blood cholesterol levels. In 1980, Sankyo finally agreed to support further studies of compactin in people. But by then, another pharmaceutical company was interested in drugs that lowered cholesterol.

Endo had spoken at an international conference on new medications in Philadelphia, Pennsylvania, in 1977, and his talk gained the attention of the company he needed to promote his discovery. In the sparse audience was P. Raymond Vegalos MD (1929-), the CEO of Merck Sharp and Dohme. Intrigued by Endo's work, Vegalos negotiated with Sankyo to obtain samples of compactin and some of Sankyo's data. Merck was going to push this drug development with great vigor, seeing the enormous market opportunity. Vegalos hoped he was not sinking money into another Triparanol. Although Endo's fearless determination and work ethic set the stage for a successful statin drug, without Vegalos' involvement, it is doubtful that the breakthrough would have happened at all. It was Merck that would need to overcome another major hurdle.

Through the work of Alfred Alberts (1931-2018) at their company, Merck had already discovered another drug, another statin, found from the fungus *Aspergillus terreus*. First named mevinolin, Merck renamed its new entry into the drug battle "lovastatin." A new class of drugs was created; now there were two statins. Doctors trying to treat patients with severely elevated cholesterol levels and a history of heart attacks were already clamoring to get their hands on the new drugs. But they were going to need to wait again.

Word that Sankyo had stopped its work on compactin reached Vagelos and made him rethink his own investment. The people at Sankyo had found that the drug might be causing lymphoma, a serious form of cancer of the white blood cells, in its experimental animals. Worse yet, the company would not even talk to Vagelos about their data. Vagelos immediately told his research people to stop all work on lovastatin and compactin. If compactin might cause cancer, there was a good chance lovastatin might do so also.

Vagelow needed to quickly discover what had happened at Sankyo. He tried to make another deal with Sankyo, to allow them to market and sell lovastatin in Japan, if Sankyo would share their data—but the company refused. In spite of Sankyo's refusal to reveal their data in the animals, the story did come out: they had given the animals a dose of compactin that was two hundred times the doses they were going to use in people. If Sankyo was trying to hide the possible cancer story to protect its investment is uncertain, but it is a logical conclusion. The company was likely aware of what had happened with Triparanol. But ironically, when the secret was revealed, independent pathologic reviews of the dog tumors questioned whether or not they were even cancerous growths at all. Sankyo's grossly unethical behavior wasn't even necessary.

Armed with Sankyo's secretive findings and able to contest them, Vagelos convinced the FDA that his lovastatin was safe to use in people, especially those with the very high risk of death from heart attack, the patients with genetic forms of elevated cholesterol levels. The first trials of statins began in earnest.

LOOKING AT LARGE NUMBERS: THE STATIN DRUG TRIALS

Problematic as the process had been, the statin drugs still needed to overcome their greatest hurdle: time. When penicillin was invented, it didn't take too long or too many patients treated for pneumonia or other infections to realize that penicillin worked as advertised. The results were dramatic and easily documented. But a drug that lowered cholesterol? This was a long-term process. It would take years to see an effect, thousands of patients would need to be studied, and the data subjected to stringent statistical analysis before the medical world was convinced that this therapy was effective and safe.

Time also provided the answer to another plaguing question. In the research trials done before its use was widespread, lovastatin lowered cholesterol levels by only about thirty percent, not eighty or ninety percent. Would the inhibition of one enzyme, even the "rate-limiting" one, be enough to eventually save lives from heart attacks? In a climate of skepticism about the effectiveness and side effects of cholesterol-lowering drugs that had already been tried and failed, this was a legitimate question. No one was sure.

The wait was over when the results of the first large-scale research study arrived from northern Europe—the Scandinavian Simvastatin Survival Study (the 4S study). Researchers studied the effect of simvastatin, Merck's second statin discovery. This massive effort followed almost 4,500 patients with a history of a myocardial infarction or angina pectoris due to severe coronary artery atherosclerosis for a median of 5.4 years. The result: the average cholesterol level was reduced by twenty-five percent and the LDL particle levels reduced by an average of thirty-five percent. Of the patients in the placebo group, 258 (twelve percent) had died and only 182 (eight percent) in the simvastatin-treated group.

These results were not overwhelming but still significant. It did represent a thirty-three percent reduction in the risk of dying when patients took the simvastatin. The statisticians also told the researchers that the chance that this was just a random effect, and not a "real" effect of the drug, was less than one in a million. The drug worked. Other important findings of 4S were that simvastatin lowered the heart attack risk in women and people over the age of sixty. Compared to any other study done prior to 1994, the 4S study solidified the belief that cholesterol in the bloodstream was the first step toward a heart attack. Even in the 1980s, some experts still questioned this now-fundamental fact. They were rendered silent as the drug companies and cardiologists enrolled more and more heart attack patients into studies with eventually thousands of patients.

The more time that went by, the more the results proved worth the wait. The studies between 1980 and 1987 were unanimous: all of the new statin formulations not only reduced blood cholesterol levels significantly but also reduced the incidence of heart attacks and death.

After the data from 4S was known, a crucial next step took place—addressing whether statins could stop a first heart attack from occurring at all. Millions had elevated levels of blood cholesterol and LDL particles but no history of a heart attack. If statins could reduce the risk of a myocardial infarction in those people, that would be a magnificent achievement, proof that the Widowmaker could be completely thwarted. Prevention, not just treatment, would become real and available, not just an unfulfilled goal.

By 1986, there were fourteen trials conducted that all pointed in the same direction: the drugs worked and were safe. In over ninety thousand patients studied, for each reduction of LDL levels of 40 mg/dl, there was a two percent reduction of risk of death from atherosclerotic heart disease. Because the statins affect the cells of the liver, there was anxiety that liver side effects would be a problem, but the incidence was vanishingly low. Muscle aches and pains, usually mild, did happen to some patients, and very rarely statins caused major muscle breakdown. But the side effects on the liver and the muscle resolved within weeks when the medication was stopped.

In August 1987, the FDA approved Merck and Co.'s Mevacor (lovastatin) for use not only in patients with atherosclerotic heart disease but also those with elevated cholesterol and LDL levels only, use as "primary prevention" for people at risk but who had never had a cardiac problem. Now there was strong evidence not just from animals fed high cholesterol diets as Anichkov did in the 1910s; not just from Gofman's discovery in the 1950s that it was the LDL particle cholesterol that was doing the damage; not just from Brown and Goldstein's discovery in the 1970s of the LDL particle receptor and the metabolism of cholesterol; and not just from Endo's discovery of statins in the late 1970s. Here were data in real live people, those who had already had a major heart problem from cholesterol and also those at risk. Reducing cholesterol levels with medication saved lives and did so with great safety and minimal side effects.

Pursuit of the Widowmaker sped up considerably. Statistics of the number of deaths from heart attacks in the United States show that the death rate from this epidemic began decreasing steadily by the late 1980s. The release of Mevacor, followed in the next two decades by additional and more powerful statins, and these data are no coincidence. By the early 1990s, for the first time, therapy for acute care was now coupled with very effective treatments of prevention. The researchers of the Framingham Heart Study were gratified that their persistent work of epidemiology had gone far beyond just pointing out the causes of the Widowmaker's epidemic.

DAMAGED—BUT THE WIDOWMAKER CONTINUES

The epidemic was starting to decline, but people were still smoking, eating badly, getting fat and then acquiring diabetes, and not controlling their high blood pressure. In addition, there was still tremendous uncertainty about what level of blood cholesterol was optimal. More studies were conducted asking the very simple question: should the level of cholesterol be even lower than we thought? The answer was always the same, that lower is better, so the guidelines for treatment changed, urging higher doses of statins, especially in people with known atherosclerosis and those with a disease strongly associated with the development of arterial disease: diabetes, a disorder that has dramatically increased in the last three decades.

All the evidence confirmed that the warnings from old data should have been taken more seriously. Atherosclerosis was found in young men killed in the Korean War in the 1950s. Yet there was little recognition that atherosclerosis was a very long-term disease and that the risk was not just from a cholesterol level found in one blood test at a particular point in time. The risk was more about the years and years of chronic high cholesterol levels that increased the chances that more and more plaque would end up inside the heart's arteries.

The guidelines for more aggressive and widespread use of statins came slowly. It took several decades for some cardiologists to accept the "Lipid Hypothesis" of the cause of coronary artery disease. Throughout the last two decades of the twentieth century and the beginning of the next, most cardiologists were infatuated with their new tools to deal with the most severe problem of severely blocked coronary arteries—care in the Coronary Care Unit, angioplasty procedures, and bypass surgery. Giving patients statins in the clinic and checking blood cholesterol levels every six months just wasn't that exciting.

But the most confounding phenomenon in the statin story concerns the explosion of computer technology and the internet. One of the favorite topics for these internet "experts" is to not only doubt that statin drugs are effective but profess that they are dangerous and should never be taken by anyone. Perhaps these dire warnings about statins are a vestige of some of the problems and side effects of the earlier drugs used to lower cholesterol, but the vigor of these websites suggests there are some deep-seated conspiracy notions about the drug companies and doctors in general. People write about memory loss and dementia, severe muscle problems and kidney failure, and a risk of diabetes from the statins, yet there are no data (and these potential side effects have been looked at) to support these claims. For unknown reasons, the doubters don't question the benefits of lowering blood pressure with medication or lowering blood sugar with pills or insulin.

Another problem comes from the patients themselves. Noncompliance with all medications is a major problem that has been well-studied, and statins are no exception. The number of patients who actually continue to take statin drugs on a long-term basis is many fewer than it should be. Perhaps cost is a problem, although by 2015, all of the FDA-approved statins were generic drugs with a much lower cost than when they were first introduced, and medication insurance has little problem in helping with payment for the statins.

By the beginning of this century, the use of statins in millions of patients at risk or with a history of coronary artery disease was the standard of care to try to abort the Widowmaker's job. The data all point in the same direction, whether used chronically or in the acute setting after a heart attack, or in patients with diabetes, high blood pressure, and kidney problems. The statins work effectively in both men and women, and in all races. In the United States, there are seven different statins one can use and all are effective.

Akira Endo started his search for a safe drug to lower cholesterol levels in the blood, and P. Roy Vagelos and Alfred Alberts of Merck and Co. finished the project, an endeavor that for the first time made prevention an effective form of treatment for those at risk for the ravages of the heart attack. We humans owe a debt of gratitude to the "blind watchmaker" of evolution, who set up the life force that led the lowly fungi to produce "wonder drugs" for creatures much higher up the evolutionary chain (at least from the human perspective). Penicillin from fungi cured pneumonia, the first thrombolytic medication from bacteria stopped heart attacks, and now other fungi-based drugs are preventing millions from suffering heart attacks. There is a medical bounty from nature.

But there was still much more to do before the Widowmaker was truly in our grasp. A thirty percent reduction in death rates, like in the 4S study, is a great achievement, but that leaves seventy percent more to do. The Widowmaker's shop has not closed up yet. Heart attacks continued, and although many more were surviving, too many were dying suddenly within a few years of going home after their hospital stay. Another form of prevention was needed.

CHAPTER 22

KEEPING THE BEAT: THE PERSONAL DEFIBRILLATOR

So often the doctors send their patients back into battle defenseless against a new attack. Since they have not found a way to prevent me from starting the job, they have to settle for keeping me from finishing it.

Yet this new invention is like a shield and, if successful, could stop me in my tracks. At least for a lucky few.

A GRIM AWAKENING—SUMMER 1985

I never got used to the jolt to my brain—the loud ringing of a telephone that woke me up and instantly causes a surge of adrenaline and a fast heartbeat. I don't care how little sleep you think you need; three thirty a.m. is a tough time to be awakened, but being on call was a big part of my job.

"Hello," I said.

"Dr. Meshkov, this is one of the nurses in the ER at Abington. We have your patient Richard S. here."

"What happened? Is he okay?"

"He's dead. Can we send the death certificate for you to sign to your office tomorrow?"

I sighed and needed a moment before I could respond. "Tell me the story, please."

"His wife got up to go to the bathroom and realized he wasn't breathing. She called 911, and the EMTs gave him some meds in the field, but he was asystolic—no rhythm or blood pressure. We pronounced him dead when he got here. His wife said he had heart problems and that you were his cardiologist."

"Yes. He was a young guy with a cardiomyopathy. But he was doing great, no shortness of breath, taking his meds, and back at work. Damn it."

"I guess I know how you feel." The nurse waited a moment and then asked, "About the death certificate, okay for you to sign it?"

"Sure," I replied, and that was the end of the conversation . . .

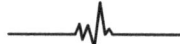

THE HOLOCAUST SURVIVOR'S TALE: COMING TO AMERICA AND SAVING LIVES

By the mid-1980s, there were many great advances in the diagnosis and treatment of coronary artery atherosclerosis and its complications of angina, heart attacks, and even congestive heart failure as a result of permanent damage from the Widowmaker. Even drugs for prevention were available. In addition, there was also progress in the treatment of abnormal heart rhythms after a heart attack, especially in the CCU. Progress was made on many fronts from many different sources worldwide. But there was still one huge terrible threat that had defied good prevention: Sudden Cardiac Death. A man who had barely survived his youth would soon try to deal with this tragedy that each year takes hundreds of thousands of Americans and untold millions worldwide.

Michel Mirowski was not his real name. Mordecai Frydman (1924-1990) knew that times were desperate for him and his family. The son of a well-to-do Jewish family living in the capital of Poland, Warsaw, in 1939, the fifteen-year-old Mordecai was told by his father that his new name was to become a Polish one—Mieczyslaw Mirowski. The change was an attempt to protect him from the virulent anti-Semitism that existed in Poland for many years and became ominous when the Nazi Wehrmacht invaded Poland in September of that year.

After years of great upheaval in the young man's life, including fleeing Poland, he finally attended medical school in Lyon, France, and ultimately settled on a medical career at Assaf Harofeh Medical Center in Israel. His mentor there, a Professor Heller, developed a condition that would have a huge impact on the young doctor's career. Dr. Heller unfortunately began having episodes of a malignant arrhythmia, ventricular tachycardia, and died suddenly at home with his family as witnesses. Mirowski was well aware that so many patients with heart disease, and especially those who had recovered from heart attacks but had badly scarred heart muscle, full of dead and damaged cells with erratic electrical properties, were dying suddenly as his mentor had, but couldn't something be done about this?

Mirowski also knew that rapid defibrillation could restore a normal heart rhythm and save lives when a malignant arrhythmia was identified in a hospital, especially in a Coronary Care Unit. But what if he could produce a defibrillator that was small and powerful enough to deliver a shock when necessary and could be put into place by a surgical procedure? Naturally, other cardiologists who had more experience with defibrillators, large devices weighing over thirty pounds, told him to forget this idea. It just couldn't be done, they warned.

Realizing that only an innovative medical center in the United States could provide him with the support he needed to pursue such a device, he took a position as the director of a Coronary Care Unit in Baltimore, at Sinai Hospital, an affiliate hospital of Johns Hopkins

School of Medicine. In 1969, Mirowski pitched his idea to Morton Mower MD (1933-), another cardiologist, and William Staewan, an engineer, both of whom recognized the significant difficulties with bringing this idea to fruition. This project would be an engineering challenge; the basic science was clear: if you could deliver a strong enough shock to a heart in ventricular fibrillation, the electricity would cause all of the heart cells to "depolarize" and, after a short recovery time, allow the normal pacemaker cells of the heart to start up again, restoring a normal cardiac rhythm and blood pressure. The Hopkins team needed to first decide how to deliver the shock inside the body of experimental animals. To be successful, a shock must pass strong electrical current between two metal sources, one generating the electricity and the second receiving it. In between the two ends of the electrical path is the heart, the target of the therapy. The procedure would be an electrocution that they hoped their subjects would survive.

Though they were ready to test on animals, there was still the question of the size of the charge. Mirowski and his two colleagues decided to try putting the electrical source connected to the battery in the vena cava, the large vein that carries blood into the heart, and the second electrode at the tip of the right ventricle. They created a path of electricity from outside of the heart, but inside a large vein, to the inside of the heart. But how much current was needed to actually defibrillate the heart using this internal pathway? Defibrillation done through the chest wall required up to 300 watts-seconds of energy, an amount that no small internal battery could come close to delivering even once, let alone remain able to recharge and deliver another shock at another time. Mirowski and Mower thought that an internal battery, with an electrical path to the heart much shorter, might require less than ten percent of the charge needed externally. But they needed to prove that they were right.

By the early 1970s, Mirowksi and Mower were publishing articles about their work in animals, but the skepticism by the major thought leaders in cardiac electrical disease was widespread. Even Bernard Lown of Harvard, the man who championed the use of external defibrillation, had his doubts. He questioned just about everything about internal defibrillators and published his thoughts in 1972. His concerns seemed quite legitimate. Wouldn't an internal shock damage the heart muscle, perhaps creating a scar, an iatrogenic heart attack? How could Mirowski and Mower be sure that their electrical "sensing" device, whatever that would be, could tell accurately when in fact a patient's heart rhythm was so abnormal that a shock was necessary?

Finally, there was a strong moral consideration. How would you test such a device to make sure it was working in an individual patient? You couldn't wait for them to have ventricular fibrillation on their own; would you then need to use a pacemaker wire to stimulate the heart and produce another iatrogenic problem, ventricular tachycardia or fibrillation, just to see if your machine was able to do its intended job? What were the ethics of that? A doctor was going to induce a deadly arrhythmia in someone when it wasn't present to begin with? What if the device didn't work? Would the patient survive a standard external shock to try to restore a normal heart rhythm? These were not simple problems with straightforward answers.

Undaunted, Mirowski and Mower continued their work. Using an external battery with a charge of less than 20 watts-seconds, they were able to correct ventricular fibrillation in animals, using their system connecting the two poles of the battery to an electrode wrapped around a catheter in the vena cava and an electrode inside the right ventricle. They even made a short film of their successful experiment in a dog, showing at first the dog standing normally, collapsing, being shocked, and standing up again after a second shock. So they knew much smaller energy was needed to do the job if the electrical path through the heart was much shorter, at least in dogs.

But how to try this out in humans and do the experiments ethically? Mirowksi and Mower finally thought of an idea that might work. When patients undergo coronary artery bypass graft surgery or a valve replacement operation, the heart is shocked to get it to stop completely while the patient's circulation is replaced by the heart-lung machine. When the surgery is over, the heart, needless to say, needs to be restarted. A tiny defibrillator is used to shock the heart as it is taken off the heart-lung machine, and most of the time, it starts right up. This is a major miracle, but it does occur easily unless the heart muscle was severely damaged prior to the surgery. However, sometimes when the defibrillation is completed, the heart will start to beat but will be in ventricular fibrillation. This requires an immediate second shock to be delivered and fortunately is also successful most of the time in restoring normal cardiac function. This random occurrence of ventricular fibrillation of the heart of a patient coming off the heart-lung machine circulatory support was the opportunity Mirowski and Mower were looking for.

The pair convinced their cardiac surgeons to participate in a study, experiments during which electrodes were placed into the superior vena cava and the apex of the right ventricle in humans, just like they had done in animals. Then if some of these people went into ventricular fibrillation after their heart-lung machine time, the Mirowski-Mower electrical circuit could spring into action, again using an external battery source. If their contraption failed, the surgeon would very quickly use the standard defibrillator to get the heart restarted. Sure enough, eleven patients developed ventricular fibrillation. In nine of eleven, the Mirowski-Mower electrical circuit worked, using only 5 to 15 watt-seconds of electrical energy. By 1973, the Sinai collaborators had a proof of concept in humans.

Now was the time to address Bernard Lown's unanswered questions. The abnormal cardiac rhythm detection problem was still unconquered, but the electrical engineers came to the rescue, developing very sophisticated electrodes that could detect changes in the electrical signal coming from the heart, focusing on the heart rate. Next, the concern over damage of a shock to the heart muscle turned out to be a minor issue as the very small amount of cell damage was completely tolerated by the heart. Two down, one to go.

Bernard Lown's final concern about testing, that proper function of a device in a human being could only be determined by inducing ventricular fibrillation and then shocking the heart back to normal, was still a major obstacle. The safety of this iatrogenic cardiac arrhythmia did not come from Mirowski and Mower but from other cardiac specialists from a new subspecialty of the field, the electrophysiologists who were regularly inducing ventricular arrhythmias with special electrode pacemaker wires in their laboratories. They knew from animal experiments that if ventricular arrhythmias were corrected by a shock within seconds, the animal would survive. Human hearts had the same response.

With these questions addressed, the team turned to the final challenge, which proved the most daunting—the engineering design of the device. Mirowski and Mower needed a small, very powerful, and long-lasting battery. The battery also needed to be insulated enough so that external electricity sources, such as from a microwave oven or surgical electrical tools, would not mess up the circuitry with signals that were not from the heart. The Sinai cardiologists found a small battery company in Pittsburgh, Pennsylvania, and the owner of Medrad, Stephen Heilman began work on the battery problem. Another source of help came from Honeywell in Horsham, Pennsylvania, where experts were able to produce a battery that delivered only a maximum of 25 watt-seconds of energy with each discharge. But would it work as needed?

PROOF—LIVES SAVED

By the late 1970s, Mirowski and Mower were finally ready, but they needed the right subject to test it. They and their colleagues had produced a three-part device—a lithium-powered battery weighing 250 grams, slightly more than half a pound, sized at 150 ml (about five ounces), an intravascular catheter to place into the superior vena cava, and a rectangular electrode tip to be placed at the tip of the right ventricle. Who would be the first human being to receive this potentially life-saving device?

Mirowski and Mower had developed some allies in the medical world, including Roger Winkle MD, an electrophysiology cardiologist from Stanford. In 1980, Winkle had a patient he thought was perfect for the brand new "automatic implantable cardioverter defibrillator"— the "AICD." She was a fifty-seven-year-old woman who had had a previous myocardial infarction and survived a cardiac arrest but was doing poorly on medication to try to suppress future arrhythmias. The lady traveled to Maryland, and on February 4, 1980, Mirowski and Mower, with the great help of several cardiac surgeons, implanted their device at The Johns Hopkins Hospital in Baltimore. The vena cava electrode catheter was inserted through a jugular vein in the neck and positioned with the fluoroscope. The right ventricular lead needed to be sutured to the external wall of the heart and then both electrodes "tunneled" under the skin to connect to the battery pack placed into the upper abdomen. This was major surgery, opening up both the chest wall and the abdomen, but the skilled surgeons at Hopkins did their job smoothly, and the woman did very well afterward.

Soon the team was ready for more, and it was not long before word got out of their accomplishments. Within a few months, Mirowski and Mower did two more implants, one in a sixteen-year-old boy with malignant arrhythmias of unknown cause and in a forty-three-year-old man with heart muscle disease, a cardiomyopathy. Both procedures and the resulting impact were successes. The three cases were summarized in a publication in the *New England Journal of Medicine* in August 1980. The patients had a total of seven episodes of ventricular tachycardia and "flutter-fibrillation," both life-threatening arrhythmias. In six out of seven, the AICD restored a normal heart rhythm after only one shock. In the one situation where the AICD failed, external shock was quickly used and was successful.

Mirowski and Mower were cautiously optimistic, realizing that their work was still in its infancy and needed more testing. But what about those patients with little hope from anything else? Mirowski and Mower did point out that there was "increasing ability to identify patients at high risk," and the AICD might prove very useful in those people. Roger Winkle implanted a device at Stanford in 1982, and Mirowski went to national meetings to recruit electrophysiologists to enroll patients into clinical trials of his AICD.[143] Most of the patients had severe coronary artery disease and often-intractable symptoms of angina and heart failure, in spite of having had coronary artery bypass graft surgery. Although the surgery was daunting, the majority of patients did well, and the risk seemed worth it to try to abort a fatal disease.

By 1985, eight hundred devices had been implanted worldwide, and the Food and Drug Administration saw enough data to approve the AICD for general use; however, what was very unclear was who actually needed the AICD. The insurance companies and Medicare were skeptical about the widespread use of the new machine and insisted on more information before agreeing to pay for the device. In addition to the uncertainty of which patients would have their lives saved, the AICD batteries lasted only a few years, and even less if the device was discharging frequently. That meant the patient would require surgery again and another bill for insurance to pay.

Despite these ongoing uncertainties, the demand kept increasing as more people were surviving the initial trauma of the Widowmaker's work, left with badly scarred hearts but enough strength to go on with their lives. Ambulatory monitoring of the heart rhythm, spearheaded by the invention of a biophysicist named Norman Holter PhD (1914-1983), could determine if people were having short episodes of dangerous arrhythmias that lasted only seconds and often caused no symptoms. By the late 1970s, it was clear that these asymptomatic arrhythmias were often harbingers of major events in those with damaged left ventricles.

---

143 At one of those meetings, Mirowski met my friend and medical school classmate Peter Kowey MD. Peter and his colleagues were the third group to implant an AICD in the world and the first in the Philadelphia area, home to six medical schools at the time. Peter is a world authority on arrhythmia treatment.

When Mirowski and Mower put in their first AICD in 1980, there was already a major effort to treat malignant arrhythmias with medications, but Roger Winkle, after his first AICD procedure had succeeded, was convinced that the AICD was a better long-term option. From 1982 to 1989, he and his colleagues put in 270 of the devices. Eighty percent of the patients had severe coronary artery blockages and an average left ventricular ejection fraction of thirty-four percent, far below the normal range of fifty-five to sixty percent. Over an average of five years after the device was inserted, just short of sixty percent of the patients had received a shock, a feeling usually described by patients as being "kicked in the chest by horse," but a jolt that saved their lives. Those with the AICD implants, compared to similar people who had not gotten the device, had only an eight percent chance of dying over the course of the study. Just over a quarter of the patients without the device, twenty-six percent, had died. The drumbeat for more widespread use of the AICD was getting louder and louder.

But adding to the difficulty of knowing who really needed this surgery and who did not—after all, forty percent of Winkle's patients never received a shock, and some of the warts of the AICD and the surgery began to surface. A few patients died shortly after the major surgical procedure. Sometimes the device and the surgical pocket into which it was placed would get infected, forcing removal of the battery pack and all of the electrodes, followed by treatment with antibiotics for weeks.

Despite the fact that in time the technique was getting much better,[144] the controversy persisted. The insurance companies were still balking at paying for a procedure that they considered experimental. By the mid-1980s, Mirowski had become a celebrity in the medical

---

144   The battery pack had gotten small enough that it could be implanted into a small pocket in the chest wall rather than into the upper abdomen. The electrodes used to create the path for the shock could be implanted through veins in the chest and arm and no longer needed to be attached to the outside of the heart in most cases.

world and was asked to speak at conferences all over the Western world. He taught himself to speak many different languages, with one exception—German. Just as the real controversy heated up regarding who should or should not receive an AICD, Michel Mirowksi fell ill with a blood cancer and died in 1990. But he had left his mark. It was now up to others to try to sort out the future of the AICD.

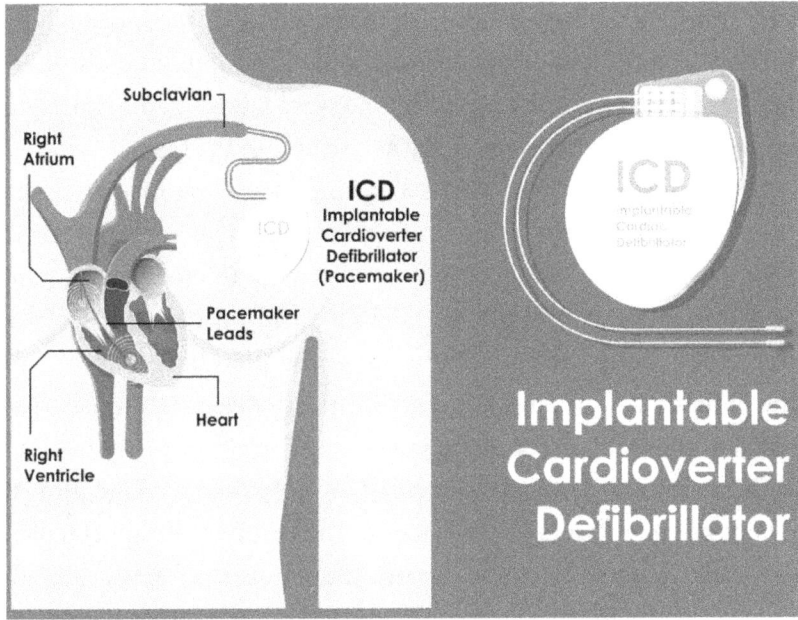

Figure 28. Technique of implantation of a defibrillator (device under the skin), leads entering the subclavian vein and ending up in the right atrium and right ventricle. (Copyright Shutterstock)

LOOKING AT LARGE NUMBERS—AGAIN

The key to AICD's future lay in the ability to answer one vital question: how do you determine a bad heart from a good one after a heart attack? The solution came from stepping back from the absorbing fascination with arrhythmias and how to stop them. In hindsight, the studies that needed to be done were not complicated intellectual endeavors. Clearly, the worse the heart attack, the worse the chances for long-term survival, and about thirty percent of the time, the death would come suddenly from a malignant arrhythmia. All that remained was to clarify what marker would indicate how compromised the heart had become.

The answer was that crucial number, the ejection fraction of the left ventricle, the LVEF. When that number drops to thirty-five percent or less, the research was clear: people did much worse over time. Fortunately, by the 1980s, the ejection fraction could be measured accurately by nuclear imaging techniques and also by a new method, echocardiography, sound wave images of the heart and left ventricle. All that remained was to put it to the test.

Arthur Moss MD (1931-2018), a longtime leader in arrhythmia research from the University of Rochester in New York, proposed a simple study: take a group of people with an ejection fraction of less than thirty-five percent and give half of them AICDs, the treatment group, and not the others, the placebo group. All of the patients had to have a history of ventricular arrhythmias that could not be suppressed during their electrophysiology studies and with medication. A total of thirty-two hospitals enrolled almost two hundred patients into the study. The results were spectacular, especially for treating sudden death. There were twenty-six cardiac-related deaths in the placebo group and only eleven in the AICD group, a drop of over fifty percent. This one study, the MADIT, the acronym for "Multicenter Automatic Defibrillator Implantation Trial," proved the efficacy of the AICD in a group of very sick people, making a major dent in sudden deaths. But it was still a small study of two hundred people.

More data were needed, and two new studies addressed whether AICD was more effective than anti-arrhythmic medication. First, a group of electrophysiologists, led by Alfred Buxton MD of the University of Pennsylvania, set up The Multicenter Unsustained Ventricular Tachycardia Trial (MUUST). MUUST enrolled a much larger number of people than MADIT—704 patients. The results were reported in 1999. More people who received the AICD survived, and the medication treatment group had no reduction in the chance of dying from a ventricular arrhythmia. Next Arthur Moss organized an even larger study, MADIT-II, that enrolled over 1,200 people and followed them for an average of four years. Remembering that these were people with bad hearts, just short of eighty-six percent of the AICD recipients were alive, as opposed to eighty-one percent of the patients treated with standard cardiac medications appropriate for their condition.

These results in such a large trial might not seem that impressive at first glance, but one must consider the disparate risks after a heart attack. The two threats to life after a major heart attack are the malignant arrhythmias, as well as the further weakening of the heart muscle and the development of congestive heart failure, a disease with a very high mortality rate over years. The AICD had no effect on this second problem, a condition that more modern medication is improving but not eliminating. But now three studies showed that the sudden death problem was much less common in the people who received Michel Mirowski's AICD.

Because of the powerful results from these studies, the number of AICD implantations rose significantly, and they started to be used in not just patients with coronary artery disease, heart attacks, and other cardiac conditions but not without problems.[145] As happens with almost all new drugs or devices, the more that are done, the more complications occur. With larger numbers, the chances of seeing a problem that was either not seen at all or very rarely increases,

---

145 AICDs reduce the risk of sudden death in several structural and electrical problems of the heart, usually inherited disorders such as hypertrophic cardiomyopathy. They have also been used widely in patients who have poor heart muscle function of uncertain cause, called a "non-ischemic cardiomyopathy," disease not due to coronary artery atherosclerosis and heart attacks. These people are also at high risk for sudden death if their ejection fraction is less than thirty-five percent, just like my patient Richard was in 1985. Currently, there is some controversy as to whether or not AICDs are as effective in those with a non-ischemic cardiomyopathy than those with damaged hearts from coronary artery disease and heart attacks.

and the AICD was no different. Infection in the surgical site around an AICD can be a major problem. There is now a small cadre of electrophysiologists who are known for their expertise in removing the stubborn infected AICD electrodes, using unique tools to cut the electrodes and free them from the spots tightly embedded in the heart muscle. Recently, AICDs have been produced with coatings of antibiotics to try to decrease the chances of infections.

There are other problems with the ACIDs that persist. First the sensors of the heart rate cannot determine if a rapid heartbeat is from the ventricle, and thus a shock appropriate, or from the left atrium, one the upper chambers of the heart. Usually rapid heart rates from the atrium are from a common disorder called atrial fibrillation. If the rate is fast, the AICD will respond with a shock, a discharge not usually necessary to treat atrial fibrillation, but a shock that will stun the patient and also use up battery charge.

The second, and perhaps less solvable, problem are the ethical dilemmas posed by the AICD in an ever-aging, condition-laden population. Is the AICD indicated in someone who is ninety-three years old and found to have a low ejection fraction? Should a patient with advanced cancer receive an AICD? What about someone who develops end-stage congestive heart failure, a situation where the malignant arrhythmias may become very common, causing multiple powerful shocks to the chest in a dying patient? There have been situations in which patients or their families have asked that the AICD be disabled, allowing someone to die peacefully.

In spite of its flaws, the AICD has given hope for those with bad hearts who are at risk for a sudden demise, a death due to a cardiac electrical disturbance that can be aborted with a shock delivered within seconds. Sudden Cardiac Death remains a huge problem, claiming an estimated 300,000 to 500,000 human beings in the United States each year and many more worldwide. Many of these people never knew that they had a heart problem or were not informed of their risk. Much more progress needs to be made before the sudden death issue is resolved, but there is at least now a tool that works.

Michel Mirowski was a medical-scientist whose idea and work will stand the test of time. The AICD stimulated so much more interest, ideas, and research into the cause and treatment of the most feared residua of the work of the Widowmaker. He took a fundamental truth, that the heart could be shocked back to life, and created a device that was a technologic tour-de-force. A modern version of the Frankenstein story has come true.

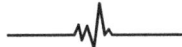

AICD EPILOGUE

... Richard had come to see about a year before his sudden death. He was very short of breath, and his tests showed that the function of his left ventricle was very poor, with an ejection fraction of about twenty-five percent, much less than the fifty to sixty percent normal range. Richard had congestive heart failure. A cardiac catheterization showed that he had an unknown disease of his heart muscle and that the muscle problem was not due to atherosclerosis and previous heart attacks, which would have been unusual in a twenty-seven-year-old man.

I did what I could by starting him on medication to get the fluid out of his lungs and two medications that had just recently been proven to improve the prognosis in people like Richard, beta-blockers and angiotensin-converting enzyme inhibitors. He was a great patient, a thin quiet man who took his meds and soon began feeling better. He had a wife and two small children. My medicines were able to dramatically help one part of the problem with severe heart muscle disease, the shortness of breath. But the other part of the risk was much more challenging in the mid-1980s for most cardiologists: trying to prevent Sudden Cardiac Death.

I can still see his face and hear his voice even after all these years. I was angry; there was in fact a treatment that might have saved Richard's life, but at the time, there were no agreed-upon reasons to implant an AICD and, worse, no insurance coverage for someone who had never had a previous cardiac arrest or documented malignant arrhythmia. His death still weighs on me.

But many others have been saved since then, and many more in the future will also benefit. Great advances had arrived by the early 1990s. But there was still a huge "blindspot" in the cardiology world, a negligence that impacted just over fifty percent of the human beings on earth.

CHAPTER 23

SHATTERING THE THIRD SHIBBOLETH: HEART DISEASE IN WOMEN

There is a theory that one cannot see what one does not know exists. Whether this is truth or fiction, the willingness of doctors to be blind to what appears in front of them serves me well.

In this way, half my victims remain invisible.

STAT TO THE OR: MY LADY IS IN TROUBLE

My day was busy enough. I didn't recognize the four-digit extension number on the text message. I called back in just a few seconds. "Dr. Meshkov, we need you STAT in the OR." You might think as a cardiologist this was not an uncommon request, but for many of us, it actually is, especially at a large academic medical center with all kinds of other specialists on site.

"What? Which OR and what's going on?" I asked.

"Your patient, Ms. J in OR #4, is having a problem, and the anesthesiologist wants you up here right away."

"Okay, but what problem?"

"She's getting her kidney transplant today, and she went into rapid atrial fibrillation. The anesthesiologist wants to cancel the surgery."

"That's nuts. I'm running up there right now. I know the transplant was scheduled for today."

My patient Carla was in her late thirties, and I had first seen her when she had a seemingly shocking event for a young woman: a myocardial infarction at age thirty-three. The heart attack damaged the bottom wall of her heart, the inferior wall, and also caused some leaking in her heart valve, the mitral valve, on the left side of her heart. A few years after the heart attack, she developed kidney failure from high blood pressure and started dialysis.

We worked together to create a plan for a kidney transplant so she could live a long life. I needed to fight with the transplant surgeon to convince him that her heart was strong enough to survive the surgery and get her on powerful immunosuppressive medications to prevent the rejection of the kidney she was going to receive from her sister. And after years of persistence to get her to that point, it was all going to be wiped away. But not if I had anything to say about it.

I entered the OR and saw the frantic anesthesiologist yelling that they were going to stop the anesthetic and wake Carla up. I took a deep breath and said, "You're not going to do that . . ."

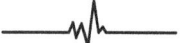

BIAS: A PARTICULAR TENDENCY, TREND, INCLINATION, FEELING, OR OPINION, ESPECIALLY ONE THAT IS PRECONCEIVED OR UNREASONED

—Dictionary.com

Atlanta, Georgia 1958

When Nanette Wenger MD (1930-) moved to Atlanta in the late 1950s, there was culture shock for a young doctor coming from New York City. She took the position as the Chief of Cardiology at Grady

Memorial Hospital, the large public hospital and major teaching center at Emory University School of Medicine. This was the American South, and there she soon noticed that in the treatment of patients the traditions of Jim Crow were still very active.

Wenger was taken aback by these norms at her hospital, where she discovered that white patients and nurses were all addressed as "Mr.," "Miss," or "Mrs." African Americans were all called by their first names only. Hospital charts all had letter designations clearly attached to the front of them—"W" or "C" right next to the patient's name. There were even separate blood banks for black and white patients. She expressed her frustration in an interview in 2011: "You come with a set of core values. I had never lived in the segregated South. I couldn't accept people not being treated as equals."

Wenger was from a family of Jewish-Russian immigrants and grew up in New York, a childhood full of educational opportunities and culture, and her parents raised their children to believe that they could become anything they wanted if they were willing to work for it. After graduating from Hunter College in Manhattan, she gained acceptance to Harvard Medical School, a great accomplishment in any age but especially for a woman in the early 1950s. When she graduated in 1954, her class was only the sixth class at Harvard to have female graduates. That year was the end of a ten-year probationary time period that Harvard had established to see if women could actually thrive at the university.

Soon, her career would pull her southward. After training at Mt. Sinai Hospital in New York, captivated by cardiology and the explosion of new procedures available, she and her husband, also a physician, decided to move to Emory and Georgia. Wenger fell in love with her work at Grady Memorial; she saw it as a "chance to take the physiology I learned in my training and see it play out at the bedside." She became a consummate physician and educator of her younger colleagues. Her patients at Grady were often poor, but they were very willing to participate in the research and teaching at the medical school hospital. Though she was often referred to as "lady doc" or "sweetie," she viewed these as terms of admiration and respect. Even given her growing prestige, she was often asked by the wives in their Atlanta social circles, "Why are you working?" After all, her husband was a successful doctor. It was the 1960s.

In numerous ways, Wenger began changing the culture at Grady. Following the lead of Samuel Levine and Bernard Lown at Harvard, she got patients out of bed after their heart attacks, much to the consternation of many of her colleagues. She pushed the envelope even further by starting an exercise program for heart attack patients, the first cardiac rehabilitation treatments in the world. These were radical ideas for the 1960s, a time for many culture-shattering concepts.

Besides the use of psychedelic drugs, marihuana, rock music, long hair, bell bottom pants, Woodstock, and protests against America's war in Vietnam, there were other new shifts in Western culture; one of these changes was to have an impact on women and their hearts. In 1968, Phillip Morris used "You've come a long way, baby!" to publicize its new cigarettes—Virginia Slims, made specifically for the smaller hands of most women. The implication was that here was one example of how a woman could distinguish herself from the constraints of previous eras: by smoking Virginia Slims.

Though the regulators were becoming wise to the effects of cigarette smoking, the rising number of women smokers had already begun. After being forced to stop advertising on television in 1970, the Virginia Slims campaign became entrenched in magazine and newspaper advertising, even becoming the major sponsor of women's professional tennis, where free cigarette samples were given away at the tournaments. By the 1990s, the ad campaign had changed the slogan to "It's a woman thing," and it was no coincidence that the incidence of coronary artery disease in women was rising.

In addition to the cultural bias against black people in the South, Nanette Wenger was also upset about the medical bias she saw affecting women. She witnessed the fact that the coronary artery disease epidemic was spreading to women as well. Why did no one else notice that atherosclerosis and coronary heart disease could also afflict women? Were there more medical shibboleths to topple? This was going to be a difficult battle.

While bias often hinders our thinking, medical students are taught that bias can be valuable in specific situations. Many diseases afflict certain ethnic groups more than others, especially genetic diseases. For example, sickle cell anemia is a disease of those of African descent, Tay-Sachs disease (a deadly neurologic disorder in children) is a disorder of Jewish people, and hemochromatosis, a chronic liver and heart disease, is a problem in those of Northern European ancestry. These are helpful facts to know in order to establish a diagnosis and treatment. These taught-biases can apply to gender as well; autoimmune diseases like rheumatoid arthritis are much more common in women than men. But for generations, students were taught that the epidemic of coronary artery disease and heart attacks was a disease of men.

The bias against women having coronary artery disease went back many decades. By the 1930s, it was clear that the prevalence of coronary artery disease was rapidly increasing in the United States. Two New York City heart specialists saw many, many patients with chest pain and thought that they were very good at picking out those people who had coronary artery disease and those whose chest pain was due to something else. Ernst Boas MD (1891-1935) and Hyman Levy MD (1906-1998) had a large cardiology practice in Manhattan. In the days when esteemed medical journals published descriptive accounts of practice experience, in 1936, the *Journal of the American Medical Association* published Boas and Levy's office practice findings in almost four thousand patients over seven years. Boas and Levy were convinced that although angina pectoris was common, "it is often overlooked again and again in daily practice and many mistaken diagnoses result." But the two cardiologists were convinced that coronary artery disease was overwhelmingly a male problem. Clearly, they themselves were not among those making mistakes, they thought.

Ironically, the patients they saw confirmed this bias. In the 2,135 men they saw, they made a diagnosis of coronary atherosclerosis in just short of fifty percent, based on what they considered to be a typical history of cardiac chest pain and abnormalities on the electrocardiogram consistent with a previous heart attack or chronic myocardial ischemia, lack of blood flow. In their female patients, 1,672 to be exact, a diagnosis of coronary artery atherosclerosis was made in only 10.1 percent, based on their assessment of the women's description of their symptoms, usually when their symptoms were identical to the chest pain described by men. They also noted that almost all of the women who they felt did have coronary artery disease had two suspected risk factors for atherosclerosis, diabetes and hypertension (relationships later confirmed in the Framingham Heart Study in both women and men). Boss and Levy had no appreciation of the possibility that the symptoms of coronary artery disease might be *different* in women than in men or that the different symptoms might be much more common in women than the typical symptoms of men.

The cardiologists also went on to describe some of the symptoms in those women who they felt had chest pain not due to heart disease. Their description seems medieval today: "First of all the personality of the patient gives a clue. Women with benign precordial chest pain are usually anxious and high strung, in contrast to the stolidity so often encountered in men with coronary artery disease. The symptoms are very prone to follow emotional or economic disturbances at home, such as the illness of a child, marital difficulties or financial stress." We will never know how many of the women that Boas and Levy saw did have coronary artery disease and went on to have heart attacks or die from atherosclerosis. For decades, the opinions of cardiologists closely followed the conclusions of Boas and Levy. While for some time it was true that more men had coronary artery disease than women, that did not mean that women were immune from the increasing scourge.

It is not a surprise where the term Widowmaker came from. When millions of American men returned from World War II as meat-eaters and cigarette smokers (and to a lesser degree women), the firm conviction that coronary atherosclerosis was largely gender-specific was taught to generations of medical students. It was another milieu of thought and bias that Nanette Wenger was going to try to destroy.

DESTROYING THE BIAS

Wenger was struck by the fact that very few women were included in studies done on the prevalence of coronary heart disease. William Heberden's original report on angina in the early nineteenth century included only three women in his analysis of one hundred cases! There hadn't been much progress in studying females in over 150 years. This needed to change, and the impetus came from that study in Massachusetts, the Framingham Heart Study.

By the mid-1980s, the Framingham people had twenty-six years of follow-up on both the men and women in their study. In the over five thousand people they had been studying, there were 1,240 deaths from coronary heart disease. Although 752 (sixty percent) were men, 488 (forty percent) were women. Boas and Levy would have been shocked. The Framingham doctors concluded that coronary heart disease was a "major force" in death and disability in both sexes.

There were significant differences between the men and the women in Framingham data. The men had a higher incidence of heart attacks and the women a higher incidence of angina, chest pain from coronary artery disease not complicated by a myocardial infarction. But the women also had a higher chance of having a myocardial infarction detected on the electrocardiogram alone, that is a silent heart attack. To the researchers, it was evident that women had a sharp rise in the incidence of coronary artery disease as they aged, an increase much greater than that seen in the men. There was a gap of about ten years between the men and women, a time period after the age of fifty-five where the women would catch up to men in their chance of dying from atherosclerosis. The obvious but unanswered question was whether or not this phenomenon was due to menopause and lack of the possible protective effect of estrogen against atherosclerosis in the women.

Throughout the 1980s, Wenger and by then others did the difficult and often tedious work of pouring through epidemiologic data of death rates, causes of death and disability, the use of cardiac tests and treatments, and the response to medication or surgery for coronary artery disease, comparing the numbers in women versus men. The results were startling.

To help organize and publicize the torrent of information being synthesized, the National Heart Blood and Lung Institute in 1992 sponsored an invited conference entitled "Cardiovascular Health and Disease in Women." Nanette Wenger was an interested participant. This groundbreaking meeting presented data indicating that 2.5 million women were hospitalized each year in the United States for cardiovascular illness and that there were 500,000 deaths annually in women, fifty percent of the deaths from coronary heart disease.

The conference had many other important data to report to the medical world. The participants pointed out how incomplete the known data were at that time; little was known about the best way to diagnose and treat coronary atherosclerosis in women, and whether or not the same treatments, either medication, surgery, or angioplasty, were as helpful in women as in men. Prevention in women was another huge black hole of knowledge. One of the things that was known was that the use of cigarettes in men had decreased much more than the use in women in the twenty-five years prior to 1992. Was the rise in women's incidence of coronary artery disease the "Virginia Slims effect"? It likely was an important one, but in addition, other risk factors for coronary artery disease were also on the rise, especially after menopause.

There were other considerations. People were just living longer, and with age came more high blood pressure, obesity, inactivity, diabetes, and "the metabolic syndrome," a collection of risk factors including increased waist size, low levels of HDL cholesterol and high levels of triglycerides in the blood, diabetes, and high blood pressure. After menopause, even fat distribution in women changes; it settles more in the abdomen than in the hips, creating "android" fat distribution, another previously unrecognized risk factor for coronary artery disease. The prevalence of these problems was not limited to the older women, however; younger people were also affected. Perhaps it was no wonder that the Widowmaker was indeed earning another name as "Women's Affliction."

In spite of these changes in risk factor prevalence, doctors just weren't informed very well or they just stuck to the old notions. In spite of epidemiologic data from the three decades, as late as 2012, a survey indicated that only a small percentage of physicians knew that the risk of death from cardiac disease was greater in women than in men. Only one-third of women remembered discussing the risk of heart disease with their family doctor. As a group, women were much more worried about the risk of breast cancer than a heart attack.

Additional surprising findings were uncovered. One was that women as a group underwent less intensive evaluation for chest pain; they were less likely to have stress tests done and fewer cardiac catheterizations, angioplasty, and coronary artery bypass graft procedures than men. These differences were in spite of the fact that women were twice as likely as men to come to a hospital for evaluation of chest pain. Another was that the most common test to diagnose coronary artery disease, the exercise stress test, was less accurate in women. Their electrocardiograms were often different from the patterns seen in men, making interpretation after exercise more prone to false positives, that is an electrocardiogram that suggests coronary artery blockage is present but then not seen at the time of a cardiac catheterization. Imaging with nuclear isotopes was more often necessary in women to clear up the uncertainty about the EKG changes.

There were other differences that doctors needed to learn. Some of the symptoms in women were unique, causing a major problem for most doctors, just like the differences noted by Boas and Levy in the 1930s. Before coming to a hospital with chest pain, women often reported "prodrome"[146] symptoms weeks before, complaints of fatigue, change in sleep patterns, shortness of breath, and often fleeting chest pain very different from that reported by many men. When they were having a heart attack, however, they complained just as the men did of severe chest pain. Although women were coming to the emergency rooms more often than men, the women with confirmed heart attacks were actually waiting longer than men to seek care. That meant that if they were having a major heart attack, the ST segment elevation on the electrocardiogram kind, the one with a sudden blood clot occluding a major coronary artery, that even when they were given the thrombolytic drugs, the "clot busters," more damage had already occurred than if they had come for treatment hours earlier.

The risks of doctors not appreciating these disparities could be dire. Women had a higher rate of death after a major heart attack than men, and a higher death rate also after angioplasty or coronary artery bypass graft surgery, in spite of the fact that drugs like aspirin appeared to be working as well in women as in men. Particularly in older women, often their coronary artery blockages were more severe and widespread than in men. Discouraging results to be sure. In addition, the women who needed bypass graft surgery more often required emergency surgery, which always carried higher risk of not surviving the procedure. Were their doctors referring them for advanced care later than they would men? If so, why? Was the old Boas and Levy bias in the minds of their doctors? Clearly angina pectoris was not a benign disease in women.

The results in women after angioplasty were also different; they were twice as likely to have recurrent or persistent chest pain than

---

146   An early symptom indicating the onset of a disease, such as nasal congestion prior to a viral illness.

men after a year. Their arteries are usually smaller in diameter than men, and the balloon angioplasties of the 1980s and early 1990s had an almost fifty percent restenosis rate in women, a problem that decreased only with development of stents inserted after angioplasty and the discovery that taking two anti-platelet drugs together after the procedure reduced this restenosis problem dramatically in both women and men.

Lastly, even after a heart attack and treatment, women were less likely to go to a program like Dr. Wenger's at Grady, outpatient cardiac rehabilitation. Was this due to family commitments or was the exercise just not being recommended to the women? There were many unanswered questions, but the tide was turning.

By the early 1990s, the academic cardiology world had awoken to these major differences between the genders. Again, the National Heart and Blood Institute came forward with the funds to continue more research—the Women's Ischemia Syndrome Evaluation study (WISE). Led by two women who were to become Wenger's collaborators and also international stars in women's heart health, Leslee Shaw PhD and C. Noel Bairey Merz MD, with the input of Carl Pepine MD, already renowned in cardiology circles, the WISE study wanted more detailed information about what happens when women are evaluated for chest pain. Their findings were surprising.

Even more differences between the genders were discovered. The study involved four medical centers around the United States and recruited slightly more than nine hundred women with chest pain, 888 of whom underwent the "gold standard" test, coronary angiography. To the shock of the investigators, less than forty percent of the women had obstructive coronary artery disease, that is a blockage that was greater than fifty percent of the diameter of the artery. But it had always been assumed that before chest pain could result, a coronary artery needed to have at least half of its lumen obstructed by cholesterol plaque. The angina from atherosclerosis was happening to be sure, but only in less than half of the women studied.

What was going on in these other women? A foundational shibboleth about angina was about to be destroyed. There was much more going inside of these women's coronary arteries than just plaque buildup. Their heart arteries were malfunctioning at a cellular level, at the level of small blood vessels, proven by studies that obtained samples of blood coming from the veins of the heart, showing that there was a buildup of lactic acid in the heart. Lactic acid is what makes our muscles ache after strenuous exercise; its presence in the veins of the heart means there was ischemia causing the chest pain in these hearts but ischemia not just due to plaque buildup. WISE resurrected a phenomenon that had been seen on occasion previously; some patients had severe chest pain, just like those with atherosclerosis seen on an angiogram, but without any major blockages seen in their coronary arteries when they underwent an angiogram.

But this problem, usually seen in women, was felt to be rare—until now. Because no one understood the pathology of the chest pain, this disease was called "Syndrome X" (clearly no one was clever enough to think of a better name). Until WISE, no one could have imagined that Syndrome X was so common. To this day, the understanding of women with chest pain and no obstructive coronary artery disease is still poor.

Hopefully, the attention given to the special characteristics of women and their hearts has shredded the bias that existed for decades, a belief that only began to unravel in the 1980s. The persistent work of Nanette Wenger and others revealed the truth: coronary artery disease does affect women just as often if not more often than men and with the population aging will become even more prevalent in the future.

Women are indeed different from men but in many ways the same when it comes to chest pain and coronary artery disease, and doctors should have known that many years ago. More insight into what happens inside of the heart's arteries in women will be invaluable and perhaps generate more treatment options. The complex biology of the heart's arteries needed to be unraveled. Heart attacks were caused by much more than just "rusty pipes" from cholesterol buildup.

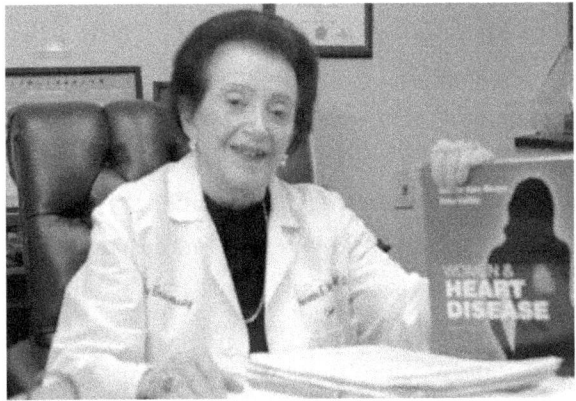

Figure 29. Nanette Wenger MD, pioneering cardiologist exploring women and heart disease. (Courtesy of Embraceofaging.com)

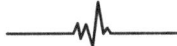

CALMING THE STORM

... The anesthesiologist was understandably agitated. "She's in rapid atrial fibrillation. We need to slow her heart rate down immediately."

I didn't say anything for about thirty seconds. The heart monitor showed that she was in atrial fibrillation with a heart rate of about 130-150 beats a minute, far above the normal range of sixty to one hundred, but her blood pressure was normal and so was the oxygen content of her blood. Two of her three "vital signs" were completely normal. This problem could be handled.

While I respected the anesthesiologist for being worried, as the cardiologist, I knew Carla's heart rate could be managed. "What if we give her some intravenous diltiazem to slow her heart rate? If that doesn't work, we'll try other medications. By the way, how's her sister doing in the next room?"

"They've already taken out her kidney."

"We are not going to waste that organ, trust me. I'm staying until that transplant is sewed in place and working well." Now my determination was fierce. The transplant surgeon nodded in approval of the plan and kept working to prepare the operative field for the new kidney.

Calm returned to the troubled OR. We needed to wait a few minutes until the pharmacy brought us the diltiazem, an uncommon drug to be used in the operating room. I began with a modest test dose and the rate slowed down, so I increased the dose. The anesthesiologist's respiratory rate and heart rate also likely slowed down. Progress was made. Over the next two hours, the medication did its job beautifully, and the transplant was a success. That was over ten years ago.

Carla still has normal kidney function. Her blood pressure and high cholesterol are much better controlled with the great medications available, and she has "almost" quit smoking. She leads an active and happy life, caring for her family. But how did Carla come to need a cardiologist in the first place at such a tender age? For most of the last century, doctors, almost all men, were sure that atherosclerosis, angina, and heart attacks were diseases of men. Women with chest pain were often felt to be suffering from anxiety and hysteria, not "real" disease of the heart. They were wrong about that, even years ago.

My patient Carla had most of the important risk factors for atherosclerosis and coronary artery disease from the time she was in her teens: high blood pressure, high cholesterol, excess weight, and cigarette smoking. Much of this was a product of circumstance. Carla still lives in the Philadelphia inner city, and her diet is pretty awful. There aren't many supermarkets near her with adequate stocks of grains, legumes, fresh fruit, and vegetables. There are many offerings of red meat, pork, and processed foods. On the streets, there are individual cigarettes you can buy without spending the money for an entire pack. Given the bias pervasive for so long, it isn't surprising that her risk factors were not addressed by any doctor earlier in her life.

It took the work of a new breed of cardiologists, mostly women, to prove to their male colleagues not just the error of their ways in thinking about atherosclerosis in females but also to point out the unique features of coronary heart disease in women. Nanette Wenger led the way, a path now taken by many brilliant women studying and treating patients with coronary artery disease. Even some of their male colleagues have helped out. Hopefully the bias of many years about women and their hearts is gone.

CHAPTER 24

THE FIRE INSIDE: TAMPING THE FLAMES OF CORONARY ARTERY DISEASE

*You know me as I am, an instant—a spark.
But this is only part of the picture, for I watch from the sidelines
with the patience of a saint as the pyre is laid, all the elements
coming together, until it is time for me to strike.*

THE CORONARY CARE UNIT—FALL 2008

Her chest pain started in the middle of the night. She knew something was wrong, and she came to the emergency room within an hour. The electrocardiogram told the story, an acute myocardial infarction due to a major occlusion of the right coronary artery. But one could not have guessed by looking at her; she was thin, appearing younger than her late forties, not like a CCU patient at all.

As soon as she had her EKG done in the ER, the "door to balloon" emergency angioplasty team sprang into action, and within ninety minutes, they had her in the cardiac cath lab. In short order, the cardiologist on call pushed open the blocked artery with a balloon catheter followed by a metallic stent. The procedure was a complete success. The patient's next stop was the CCU, where she spent a few quiet hours sleeping before the residents presented her story to me on rounds in the morning.

The resident described the onset of the chest pain and then told me about the woman's risk factors for coronary artery disease, none that he knew of: no diabetes, no high blood pressure, no elevated cholesterol, no cigarette smoking, and no family history of early heart disease in anyone. What's more, she exercised some and had a steady job. So why did this woman have a heart attack? While myocardial infarction can occur without any of the typical risks for atherosclerosis, there had to be more to this woman's story.

I stopped the resident's report after he described four different areas of atherosclerosis that had been found, not including the severe blockage of the right coronary artery. We were going to review the angiogram anyway, but I wanted to see her images for myself immediately. Pictures would help to fill in the story.

We walked over to one of the computers in the CCU, and I pulled up the images. Before her angioplasty procedure, the right coronary had an almost one hundred percent occlusion from a clot and a plaque in its top or proximal portion, but there was a slow flow of the contrast dye down the right coronary artery, and I could see several more areas of atherosclerosis in that artery. The plaque was not just limited to the proximal portion of the artery. I almost gasped when I saw the images of the left coronary artery—this young woman's entire coronary artery tree was studded with areas of plaque formation, some much larger than others. Sometimes we called these focal plaque growths "lumpy bumpies," but these were much more severe than the usual. This artery was not even the one that caused her heart attack, but her left coronary artery looked awful.

If we could have seen her coronary arteries under a microscope, we would have seen a combination of white blood cells, smooth muscle cells, and clotted blood in multiple spots throughout all of her coronary arteries. Although a large blood clot caused the final severe obstruction to blood flow that propelled her to the emergency room, this event was due to a complex, long-standing pathology.

We walked into the room, and I again looked at the woman and saw some gnarled joints in her hands. The resident noticed where my eyes were going and offhandedly mentioned to me: "Oh yeah, she has rheumatoid arthritis." Finally, I knew what was happening to this lady: her coronary arteries were on fire...

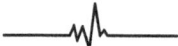

BACK TO THE LAB: SMOLDERING ARTERIES— A NEW SPIN ON OLD KNOWLEDGE

In the 1970s, the dogma of what happened to patients with coronary artery blockages was pretty simple: angina and heart attacks were directly related to flow. The plaque built up gradually over years, and when the lumen of the artery was blocked over fifty percent, the flow dropped, and the patient had angina with exertion and was at risk of a heart attack.

Much about coronary artery disease *is* about hydraulics and physiology; those are scientific terms for plumbing, but they don't explain everything. It is true that the same ideas about flow of liquid apply to the blood flow in small coronary arteries; the heart relaxes, the blood flows by gravity from the aorta into the two openings of the coronary arteries, and the blood gets into the heart muscle. Pretty straightforward, right? But there was a huge "elephant in the room." The rusty pipe idea didn't explain the acute heart attack at all. There were inconclusive ideas about blood clots as the cause, but most authorities at the time didn't subscribe to these ideas. It was never clear to students at the time what the experts did think caused heart attacks. The discovery of Dewood and the work of Rentrop in the early 1980s settled the blood clot question, but there was much more to learn.

Cardiologists needed to turn to their basic science colleagues to try to get some fundamental facts straight before better treatment or even prevention would make any sense at all. What cells cause atherosclerosis and heart attacks besides cholesterol and LDL particles, and why do they predispose to blood clots? How did these cells know to get involved in the plaque "play"? Were there medicines that could stop the performance? These questions were daunting, but there was a starting line of knowledge to use. Modern researchers could follow the path first laid down by two of the great medical scientists of the nineteenth century, a Ukrainian and a German. Their ideas, long applied to many other human diseases, were about to resurrect attempts to understand the still befuddling work of the Widowmaker.

THE CELLS REVEAL THEIR SECRETS

Not that many people wanted to do research into pus, but it is a rather ubiquitous and scientifically intriguing substance. It had been noted for millennia that when injuries and infection occurred, the body responded with a yellow-white liquid flooding the area. With the invention of the microscope, it was clear that pus was made up of white blood cells. What was unknown was what the white cells were doing; were they helpful or harmful? Did they attack bacteria or just help carry them to other parts of the body? Such questions plagued those scientists interested in this strange fluid.

But help was on the way. The Ukrainian man who discovered what white blood cells do was Ilya Metchnikov PhD (1845-1916). He received a degree in the natural sciences at the University of Kharkov and then moved to Germany for more research into an area far removed from medicine, the biology of marine animals, like starfish and their larvae. During his work, he noticed a very strange phenomenon under the microscope; one of the flatworms he was studying was eaten up by some cells. Metchnikov thought that the cells he saw ingesting the flatworms might have something to do with defending organisms from injury and infection. He wondered if stimulating his study animals, the larvae of starfish, with some form of injury might reproduce the same defensive result.

Solutions sometimes come from the strangest places. He bought a Christmas tree for his children and noticed the menacing thorns. One December night, he put some of them into a dish containing the starfish larvae. The next morning, he saw a group of white blood cells from the starfish swarming around the thorns. Those leucocytes were indeed coming to the rescue, saving the tiny organism from potential damage. When he explained his findings to a colleague in Vienna, they came up with a new term to describe white cells ingesting other cells: "phagocytosis," the term still used to explain the body's immune system's cells gobbling up strangers and digesting them with their internal enzymes.

Metchnikov for certain didn't think these cells had anything to with heart disease and atherosclerosis. The scientists of the time saw only the link between white blood cells and infectious diseases. Atherosclerosis research was not an attractive area for a career in pathology. But there was one giant in the field who thought otherwise.

Rudolph Virchow MD (1821-1902) created a new fundamental paradigm in medicine and science that has stood the test of time and would impact those studying heart disease. His work stood on the pillar of one concept—Virchow believed that all diseases were related to "sick cells." Like Metchnikov, his tool was also the microscope.

Virchow was fascinated by arteriosclerosis.[147] Under Virchow's microscope, this disease was a mysterious accumulation of abnormal-looking cells and fatty material that invaded the inner lining, the intima, of the walls of arteries. Virchow meticulously outlined the phases of this arterial disease, believing that the first step in the process was due to the "imbition of blood elements" of some kind, followed by softening of the structural support molecules of the outer wall of the artery. This was followed by the growth of abnormal

---

147 The term atherosclerosis only came about years later when the role of cholesterol was established in this disease.

cells inside of the intima, ultimately resulting in marked thickening of this layer of previously normal cells of the artery. Virchow termed this process "endarteritis deformans," some kind of repair process from the initial intake of some blood element into the arterial wall. The great pathologist did not believe that endarteritis deformans was a "passive process." He noted that: "In some particularly violent cases the softening manifests itself even in the arteries not as the consequence of a really fatty process, but as a direct product of inflammation." Under his microscope, Virchow recognized the "fire" in the arteries.[148] His work was done in the 1870s.

RESEARCH SILENCE—AGAIN

But for close to a hundred years, the discoveries of Metchnikov and Virchow hibernated away from research that could have linked their findings to atherosclerosis and heart disease. Finally, in the 1970s, a renaissance into the cells of atherosclerosis began. Scientists in the mold of Metchnikov and Virchow, not doctors who care for patients, led the way.

One of those science "lab rats" was Russell Ross DDS PhD (1929-1999) of the University of Washington, who took a keen interest in the cause of heart disease. Educated initially as a dentist, Ross changed his career and became a pathology professor. He was fascinated by atherosclerosis, and he unearthed the insights of Metchnikov and Virchow. Determined to find what caused atherosclerosis, Ross believed he could take advantage of the modern tools, not just light but electron microscopes, allowing far more detailed examinations of arteries. Ross and his collaborators went to work on human specimens of atherosclerosis from all kinds of blood vessels, not just the coronary arteries.

---

148 When Rudolph Virchow died in 1902, he had over two thousand publications in scientific journals. One of his biographers wrote that when he died, "Germany would complain of having lost four great men at once: her leading pathologist, her leading anthropologist, her leading sanitarian, and her leading liberal."

Ross agreed with Virchow. Atherosclerosis was not just the passive accumulation of lipid material into the artery wall, but it was the result of a multi-pronged "response to injury" of the artery, choreographed first, he thought, by the smooth muscle cells in the arterial wall. By the 1970s, previous work confirmed that there were multiple stages of atherosclerosis, the earliest abnormality called the "fatty streak," often observed in the arteries of many of the young Americans in their twenties who died during the Korean War of the 1950s. Under his microscope, Ross saw that these nascent lesions were made up of smooth muscle cells that had migrated into the intima and engulfed lipid particles. He observed Metchnikov's phagocytosis, performed by the cells that Virchow and Anichkov saw in the distant past, this time under an electron microscope.

In addition, in more advanced lesions, Ross saw that the lipid-laden smooth muscle cells seemed to recruit other cells to join the microscopic performance. He saw a buildup of collagen, and another structural protein called elastin, coalescing with the smooth muscle cells to form a "fibrous cap" over the lipid buildup. To Ross, this phenomenon clearly was a "response to injury" on the part of the body, covering over a material that didn't belong in the wall of the artery, and "walling" it off from the bloodstream—this was a microscopic "cover-up."

Ross also described a more ominous appearance of atherosclerosis, a microscopic view of the progression of the lesions from fatty streaks to clinical events like heart attacks. These "complicated lesions" were a chaotic mixture of dying cells (*necrosis*), accumulation of blood and blood clots (*hemorrhage and thrombosis*), and finally a buildup of calcium, a rock-hard element in the wall of a diseased artery. These "end-stage" lesions were dramatically different from just fatty streaks. In exploring all of this, Ross documented the life-history of atherosclerosis and its progression to a heart attack.

As is always the case with good science, Ross' observations raised more questions than they answered. Did the smooth muscle cells, Ross' primary actor in the atherosclerosis play, come from the inner or the middle lining of the blood vessel wall?[149] What stimulated them to react as they did? Were other cells involved in the process? This was not a response to foreign invaders like bacteria but a response to one's own molecules. This was a form of autoimmunity, suggestively similar to the pathologic findings in the joints of someone with rheumatoid arthritis.

After doing studies initiating injury to the arteries of the legs of animals and watching the results, Ross and his colleagues turned their attention to the heart to answer the question of what was causing the injury in atherosclerosis. Atherosclerosis was not due to physical trauma such as a contusion to an artery from a catheter, so Ross' experimental model didn't mimic closely what happens in people. He knew that the lipoproteins were closely associated with atherosclerosis. He then moved his work into the in vitro world, growing smooth muscle cells in tissue culture containers, exposing them to different stimuli, and seeing how they responded. When exposed to lipoproteins, especially high concentrations of low-density lipoprotein, LDL, the smooth muscle cells became voracious, engulfing the LDL. Was this the start of the sequence of events that caused atherosclerosis and inflammation in people?

Russell Ross went on to do much more work in atherosclerosis throughout his career and helped contribute to the next stage of the work—the use of specific "cell markers" and molecular biology techniques to find out not just what the cells were doing inside of atherosclerosis plaques but also what strange molecules were "signaling" to the cells what to do. The smooth muscle cells were only one actor in the play of atherosclerosis. What was commanding the performance that led to heart attacks? Could this process be stopped? Ross had uncovered some clues that needed to be followed.

In his important publication in the journal *Science* in 1973, Ross outlined his discoveries and included references to work done by

---

149 Blood vessels have three distinct layers of cells: the innermost called the intima, the middle layer the media, and the outer layer the adventitia.

others in the field in the 1960s, but he also cited a paper written in 1856 by Virchow. Ross was like a scientific archaeologist; he dug down into the old debris of research and took another look, this time with much better tools. The key idea was that atherosclerosis was *not* just due to the lipids getting stuck to the artery walls, like rust accumulating gradually in a water pipe. This disease was a complex creation, with many cellular partners, all playing a role—the white cells, the smooth muscle cells, the platelets, the endothelial cells, the clotting proteins, and the molecular signals. The body was trying to do the right thing, cover up or destroy the LDL in the artery walls. But perhaps it too often got carried away and made the situation worse over time. This disease was daunting to unravel, and treatment was a distant dream in the 1970s.

CELLS THAT ATTACK

> "Atherosclerosis is an inflammatory disease."
>
> —*Richard Ross MD (1924-2015), Dean of Johns Hopkins School of Medicine, New England Journal of Medicine, 1999*

At the time that Ross was implicating the role of the smooth muscle cells of the arterial media in the genesis of atherosclerosis, others were looking closely at some of the other bad actors, the white blood cells and the platelets. Atherosclerosis was not just an attack of the smooth muscle cells that led to plaque in arteries; the process was inflammation, and that involves white blood cells and the immune system. Inflammation is like a "crowd" of cells that gather around a car accident on a crowded street in the city. This crowd of rowdy cells does generate heat—arteries on fire.[150]

---

150   In 1999, a group of Greek cardiologists actually measured the temperature of the inside of coronary arteries in normal people and those with active coronary artery disease like unstable angina or acute myocardial infarction. To no one's surprise, the heat from the plaque lesions of the coronary artery disease patients was higher than in the normal group.

It was discovered over a century ago that it is the lymphocyte population of the white blood cells that contributes so many of the key players to the immune system and that the monocyte type of lymphocytes are the real champions of phagocytosis.[151] They ingest bacteria easily, and they also like to swallow up the molecule that causes atherosclerosis, the LDL particle. When they do, the lipid causes the monocyte to bloat up and gives it a characteristic appearance under the microscope; it looks like the cell is filled with foam. When the monocytes reach this stage, they are called "macrophages," or "foam cells." The final player to enter the atherosclerosis stage are the blood platelets, those tiny particles[152] made by the bone marrow that respond to a break in tissue almost immediately, releasing granules of molecules that signal to other platelets floating by in the bloodstream to join the party and start a blood clot.

There were multiple roles in this microscopic play, a collection of different types of white blood cells, smooth muscle cells, platelets, and clotting proteins, a performance initiated by the entry of LDL into the inner wall of an artery. The result is a group of pathologic lesions, first a fatty streak, then a mess of lipid-filled cells covered over by a fibrous cap of cells, and then finally a chaotic mass of all of the actors, with scattered blood clots in the mixture, indicating that often clots formed, were broken down, and then healed over.

THE MOLECULAR DIRECTORS OF INFLAMMATION

But why is LDL so toxic to the walls of arteries? It was time for the molecular biologists to enter the research scene. Other participants were directing all of these cellular players, and if you could discover who they were, then maybe you could defeat their malignant effects.

An outstanding physician-scientist from California has had a leading role in discovering the intricacies of atherosclerosis and the

---
151 Monocytes are easily identified under a microscope because of the typical appearance of their very large nuclei.
152 Platelets are not cells because they don't have nuclei.

role of the molecules that order the many cells involved to enter the stage. Peter Libby MD was born in Berkeley, California, in 1947 and received his medical degree in San Diego. Currently, he is a chaired professor in the Cardiovascular Division at the Brigham and Women's Hospital. Dr. Libby has a passion not just for clinical medicine but research into the basic nature of the Widowmaker's work, insights that will hopefully lead to better treatment and saving lives. When I asked him in December 2019 how he became interested in atherosclerosis and inflammation, he said, "I just listened very carefully when I took pathology in medical school." Virchow would have been glad to hear that.

Libby and others in the field wanted to know what was driving different cells to infiltrate the plaque, creating the milieu that could lead to a clinical event—a heart attack. They were convinced that the culprits were specific molecules that didn't just affect atherosclerosis but also cancer and diseases of the immune system like rheumatoid arthritis. It was painstaking work, but they were dedicated to finding these bad actors and understanding their role in heart disease.

By the mid-1980s, the research found a culprit: LDL stimulated the cells of the intima to pour out molecules named Vascular Cell Adhesion Molecules (VCAM-1), proteins that attract the T lymphocytes to the area and induce monocytes to become those ferocious macrophages.[153] Once the T cells enter the fray, they go to work making molecules called "cytokines," small proteins that engage in signaling between cells and the pathologic process really accelerates. Dr. Libby, a classical music fan, prefers the "orchestra" metaphor for atherosclerosis. He described the T cells in this way: "Armies have more foot soldiers than generals and orchestras many instrumentalists but only one conductor."

It was now clear that specific molecules, especially the cytokine

---

[153] The immune system has two types of cells, T cells that gain their specific characteristics by contact with the small thymus gland in the neck, and B cells from the bone marrow that manufacture antibody proteins. The complexity of the immune system requires an entire new book to explain in detail.

interleukin 6, signal the inflammation to other organs, like the liver and also adipose tissue, the fat cells, to release other markers of inflammation. These fat cells make so many different cytokines that as a group they are called "adipokines." The "cytokine cascade" goes into full operation when LDL particles infiltrate the walls of arteries. The research had now discovered a sequence of events all leading to atherosclerosis and the heart attack: cholesterol carried into the cell wall by LDL particles, followed by activation of numerous types of cells responding to molecular signals telling the body to try to protect itself from an invader.

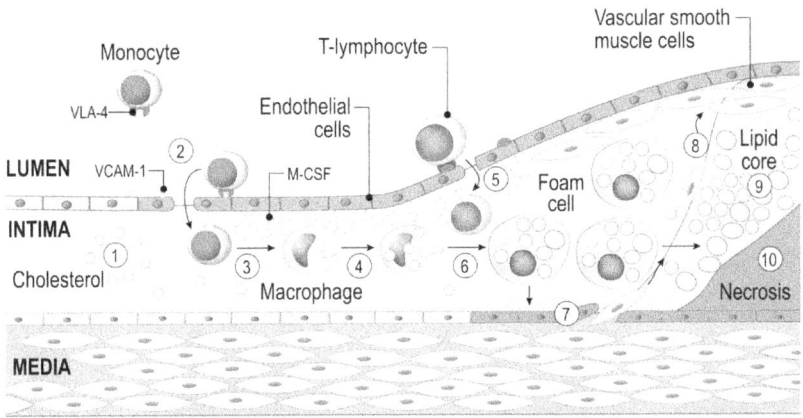

Figure 30. Pathogenesis of inflammation and atherosclerosis. 1—cholesterol enters intima of artery; 2—"Signal molecules" (VCAM-1, etc.) activate monocyte white blood cells; 3, 4—monocytes become macrophages and ingest cholesterol; 5—T-lymphocytes interact with macrophages to form "foam cells"; 6-7, 8—vascular smooth muscle cells form barrier of cells over "lipid core"; 9, 10—breakdown of cells leads to tissue necrosis and chance of "plaque rupture" followed by acute myocardial infarction.
(Copyright Shutterstock)

THE PLAQUE COVER-UP

Once fully engaged, the cellular actors begin a repair process, an attempt to cover up the LDL and their own work, the response to injury seen by Russell Ross. A firm layer of collagen and new endothelial cells provides physical cover for the plaque components from the bloodstream. This process is not dissimilar to forming a scar after surgery or trauma, and with heart disease, it is key.

Why is this so important? Because without that protective cell layer, all of these inflammatory cells and the lipid particles attract more platelets into the plaque and the platelets then attract clotting proteins. Then a person suffers a heart attack. But as long as that plaque cover remains intact, an acute myocardial infarction due to a blood clot will not occur. A patient with a severe blockage from plaque inside a coronary artery often has angina, but not a heart attack. On the other hand, in a patient with a mild blockage from plaque, if that protective layer of cells opens up and the platelets and clotting proteins gather, a mild blockage changes in a matter of hours to one hundred percent and the Widowmaker is fully engaged. *So what compromised the protective covering?*

The molecular biologists have discovered that the macrophages and T lymphocytes play the largest role in eroding the protective collagen cover over plaques, resulting in fissures or erosions into the plaques. Their weapons of choice appear to be specific proteins they secrete called "matrix metalloproteinases" (MMPs) and "cysteine proteases"[154] that damage the protective cover over the plaque. But the entire data are still incomplete.

One of the key questions needing research is why do these "plaque cover-up" cells and molecules destroy their own work? Atherosclerosis takes years to develop and people can die in their nineties, have severe coronary artery disease, but never have a heart

---

154   The suffix "-ases" indicates that a protein molecule is an enzyme that interacts with other molecules, breaking them up into smaller molecules in a metabolic and biochemical sequence.

attack. In contrast a forty-year-old with only mild atherosclerosis of a coronary artery, a blockage of far less than fifty percent of the diameter of the lumen of the vessel, can have acute plaque rupture and suffer a very large heart attack. What is the difference? No one is sure. It is the "holy grail" of atherosclerosis research. I believe that the person or group that uncovers this final secret of the Widowmaker will surely win the Nobel Prize in Medicine.

But all of this work on inflammation as a key part of atherosclerosis and the heart attack has not been for naught for patients and their doctors. Knowing that inflammation was a crucial part of the pathology, researchers began looking for blood tests or imaging of arteries that might identify people with "vulnerable plaques," lesions at high risk of plaque rupture and acute heart attacks. If you could select those at most risk, more aggressive treatment, drugs to decrease cholesterol levels and inflammation, or angioplasty or even bypass surgery might prevent the final stage of the work of the Widowmaker.

WHOSE PLAQUES ARE "VULNERABLE"?

The best that any doctor can say about a cardiac event in someone with atherosclerosis is that they have a greater chance of developing angina or a heart attack over time. It's a matter of statistics—probability. But in the last two decades, there are now ideas and techniques that may help to find people at the most risk of a heart attack.

Inflammation was the scientific link between a very old blood test and coronary artery disease. Medicine is again indebted to William Tillett, the discoverer of streptokinase. In 1930, Tillett was trying to find molecules that were important to the immune system's reaction to infection, and he found one he named C-reactive protein, CRP. CRP is a protein made by the liver. Its synthesis increases dramatically in response to inflammation. CRP levels were measured for many years as a marker for inflammation, and there are many reasons for increased levels of the CRP in the blood, including infections, cancer, and autoimmune diseases like rheumatoid arthritis. But if inflammation has an important role in atherosclerosis, might these levels also rise in people at risk for heart attacks? It was easy to show that patients in a hospital with angina or a myocardial infarction have elevated CRP levels. These results suggested that inflammation had a role in coronary artery disease, but these findings did not help identify the people with vulnerable plaques, those with atherosclerosis yet feeling fine.

Enter Paul Ridker MD, a modern Harvard professor, who was intrigued by inflammation, and he and others knew that fifty percent of the time, people who had heart attacks had what was thought to be normal or even low levels of cholesterol in their blood at the time of the myocardial infarction. One explanation is that the normal levels are too high, and that likely has merit. But if inflammation was also playing a key role, was there a simple way to check the level of inflammation, that is, how much smoldering fire was going on in the arteries of the millions who had never had a heart attack?

In the 1990s, Dr. Ridker had an idea concerning CRP that would rely on resources from a previous study. In the late 1970s, a study was organized to see if medication could reduce the incidence of a heart attack. This was a "primary prevention" trial, conducted in people who had never had any previous diagnosis of heart disease. The study participants were all male doctors[155] and was called the Physicians' Health Study, and it began in 1982. For Ridker's purposes, the study had a priceless resource: during the course of the trial, the twenty-two thousand doctors studied were asked to provide a blood sample that would be frozen at -80 C, just waiting for some future use. Almost fifteen thousand (sixty-eight percent) did send the blood tubes as requested. Ridker was going to see if the CRP levels in these blood samples predicted the risk of a future heart attack.

The frozen blood samples were incredibly telling. Using the new high sensitivity test for CRP, Ridker and his colleagues showed that

---

[155] The decision to enroll only men in the study was likely still due to the bias that coronary artery disease was much more common in men.

the levels of CPR was just short of fifty percent higher in the doctors who went on to have heart attacks than those who did not. In addition, the higher the level, the greater the heart attack risk. Those with levels in the highest twenty-five percent of the entire group had just short of three times (2.9) the relative risk of a heart attack.[156] Higher CRP levels were associated with a higher risk of the stroke as well as a heart attack. A most interesting finding was that taking aspirin reduced the heart attack risk most in the people with the highest levels. Evidence of inflammation detected on a simple blood test *was* a long-term risk for a heart attack, just as the pathologists and molecular biologists would have predicted.

However, the Harvard researchers had done their work using only samples from men. What about women? Fortunately, there was also an ongoing study in women after menopause—over thirty-nine thousand of them. The Women's Health Initiative was organized in the early 1990s, and participants provided over twenty-eight thousand blood samples frozen with liquid nitrogen. Perhaps these samples could be used to see if the same CRP/heart disease connection existed in women.

Again, the samples provided the suspected link. Just as in the Physicians' Health Study, the results in the Women's Health Initiative showed that the higher the CRP level, the higher the risk for a future heart attack. Identical to the findings in men, the CRP levels were not tied to the levels of total cholesterol and its collection of different lipoproteins. *An elevated CRP level was an "independent" risk factor for heart attacks in both men and women.*

By the early 2000s, conversations and ideas about CRP were widespread in the world of cardiology, yet there were so many more questions to answer. Is CRP a major contributor to the acceleration of inflammation and atherosclerosis, or is it just a secondary bystander,

---

156 Relative risk is a statistical term of the ratio of the probability of an outcome (a heart attack in this case) in an exposed group (i.e., a higher CRP level) to the probability of an outcome in an unexposed group (i.e., a lower CRP level).

a byproduct of the liver in response to inflammation in general? Can you treat high CRP levels with aspirin, statins, or new medications to lower the levels and reduce the risk of heart attacks?

The answers to these questions have major real-world implications for prevention, the ultimate goal in finally overtaking the Widowmaker. The research needed to go on, now seeing if medications known to decrease inflammation in other diseases could affect the risk of a heart attack.

DOUSING THE EMBERS: DRUGS AND INFLAMMATION

Aspirin is a fascinating drug with a remarkable, very long history. Hippocrates used willow leaf tea, from which aspirin was later found, to relieve the pain of childbirth in 400 BCE. By the 1980s, it was clear that this ancient compound, chemical name acetylsalicylic acid, could stop platelets from aggregating and decrease the chances of major heart damage when given shortly after the onset of chest pain from an acute myocardial infarction.

Pertinent to the connection between CRP and heart disease, aspirin also has other effects, like interfering with some of the molecules that stimulate inflammation. For years, extremely high doses of aspirin were the foundation of chronic treatment of rheumatoid arthritis. But could the drug also reduce inflammation in the coronary arteries and prevent heart attacks? Aspirin does reduce the risk of a second heart attack in someone who has already had a first attack and does slow the formation of blood clots in coronary artery bypass grafts in people who have had that type of surgery. Then the Physicians' Health Study, the one that provided Ridker's blood samples to measure CRP, showed that it could reduce the risk of a first heart attack and was the first drug of benefit for primary prevention. The Women's Health Initiative, however, did not give as clear an answer, although the risk was reduced in women over sixty-five years of age.

The most recent information paints a confusing picture about the value of aspirin to prevent a first heart attack. More research will continue, but as of 2020, aspirin seems to be valuable only in people with many different risk factors for a heart attack and not the general population. Aspirin's role as a way to stop inflammation in coronary artery disease is modest; its major effect is on blood platelets. As doctors sometimes say about drugs that might be used in millions of people, "Let's not put it in the drinking water."

The next choice of a drug to combat inflammation was also logical—a statin, one of the drugs that reduce LDL levels and by the mid-1980s had unequivocally been proven to reduce heart attack risk across the board, those with an atherosclerosis history and those without. But maybe the statin drugs could be of even more value if they were given to people with blood tests indicating inflammation, a high CRP level. Was there a hidden effect of statin drugs on heart attack risk that has nothing to do with their effect on LDL and cholesterol levels?

Organizing and conducting such a trial of a drug in people without a history of a heart attack is a massive undertaking. Designing the protocol, calculating how many patients are needed to increase the statistical chances of showing a real treatment effect, and considering the ethics of randomizing human beings to a treatment group or not: these are real challenges. This was to be research into heart attacks, not the common cold. Fortunately for the field of heart disease, Paul Ridker and his Harvard colleagues were up to the test.

In 2003, the Harvard group began its trial, the Justification for the Use of Statins in Prevention: An Intervention Trial Using Rosuvastatin[157]—the JUPITER trial. Imagine recruiting almost eighteen thousand patients from twenty-six countries, all of whom had never had evidence of atherosclerosis, had low LDL levels but also had a CRP level of greater than 2.0 mg/dl, a level shown to increase the risk. The investigators needed to screen over eighty thousand people first, and then the real work began.

---

157 Rosuvastatin is a powerful statin, trade name Crestor, manufactured first by AstraZeneca. Now a generic medication.

The results were very surprising in a short time for this kind of research. Half of the group, the treatment group, took 20 mg of rosuvastatin each day. The idea was to see how many in each group reached a "primary end-point" of a heart attack, angina, an angioplasty, or death from cardiovascular cause. The trial intended to follow-up all of the patients for five years. But in March 2008, the study monitors put a halt to the trial; the group receiving rosuvastatin had a major decrease in the incidence of heart attack, angina, and death, a forty-four percent decrease. The group not taking rosuvastatin had 251 end-point events; only 142 were seen in the treated group. The rosuvastatin treated people saw their mean CRP levels fall from 4.2 mg/dl to 2.2, almost in half. This dramatic result was found in just short of two years average follow-up. Even the statisticians agreed—the chance that this was a result due to random chance was less than one in a thousand.

Ridker and his colleagues were thrilled by the results. In their minds, this was proof of the hypothesis that inflammation has a key role to play in causing heart attacks. But they knew the debate wasn't over. It was no surprise that critics of JUPITER wrote sometimes scathing journal articles about the research. Several well-known professors argued that the trial was stopped too early and that longer follow-up might have changed the results. Others argued that doctors could assess risk of heart attack just as well using the traditional factors without the use of a CRP level.

But by 2005, the inflammation hypothesis had a foothold in the understanding and possible treatment of atherosclerosis and heart attacks. A greater challenge lay ahead: what about drugs that suppress inflammation but have no effect on lipid levels? Could using such a drug with a statin be more effective than using either drug alone?

There was no shortage of anti-inflammatory drugs used to treat diseases like rheumatoid arthritis that might decrease the inflammation of atherosclerosis. In the last several years, three different drugs have been used to see if they reduced heart attack risk in people with a history of a first myocardial infarction or angina and high CRP levels. The first one studied was canakinumab, an antibody that has an effect on the function of one of the interleukin signal molecules triggering inflammation, as well as CRP levels. Canakinumab did reduce the rate of new cardiac events by fifteen percent, and seventeen percent if bypass surgery and angioplasty events were included, a modest benefit but a fifteen percent reduction is massive if millions are at risk of a heart attack.[158]

The studies focusing on other drugs were mixed. The second drug, methotrexate, an old drug used to treat cancer and autoimmune diseases, had no effect on cardiovascular event rates and no reduction of interleukin-6 or CRP levels was seen.[159] The third drug trial did show promising results from another old medicine. Colchicine has been used for years to treat gout. This medicine interferes with the way white cells reproduce and also sends a molecular signal that interferes with interleukin and CRP levels further down the white cells' metabolic path. The Colchicine Cardiovascular Outcome Trial reported a twenty-three percent reduction in all overall cardiovascular events in the treated group, especially decreases in the incidence of stroke and the need for angioplasty or bypass surgery.[160]

The cardiology world has traveled a very long path with the inflammation story, but it is not at its end goal to stop the Widowmaker. The basic science is in place; the observations of the pathologists and the molecular biologics, with their special ways to identify cell types and molecular signals, have been groundbreaking. As of 2020, the data suggests that treating inflammation with medications and lowcring risk of heart attacks must be linked with aggressive lowering of LDL levels; but researchers have not found the right combinations of medications yet. They will keep trying. Currently, most cardiologists

---

[158] The CANTOS trial (Canakinumab Anti-Inflammatory Outcomes Study) was published in the *New England Journal of Medicine* in 2017.
[159] The Cardiovascular Inflammation Reduction Trial published in the *New England Journal of Medicine* in 2019.
[160] Also published in the *New England Journal of Medicine* in 2019.

are not ready to prescribe anti-inflammatory medications to our patients with coronary artery disease. We are waiting for more data to emerge.

Clinicians caring for patients have taken away at least one strong message from all of this work and especially the results of JUPITER: lowering LDL levels works and the lower the better. Often on rounds in the CCU, after seeing a patient admitted for a heart attack, a resident would ask should we start the patient on a statin or wait until we checked the LDL level first. I would always answer, "I don't care what their LDL level is now—it's too high for them. This patient has already shown there's significant plaque in their arteries. Start the drug." The data showing the primacy of LDL as the initiator of atherosclerosis and then inflammation is overwhelming. I don't know what a normal LDL level is in a population with an epidemic of coronary artery disease and heart attacks. I do know as children our LDL levels are very low and that children don't develop atherosclerosis until at least their twenties when their LDL levels rise.

We'll need to see what the next decade of research says about these new treatments. The battle of prevention continues. The Widowmaker is still at work, as it was in my young female patient in the CCU.

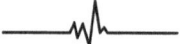

INFLAMMARE (LATIN) = TO SET ON FIRE WITH PASSION: THE RAVAGES OF LDL

... My young CCU patient suffered from rheumatoid arthritis. Her body was activating white blood cells and antibodies against its own cells, as if these cells were foreign invaders like bacteria.

In someone with rheumatoid arthritis, the white blood cells invade areas of the body, like the joint spaces, and wreak havoc, often causing permanent scarring and disfigurement of the joints. That's why this lady's hands were so disfigured.

What makes the white blood cells act so dastardly is not known, but what is known is that rheumatoid arthritis is a disease that can attack many different organs, even though its effect is best known on the joints. Patients with rheumatoid arthritis have a much higher risk of coronary artery disease, a risk that is independent of the typical risk factors for atherosclerosis.

I didn't need a biopsy and a microscope to visualize what was destroying my patient's coronary arteries. The team and I discussed the possibility of recommending coronary artery bypass surgery, but her vessels were so diseased in so many places, I doubted that bypass grafts would be able to supply blood to the ends of the coronary arteries and the heart muscle and not develop their own blood clots in short order. For this woman to live a long life, she would need some help from the basic scientists—again.

We placed her on medication to help her heart, lower her cholesterol, and two drugs to inhibit blood clot formation in her coronary arteries and her new stent. Her coronary circulation had fallen prey to the long-term effects of inflammation as a result of her rheumatoid arthritis. For now, that was all we could do, but there is real hope that the molecular biologists and the pharmacologists will come up with better treatment for not just the scourge of atherosclerosis but for the smoldering heat and fire of inflammation of the heart's arteries in millions.

CHAPTER 25

APPREHENDING THE WIDOWMAKER: HOW CLOSE ARE WE?

The weight of all these discoveries bears down on me 'til I feel that I may soon be relieved of this burden. Yet so much is known that is not shared; the victims still unable to defend themselves. It is this fact which keeps me vigilant, pursued but not apprehended.

Yes, I am but a moment in time, when all your past decisions may come together to suffocate your future.

I hope we never meet.

A CHOICE: THE END OF A DECADE OF TRAINING

A Tuesday Night—June 1981

"Artie, I just don't know if I'm doing the right thing. I've loved Yale, and the academics, and the chance to do research and teach. Maybe I was meant to be a professor, not go into private practice."

My friend and teacher Arthur Riba stared at me. Art was a terrific doctor, mentor, and human being, a junior faculty member at Yale, and he had invited me to dinner the last week of my cardiology fellowship training. It had been ten years since I had graduated college, went to medical school, and finished my training in internal medicine and cardiology. My father-in-law was happy about that; maybe I could finally support my wife and two young children.

"Are you nuts or what? You're a Philly guy; go home and help people. In a few years, if you're eating out near your home, a woman or man will come into the restaurant and tell their friends, 'Look, there's Dr. Meshkov. He saved my father's life.'"

That was all I needed to hear. I packed my bags and headed where I hoped I could do the most good. I had studied hard and saw all sorts of patients, on so many nights, weekends, and holidays, all with some form of heart disease. In my practice, I used the "state of the art" techniques at that time to help many people recover from their heart attacks.

The science of cardiac care had come so far from 1965. I thought I knew what heart attacks were, what they could do, and what caused them. Little did I know at that time how many holes there remained in the medical knowledge and that any treatments to prevent these attacks were unproven. The certainty that blood clots caused heart attacks or that a balloon on a catheter could clear out a blockage; these were ideas just evolving. There was much more to learn before we could really apprehend the Widowmaker. But I was ready to join so many others, using the tools we did have, to catch this illusive killer.

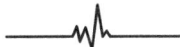

THE POWER OF ORGANIC MOLECULES AND THEIR CHILDREN

> "This is not the end, this is not even the beginning of the end, this is just perhaps the end of the beginning."
>
> –*Winston Churchill commenting on the British victory over the German Wehrmacht at the Battle of El Alamein, North Africa in 1942, three years prior to the end of World War II.*

With millions falling prey to the disease of the coronary arteries and the destruction of the heart that too often happens, chasing the Widowmaker is a long and tortuous journey. But the progress made in defining the cause, the diagnosis, and the treatment of coronary artery atherosclerosis has been astounding in the last 150 years.

The finding that nitroglycerin would relieve the chest pain known as angina pectoris was the first true scientific breakthrough in treating a disease for which there was no reliable way to relieve human pain and suffering. The drug was not a cure and could not prevent atherosclerosis from continuing its too often inexorable progression, but it greatly improved the quality of life for millions with angina, like my surgery professor Dr. Rhoads. With an even broader impact, the drugs nitroglycerin and amyl nitrite helped open the door to a new science—pharmacology, a scientific discipline that has transformed medicine from a primitive profession based on folklore and random individual observations into a marvelous endeavor that has altered the modern world. But it would still take almost a century until the biochemists and molecular biologists could finally uncover the true way that nitroglycerin works.

When Thomas Bruton and William Murrell began to use organic chemicals to treat serious heart disease and had, for the first time, tools to measure the effects of a drug on the function of the circulation, they opened the door that lead to a highway of the scientific study of potential medications brewed in the laboratories. Some of the most important of these would be variants of molecules first found in nature. Medications to prevent symptoms, stop erratic heart rhythms, soften the burden of heart failure, and retard atherosclerosis; the drug bounty continues to grow.

That road was pursued with great vigor, even though it was not until sixty years later that Eugene Braunwald and his colleagues uncovered the true nature of the circulation, for the first time understanding how the heart and the blood vessels worked in exquisite concert to adjust the heart's output of blood and then how disease of the heart caused the system to malfunction but then adapt. Braunwald's work allowed others to expand pharmacology beyond the level of the physiologists who studied blood pressure and heart rates, to now include incredibly intricate experiments on the effects of drugs on the cells of the heart and the blood vessels, discovering how organic chemistry reactions produce real changes in the function of human organs.

In the pursuit of the Widowmaker, there have been many heroes and some villains along the path, those who were determined to prove using good science that a test or a remedy would be successful and those who were violently skeptical and dismissive of the new ideas. It is natural for us to focus on the brilliant successes, but there have also been so many wonderful and creative ideas that just didn't prove to be true. Science and medicine are not easy, and if there were a medical journal named *The Journal of Irreproducible Results*, I would find that I and so many others have unknowingly contributed to its annals.

As we enter the third decade of the twenty-first century, the state of the art for treating the number one killer in the world is a long discussion, with an often-dazzling number of choices of techniques to diagnose and treat coronary artery disease. If a person can obtain skilled and rapid medical care, deadly outcomes are greatly reduced but by no means eliminated. Some concepts in cardiology are very complex, but one is quite straightforward—the heart is a pump, and the less damage it sustains from a heart attack, the better people will do.

THE JOB OF THE FIREMAN:
ON THE FRONTLINE WITH THE WIDOWMAKER

A cardiologist is always on call, every day he or she is in a hospital and every night or weekend. They are the medical "fireman" of heart disease, and it is a life of constant interruptions and juggling many tasks at one time. When the ER alarm is rung, you come.

One fact has become painfully clear: time is essential. Once a heart attack starts, when that blood flow through the blocked-up coronary artery has been cut off, the clock starts. Heart muscle cells are damaged, and within ninety minutes, many of them will die, never to spring back to life. The emergency room is the first line of defense in saving the heart, but education is essential hopefully people with chest pain will recognize the need for prompt medical attention.

Using Einthoven's marvelous machine, the electrocardiogram, the rapid diagnosis of the most dreaded form of the heart attack, the ST segment elevation kind, can be made in minutes not just by emergency room doctors but also by paramedics in ambulances. In the near future, it is also possible that personal devices, such as the Apple Watch and others, may become sophisticated enough to obtain a complete and accurate electrocardiogram that will immediately tell its wearer to get to a hospital.

Today, once an ST segment elevation heart attack diagnosis is confirmed, the cardiac cath lab team, including doctors, nurses, and technicians, will very quickly swarm to the emergency room and the cath lab, some to whisk the patient to the lab and others to get the equipment ready to go. The access artery for the catheter in the arm or the leg is prepped with skin sterilization and some local anesthetic, the patient given narcotics for the chest pain and often a mild sedative, and the well-trained and talented interventional cardiologist and the team are ready to go to work. Over the last twenty-five years, the process has become a finely orchestrated effort.

Following the lead of Werner Forssmann, Mason Sones, and Andreas Grüntzig, a superbly manufactured plastic catheter travels a blood vessel path into the aorta at the top of the heart and engages the very small openings to the coronary arteries, allowing the cardiologist to inject contrast dye that will trickle down into the artery until its flow is aborted by the buildup of cholesterol impeded in a particle called low density lipoprotein, the LDL particle discovered by John Gofman almost seventy years ago. Nikolai Anichkov's discovery has stood the test of time—cholesterol wrapped in a protein molecule causes atherosclerosis. It is tragic that the Western world didn't listen to him years earlier.

The blockage is often accompanied by a blood clot sitting on top of the plaque, a thrombus that had formed only a few hours earlier, cutting off most or all of the blood flow and sending a terrifying signal of chest pain to the patient. Marcus Dewood told us that the blood clot was the real culprit in assisting the Widowmaker when he did his study in the 1970s, resurrecting what Sol Sherry believed he had proven in the late 1950s.

Once the blockage is found, the diagnostic catheter is removed, exchanged using a guidewire technique invented by Sven Seldinger in the 1950s, and a new catheter inserted with a specific almost magical treatment wrapped around its tip—a plastic inflatable balloon, which when expanded will push the blood clot and the plaque into the wall of the artery, just as Charles Dotter described in the 1960s, like a knife through soft cheese. The entire process usually takes less than ninety minutes from the time the patient hits the emergency room until the heart's blood flow is restored.

A giant debt needs to be paid to Andreas Grüntzig, who had the nerve to perform the first angioplasty of a coronary artery, and to William O'Neill and Cindy Grines, who showed how effective the Grüntzig procedure could be for the heart attack. The successful clearing of the damage and aborting the heart muscle damage is only the first half of the treatment. Next comes a small piece of a metal lattice, a coronary artery stent to prevent that section of diseased artery from closing up again, an idea from the creativity and engineering genius of Julio Palmaz and Richard Shatz in the 1990s. And then the coup-de-grace—a newer stent, one embedded with a tiny amount of a drug used to treat cancer, a medication that has almost eliminated the chance that this particular dilated and stented artery will ever cause that patient a problem in the future.

Many times, however, the electrocardiogram is not clear-cut, and thousands of times each year, people with chest pain are admitted to that special place in the hospital, the Coronary Care Unit (CCU), where close attention to every detail of their care will save lives by treating slow and fast heart rates, blood pressure shifts, and using intravenous drugs and defibrillators if those fearful ventricular arrhythmias occur, using medications whose origin we owe to the drug used by dentists to numb your gums prior to their work.

A series of blood tests called biomarkers will often answer the question as to whether or not a heart attack has occurred, rising quickly in the blood of a heart attack patient, the source of the molecules released from the inside of damaged or dying heart muscle cells. Then choices can be made about medication to prevent more heart damage and future heart attacks, often the beta-blocker "children" of the propranolol synthesized by James Black now over fifty years ago, and to lower blood cholesterol using modern forms of statin drugs first discovered by Akiro Endo, inspired by the basic science of Michael Brown and Joseph Goldstein.

In these people with "non-ST segment" heart attacks, next a decision will be made as to whether or not to proceed with a stress test, like the one first used by Robert Bruce in the 1960s, a test often combined with the images created by radioactive isotopes to document the blood flow to the heart muscle and the function of the left ventricle, that crucial LVEF number sought by Barry Zaret and others in the 1970s.

In many cases, if a heart attack is confirmed, the doctors will then recommend a cardiac catheterization and not a stress test. Angiography reveals how many arteries are blocked, how severe the blockages are, and where they are located, providing a roadmap of the coronary artery system. That information leads to new decisions. Even though this heart attack was not the type that required an acute angioplasty, are the chronic plaques in locations that threaten large areas of the heart muscle if another blood clot forms?

These are remarkable advances, the ability to accurately define the problem and treat it, often with just prescription drugs.

Medications can control angina in the majority of people, drugs that are so effective that it has been hard to prove that angioplasty is superior in preventing recurrent heart attacks and dying. Drugs like aspirin, which inhibits the platelets from sticking together, and the statins by inhibiting the synthesis of the LDL particles that get stuck in the walls of arteries, both reduce the chances of a recurrent heart attack, with minimal side effects in the vast majority. For those who continue to have angina in spite of medication, angioplasty is a great option, improving the quality of life and reducing disability. Chronic coronary artery disease is just that—a long-term but manageable condition, like diabetes, asthma, gout, or high blood pressure.

The surgery invented by René Favaloro in the 1960s, the coronary artery bypass graft procedure, the CABG operation, still has a role to play, either when medication fails or angioplasty is not a good choice because the patient has multiple blockages that would require many stents. Modern research has told us that people with multiple blocked coronary arteries and diabetes do better in the long-term with bypass surgery than multiple angioplasties. In 2017, just short of 350,000 CABG operations were performed in the United States.

In spite of all of these options, there are still those who, while they would survive their heart attack, will end up with a badly damaged heart, one prone to the syndrome of congestive heart failure and the risk of Sudden Cardiac Death. In 2020, many of these people no longer face a short and grim future. Medications tested in the last few years, including the descendants of James Black's propranolol and a very new combination drug, valsartan and sacubitril,[161] when used together have had a major impact on the chances of being hospitalized and dying from heart failure.

The prevention of all Sudden Cardiac Death is still evasive, largely because so few people are even aware of their risk, and most of these events occur in homes, offices, or on the street, too far from the acute medical care necessary to abort the process. Much more work will

---

161 Trade name Entresto made by Novartis Pharmaceutical Corporation.

need to be done, hopefully with a better outcome for thousands. The breakthrough will be accurate noninvasive tests that identify those at greatest risk, tests that insurance companies and Medicare need to agree to pay for.

At least now there is reason for hope. For those alerted by the Widowmaker's first blow and left with a damaged heart, the automatic implantable cardioverter defibrillator, the AICD, invented by a Polish immigrant to the United States, Michel Mirowksi, has saved many lives. Secondly, first responders and those in health care, as well as thousands of the public have been trained in cardiopulmonary resuscitation, a procedure first suggested by William Kouwenhoven in the 1940s and has saved lives, although the results overall are still poor. Defibrillators are now available in many public places such as airports and gyms.

As prevention is finally possible early diagnosis of coronary artery disease is now more important than ever. The electrocardiogram and the stress test remain powerful tools. Newer imaging technologies to assess heart muscle function and blood flow, using computerized tomography (CT scans), magnetic resonance imaging (MRI), and a technique using radioisotopes, positron emission tomography (PET), have already made major inroads in improving the accuracy of cardiac imaging.

However, the financial issue may be the greatest barrier to the adoption of newer techniques. Medicare and most health insurance companies continue to refuse to pay for any "screening test" for coronary artery disease in people without symptoms such as chest pain or shortness of breath. All of the guidelines from the professional cardiology associations do not recommend such a screening test, but make no mistake—cost is a major factor in these opinions. It is a rare cardiologist who has not stretched the truth about symptoms to order a stress test on a person he or she felt was at high risk for coronary artery disease.

For the many people who suffer from the disease identified by William Heberden in the 1770s, angina pectoris, modern medication has had a great impact, markedly reducing the incidence of their frightening episodes of chest pain. There are now four different types of drugs, each with uses in particular circumstances and sometimes used in combination. These drugs all decrease the heart's need for blood and oxygen, especially with physical exertion. One of these medications is a long-acting form of nitroglycerin, that very potent chemical first synthesized by the Italian chemist Ascanio Sobrero in the 1840s.

But given all we now know, will we continue to focus too many of our resources and research in the wrong place? The modern cardiologists already have so many tools to reduce or eliminate angina, avoid long-term complications after a heart attack, and continue to improve outcomes; but we so often continue to aim our attention on those who *already have* coronary artery disease. This should change in the future.

THE NEW INSURANCE AGENT: THE CARDIOLOGIST PREVENTER

There has been a neglected "stepchild" for decades: prevention. Recent discoveries have highlighted the need for prevention of the relentless progression of atherosclerosis in the coronary arteries, in both those who have survived a Widowmaker assault, and the millions who have the early stages of a killer slowly growing in their heart's arteries.

Despite what we now know, prevention is not nearly as exciting for doctors as the rush of caring for a sick patient after a heart attack. Although the Framingham Study results identified the key risk factors for the heart attack, huge parts of the basic science were lacking. Yes, cholesterol seemed to be a major player, but we've had limited success in telling people not to eat food with too much fat and cholesterol, as John Gofman urged in the late 1950s, publishing a cookbook with barely tolerable recipes. But it was Gofman's work and the terrible fate of two children in the 1960s with a rare inherited form of elevated blood cholesterol levels that led two close friends, Michael Brown and Joseph Goldstein, to uncover the real details of the control of the metabolism of cholesterol and how disturbances of that process would lead to atherosclerosis.

Figuring out how to lower blood cholesterol levels was, and still is, the real challenge and has proven to be one of the keys to prevention. Yes, diet is helpful: it's clear that diets with lower animal fat, fewer breads, pasta, and cakes, and more fresh fruits and vegetables are of benefit. Hopefully, the next generations will be more attentive (and less dependent on K-ration-type foods) to healthier eating over their lifetimes. But cholesterol levels are not only dependent on diet. A good portion of its metabolism is genetically determined, often overwhelming the healthy intentions of a diet. After a troubled start to find medications that both lowered cholesterol and were safe, Akira Endo, with the help of the US pharmaceutical company Merck, produced the first breakthrough statin medication.

Millions of lives have been saved, and there are now several very promising non-statin medications that are both beginning to be used and further researched. A new class of drugs with the tongue-twisting name of proprotein convertase subtilisin/kexin type 9 inhibitors (PCSK9 inhibitors), drugs that slow down the metabolism of the LDL receptor that breaks down cholesterol, have been created, allowing the LDL receptors molecules found by Brown and Goldstein to work for a longer time, chewing up more cholesterol from the bloodstream. These drugs are just the latest example of translational research, careful and often frustrating work usually done in stark-looking laboratories hidden away in one of the floors of a medical school building, often with poor lighting, stained laboratory bench counters, and strange odors.

Patients receiving these new medications, even when they are also taking good doses of statin medication, have profound decreases in blood cholesterol levels, levels seen only in healthy children. These drugs prevent recurrent cardiac events and save lives. Much wider use of the PCSK9 inhibitors, even though they require self-injection every two weeks, is very likely in the next few years. Fortunately, the side effects of these drugs have been minimal.

It would be nice if more insurance companies approved the use of these medications and their price decreased. The two forms currently approved by the FDA cost just over $450 a month. When it comes to cholesterol, lower is always better, if you can afford it. There are more medications to come, one using very promising genetic manipulation science to dramatically decrease the production of the PCSK9 molecule that shortens the life of the LDL receptor so crucial to clearing cholesterol from the blood. The experimental drug inclisiran[162] is in clinical trials currently, with dramatic results so far. This medication is given as an under the skin injection once every six months. Hopes are high.

A new oral non-statin medication named bempedoic acid that lowers cholesterol was FDA approved in the last year. An exciting new entry into the lipid battle is a form of fish oil named icosapent ethyl, which targets not cholesterol, but triglycerides, a form of lipoprotein that is associated with coronary artery risk but has defied effective treatment that lower the risk of heart attack. In 2019, icosapent ethyl broke that end-point barrier of heart attack incidence, and many more patients will now have effective treatment that goes beyond lowering cholesterol levels.

In recent years, many investigators have tried to find ways to identify atherosclerosis long before a person suffers a heart attack, not just depending upon blood tests of cholesterol levels, the electrocardiogram, and stress testing. One of these tests is the coronary calcium scan. The concept is simple: the pathologists have told us that the only process that causes calcium to deposit in one of the layers of a coronary artery is atherosclerosis, and by the time the calcium accumulates in a plaque, the process has been going on for at

---

162 Inclisiran interferes with the ability of RNA in the nucleus to use the genetic code to produce the PCSK9 molecule.

least several years. Fortunately, finding coronary artery calcium does not necessarily mean that someone has a severely blocked coronary artery, at least at the time of the scan. Sometimes the calcium is in the outer layer of the artery and has not yet caused any significant blockage of blood flow through that artery. But the future can be foretold—the greater the amount of calcium seen, the higher the risk of a cardiac event in the next few years. The calcium score offers a great opportunity for prevention.

Although the coronary artery scan procedure has been available for years, too few people have had the test, a quick and easy procedure not covered by insurance companies and yet costing less than $100, a remarkably low price for any medical test in 2020. There is naturally controversy regarding who really needs the test, the argument being that a decision to give medication to lower cholesterol, almost always a statin drug, can be made by using "scoring systems" of risk that don't include a coronary artery calcium scan.

There are many such scoring systems, first introduced by the Framingham researchers, to try to determine an individual's risk of a major cardiac problem in the next five to ten years. A current popular choice is named the Pooled Cohort Equation, which anyone can access and use on the internet. However, newer and more comprehensive systems are added on almost a yearly basis. If someone's risk of a cardiac event is greater than 7.5 percent over the next ten years, then diet or medication is recommended to lower the cholesterol level. Too often diet alone fails to lower the level of cholesterol enough. So for millions, medications will continue to be necessary, usually using medications with years of track records of safety.

PREVENTING A PREDICTABLE FUTURE

In order to adequately apprehend the Widowmaker, a huge question needs to be addressed in the next few years: are the current guidelines for who should receive medication for their cholesterol just not good enough? Most of the standard risk calculators do not include age as one the major risks, and clearly the older you are, the greater the risk. But if atherosclerosis is a slow long-term process, doesn't the length of time of one's exposure to the disease matter? In the opinion of many, much earlier and long-term treatment is the only real hope to prevent the consequences of atherosclerosis as people age. Knowing at how early in life atherosclerosis can begin, I suspect the guidelines will change to urge more aggressive treatment of elevated cholesterol levels in younger people. Many of us in practice have already adopted this change in thought.

The prevention of the Widowmaker's work also requires good long-term management of high blood pressure and diabetes. Approximately thirty-three percent of the population of the United States has hypertension, a chronic disease that damages the blood vessels all over the human body, but in particular the coronary arteries, making them more prone to atherosclerosis, as well as the kidneys, the retinas of the eyes, and the brain, predisposing to the several types of strokes, the cerebrovascular accidents that killed President Franklin Roosevelt in 1945.

Though the world is quite different than 1945, the global burden of hypertension remains enormous, estimated at over one billion people. Most of them do not know that they have hypertension, and less than fifty percent of those who do know are taking medication that controls the blood pressure according to modern guidelines. The task of controlling high blood pressure is unfinished. But fortunately, there are many types of medications that can effectively lower blood pressure over the years.

The science of cardiology demands constant re-examination of even well-accepted principles, and many are hard at work doing just that. For example, a study in 2015 sought to find out whether a blood pressure of 140/90 or less was really as good as 120/80 or less. The publication of "A Randomized Trial of Intensive versus Standard Blood Pressure Control" by the SPRINT group in the *New England Journal of Medicine* in November 2015 was a bombshell to not just cardiologists, but also family doctors, internal medicine specialists, kidney doctors, and endocrinologists, all of us treating high blood pressure. The risk of the end points of the research were reduced by twenty-five percent in the 120/80 people, a major effect seen in just over three years of follow-up of the patients. The 120/80 group had fewer heart attacks, fewer hospitalizations for angina, and fewer episodes of congestive heart failure. Most importantly, their overall chances of dying was also reduced by twenty-five percent.

The control of high blood pressure is not totally dependent on medications; lifestyle plays a key role. People can greatly help the effectiveness of the drugs by doing those things that most of our mothers told us—eat healthy, exercise, watch your weight, and don't eat too much salt. The sodium in salt has long been known as a factor in retaining fluid and raising blood pressure, and most of us consume way too much on a regular basis. This final recommendation is quite challenging for many.

It is very hard to eliminate salt in our diets, as it is contained in just about every processed food and meat we eat, but a combination of moderate salt restriction and medication can go a long way toward achieving an optimal blood pressure. I always tell my patients with high blood pressure to do two other things for themselves: look at the sodium content on the packages of what they eat (or if there is no packaging, check the sodium content on Google on their cell phone), and check their own blood pressure at home. The home electronic monitors, a basic device costing about $60 (and of course not covered by health insurance), are reliable and easy to use. This is a key example of how effectively managing any chronic condition, like hypertension, requires a partnership between a patient and their doctor.

Of course, there are other significant risk factors. Cigarette smoking continues to plague too many people worldwide. The toxic products in cigarette smoke have a plethora of destructive metabolic effects on the walls of blood vessels, increasing the chance of LDL finding its way into the arteries, not to mention the damage to the lungs. The prevalence of smoking has decreased steadily over the last three decades but is still a horrible habit of fifteen to sixteen percent of the United States population of adults as of 2016. This number has decreased from 20.9 percent in 2006, and the goal of the Centers for Disease Control is to get that number down to less than twelve percent.

A new entrant into the realm of the treating cardiologist is the management of diabetes mellitus, the disorder of glucose metabolism, a process that has been known to accelerate the progress of atherosclerosis all over the body for almost a century. For many years now, it is possible to control the blood sugar of most people with diabetes, assuming a couple of things: they watch their diet and weight, exercise, and take their medications. Insulin has been available since the 1920s, and the modern forms of this hormone, of which there are many with different uses at different times of the day, are safe and effective. Until recently, none of the commonly used diabetes medications, especially the oral forms, reduced the chances of heart attacks or heart failure, even though they will control blood sugar levels.

That has changed and new diabetes medications now have a surprising effect on heart disease. There are now almost twenty newer forms of medications for the treatment of diabetes, particularly the type of diabetes that occurs as people age and become overweight, "Type II" or "adult-onset" diabetes, a modern epidemic. These new medications affect the manner in which the kidney excretes sugar and also how certain hormones secreted by the intestine interact with insulin. In addition to their effect on the blood sugar, several of these newer medications have had an unexpected and remarkable effect—they have reduced the risk of cardiac events such as heart failure and heart attacks, as well preserving kidney function, an all-too-frequent target of diabetes. Many cardiologists have taken up the task of treating diabetes because there are just not enough qualified endocrinologists in the United States.

The modern cardiologist as the insurance agent, protecting against the work of the Widowmaker, continues to be on the frontline, now not just in the emergency room, CCU, or the cath lab, but also in the outpatient office setting. Family doctors and the internal medicine specialists also have the knowledge and tools to manage those well-known risk factors for atherosclerosis and save lives.

THE FIFTY-YEAR SCORECARD

For so long it seemed that our hands were tied. Though nitroglycerin and amyl nitrite were the first drugs that changed the lives of patients with coronary artery disease, from the mid-1880s until the mid-1960s, doctors could do little else for patients. After World War II, the epidemic and deaths piled up in the western world.

But in 1965, the trajectory of the rates of death from coronary artery disease began to change. The addition of the drug propranolol to not only decrease symptoms but also the risk of a heart attack, and the CCU, with its special tools and treatments, began to make a dent in the epidemic. By the early 1970s, cardiac catheterization imaging of the coronary arteries led to bypass surgery and better testing identified people before the Widowmaker's attack happened. The epidemiologists were confirming that indeed the death rate in the United States and other high-income countries was finally decreasing, and the results were consistent year after year.

These findings were truly remarkable. The data reporting drops in overall cardiovascular death rates of forty percent to eighty percent depending upon which country's numbers were examined. These declines were far greater than the decrease in the death rate from cancer. Was the Widowmaker really on the run?

Until 2010, it appeared that the decline would continue, as the technology and treatment, as well as public health initiatives, were more available. But by the early part of the last decade, there was a change in the data. Although the absolute number of deaths from heart disease was continuing to decrease, the rate of decrease was slowing down, and the death rate even increasing in some countries of the world. The change was affecting both men and women, from an average 3.5 percent decline in the decade of the 2000s to about one percent beginning in 2010. This might not sound like a big difference, but it is a seventy percent decrease in the rate of decline. What was happening and what might be continuing to happen?

These data are coming from the richer countries around the world, while in the poor and middle-income countries, the death rate from cardiovascular disease is continuing to *increase*. Many of these countries have adopted western lifestyle patterns, like cigarette smoking and high fat, high cholesterol diets, with an end result of surges in obesity rates. It is estimated that by 2030, there will be 23.4 million deaths each year from cardiovascular disease, still thirty-five percent of all deaths. Half will occur in the West and half in Asia. Although death rates from coronary artery disease have decreased in Japan and other East Asian countries, they have increased through Central Asia.

In addition, there are two special populations of people that we now know are at increased risk of heart disease. The first are women who develop various problems associated with pregnancy, including high blood pressure,[163] diabetes, pre-term births, miscarriage, and small birthweight children. These women deserve close attention to reducing the traditional risk factors, and more aggressive treatment of high blood pressure, diabetes, and hyperlipidemia at younger ages. The second are the currently thirty-eight million people worldwide living with human immunodeficiency virus, HIV. The treatment of HIV with medications is a modern miracle, with so many people living normal lives for years with low levels of viral infection. But as more and more data have accrued, it was found that their risk of cardiac disease, especially atherosclerosis, is 1.5-2.0 times higher than the general population. Although it is uncertain, chronic inflammation from the infection, even at a minimal level, may be contributing to the

---

163 Including two serious forms of high blood pressure of pregnancy, pre-eclampsia and eclampsia.

development of atherosclerosis at a younger age. These patients also should be advised and treated more aggressively regarding prevention.

It is important to address the fact that the obesity epidemic is a key culprit for atherosclerosis in our times. For years, it was felt that being overweight itself was not really the problem because it was associated with inactivity, diabetes, and hypertension, the more important forces increasing risk. But again, those researchers have turned up something important: fat cells themselves can stimulate inflammation, that internal fire that leads to the heart attack.

The answer is once again in the numbers, and it's a relatively easy number to come up with. There is a simple calculation that determines if someone is overweight and when he or she is considered obese. The key number that we should all know about ourselves is the body-mass index, the BMI. The BMI is a straightforward calculation, although it does use the metric system unfamiliar to most Americans. You take your weight in kilograms (1 kilogram = 2.2 pounds) and divide it by your height in meters (1 meter = 39.37 inches) times itself or squared. If your BMI is over 25, you're overweight; if it's over 30, you fit the medical definition of being obese. Recent data on BMI in America paints a grim picture.

The stunning information from the World Health Organization shows that as of 2016, just short of seventy percent of Americans were overweight! Thirty-nine percent of both men and women were obese. Perhaps even worse, eighteen percent of children were also overweight or obese; that's almost one in five. Just for a moment, let those numbers sink in. The next time you can travel safely and spend time in an American airport, look around, and you'll confirm for yourself the validity of those figures.

There is a conviction that obesity, if it continues to increase, will blunt the incredible progress that has been made in dealing with the Widowmaker. So many diets and medications have been tried to combat being overweight, but none of these have proven to be effective in large numbers of people over time. For sure, many diets can result in short-term, and often major, weight loss, but sustaining that loss by converting a lifestyle is much less successful.

To reference Churchill again, the pursuit of the Widowmaker is at the end of the beginning. All of what has been so carefully learned will be needed to advise doctors about the best ways to treat the victims of the heart attack and, even more importantly, prevent so many more from ever making the Widowmaker's acquaintance. The hope is that the heart attack will be a vestige of the past someday. I am confident there will be so many more great names and achievements to report on in the rest of the twenty-first century. The rich history and tradition of the science of the heart attack will always lead the way. The chase continues.

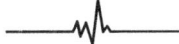

HOW FAR WE HAVE COME: ROUTINE LIFE-SAVING IN THE TWENTY-FIRST CENTURY
December 2009

"I don't think he knew what hit him," he told me. My Cardiology Fellow on his CCU rotation paged me to come see a man urgently. He had a cardiac arrest. His heart stopped, and he fell down. Somehow his heart rhythm came back.

Walking quickly, I thought about how after sixteen years in private practice, I finally had that academic job at Temple University School of Medicine and now was the Senior Attending Physician in the Coronary Care Unit that month. Arriving a minute or two later, I made a beeline towards the new patient's room, accompanied by the Cardiology Fellow and the internal medicine residents on our team. I stopped outside the room. "What's the story here?"

The Fellow spoke in the jargon. "This is Mr. Gramberg. He's sixty-seven. No cardiac history, in good health except for some hypertension. He goes to the gym pretty often, and he was there today exercising.

Then he went down. The trainers in the gym didn't know how to do anything, so they called Fire Rescue. They got there in a minute or two, and he had a normal rhythm, but they saw a lot of PVCs. Now he's good, normal blood pressure and heart rate. We started him on amiodarone, but his EKG is abnormal and his troponins are up. He had an MI. He also broke his jaw in four places because of the fall."

"Okay, let's go see him," I said.

He was a thin man, more bewildered than frightened. He said he was a little sore in the chest from the fall but more bothered by the pain in his broken jaw. "Have you had any chest pain today or in the last few weeks?"

"No, nothing at all."

"Any shortness of breath or palpitations?"

"No."

"Do you remember what happened today?"

"Not really, I was just exercising and then I passed out. That's all I remember."

I told him my recommendations, based on years of treating patients and fighting to stave off the Widowmaker. He needed a cardiac cath that day and probable angioplasty.

"Does that work?" He looked worried.

"Almost all of the time," I said. "And the arteries stay open over ninety-five percent of the time." Mr. Gramberg reflected for a minute then agreed to the procedure.

I called my colleague in the cath lab, and Mr. Gramberg was on his way there within a few minutes. He had two severely blocked coronary arteries, and angioplasty procedures successfully cleared up both of them with relative ease, pushing blood clot and cholesterol plaque into the wall of the arteries. The diseased arteries were on the right side of the heart, not a "classic" location for a Widowmaker lesion in the left anterior descending coronary artery, but potentially lethal because of the malignant arrhythmia caused by the lack of blood flow to the bottom wall of the heart.

Mr. Gramberg's hospital stay was uneventful. He had high blood pressure, and we started him on medication for that, as well as giving him medication to lower his cholesterol level, aspirin, and a drug called clopidogrel to stop blood platelets from sticking to the stents in his coronary arteries.

I still see Mr. Gramberg about every six months, and as of 2020, he has not had one single other cardiac event. He should live a long life. He takes his medications, watches his diet, checks his blood pressure at home, comes to see me on a regular basis, and long ago returned to regular exercise. He has eluded the grasp of the Widowmaker.

Mr. Gramberg and so many others owe their lives to the discoveries outlined in this book. There is so much now that doctors and patients can do, in a long-lasting partnership, to prevent and treat the consequences of the heart attack. All of us should understand what causes heart attacks, how to prevent them, and about the dedicated medical scientists who have avidly pursued and continue to chase the Widowmaker.

GLOSSARY

ADRENALINE: a hormone molecule secreted by the adrenal glands and the nervous system, especially in conditions of stress, increasing heart rate and blood pressure and preparing muscles for exertion; also known as epinephrine

AMYL NITRITE: an organic chemical synthesized in the nineteenth century; the first medication used to effectively relieve angina pectoris

ANEURYSM: an excessive localized enlargement of an artery caused by a weakening of the artery wall, with increased risk of sudden rupture and massive bleeding

ANGINA PECTORIS: pain in the chest, often also spreading to the shoulders, arms, and neck, caused by an inadequate blood supply to the heart due to atherosclerosis of the coronary arteries

ANGIOPLASTY: unblocking of a blood vessel, especially a coronary artery, by using an inflatable balloon attached to a catheter inserted into a blood vessel of leg or the arm

ANTIARRHYTHMIC MEDICATION: drugs that are used to treat abnormal heart rhythms resulting from irregular electrical activity of the heart

ARRHYTHMIAS: abnormal heart rhythms that originate from the cells of the heart muscle; usually an abnormally rapid rhythm associated with palpitations and/or shortness of breath, chest pain, and dizziness, as well as sometimes passing out

AORTA: the main artery of the body, supplying oxygenated blood to the circulatory system; it originates from the top of the left ventricle of the heart and runs down in front of the backbone

AORTIC VALVE: the valve in the human heart between the left ventricle and the aorta; one of the four valves of the heart; made of connective tissue similar to cartilage and opens and closes with each heartbeat

ATHEROSCLEROSIS: disease of the arteries characterized by the deposition of plaques of fatty material on their inner walls, composed of cholesterol, lipoproteins, white blood cells, smooth muscle cells, blood platelets, and areas of blood clots and red blood cells

ATRIAL FIBRILLATION: an irregular, rapid heart rate that may cause symptoms like heart palpitations, fatigue, and shortness of breath; occurs when the upper chambers of the heart (atria) beat out of rhythm; as a result, blood is not pumped efficiently to the rest of the body

BETA BLOCKERS: a class of medications that attach to the beta receptor molecules on the cell surface of many tissues including the heart, where they block the effect of adrenaline and cause slowing of the heart rate and lowering of blood pressure

CARDIAC ARREST: an abrupt cessation of contraction of the heart muscle resulting in absence of blood pressure and often death within minutes unless the heart rhythm is restored by electric shock, medication, or a pacemaker

CARDIAC CATHETERIZATION: a diagnostic test during which a thin hollow plastic tube, a catheter, is inserted into an artery of the leg or arm and passed into the heart to measure the pressures inside the heart chamber and often then to inject dye through the catheter to take "angiogram" images of the coronary arteries to look for atherosclerosis and/or blood clots

CARDIOPULMONARY BYPASS: a procedure during which blood from a large vein is diverted into a tube and propelled into a machine that provides oxygenation to the blood, which is pumped through a second tube back into either the aorta or an artery; a circulation of blood outside of the body using the "heart-lung" machine during cardiac surgery

CARDIOPULMONARY RESUSCITATION: using external compression of the chest and artificial ventilation to attempt to provide blood pressure and oxygen during a period of cardiac arrest

CATHETER: a small lumen plastic tube inserted into an artery or vein to administer fluid, transfuse or withdraw blood, or inject contrast dye to image blood vessels, in particular the arteries of the heart, the coronary arteries

CHOLESTEROL: an important organic molecule used to build cells walls, hormones, and bile; absorbed from the diet and produced by the liver; combines with proteins in the blood to form lipoproteins, one of which, "low density lipoprotein (LDL)," is the molecule that becomes embedded in the walls of arteries and causes atherosclerosis

COLLATERAL BLOOD VESSELS: small blood vessels normally present that enlarge and supply more blood when the major large artery supplying a portion of the heart or leg muscle becomes obstructed

CONGESTIVE HEART FAILURE: a chronic or acute set of symptoms due to a marked decrease in the pumping function of the major heart chamber, the left ventricle; often a consequence of a large acute or chronic myocardial infarction or a form of heart muscle disease; symptoms often include shortness of breath, extreme fatigue, and ankle swelling or edema.

CORONARY ANGIOGRAPHY: direct visualization on x-ray film of the lumen, the inside, of the coronary arteries achieved by the injection of contrast dye through a fluid-filled plastic catheter inserted first into an artery of the leg or arm and advanced to the edge of the opening of the two major coronary arteries at the top of the heart

CORONARY ARTERIES: the small tubes on the heart surface that carry blood and oxygen to the heart muscle; anatomically two blood vessels, right and left, but functionally three as the left coronary artery branches after a short distance into the left anterior descending coronary artery and the left circumflex coronary artery

CORONARY ARTERY BYPASS SURGERY: technique used to supply blood beyond areas of obstruction in the coronary arteries usually due to atherosclerosis; an artery from under the sternum (breastbone) or pieces of veins from the legs used to create the bypass conduits

CORONARY ARTERY DISEASE: complete or partial obstruction of the blood vessels of the heart muscle, almost always due to atherosclerosis and/or thrombosis (blood clot) formation inside of the lumen of the artery; the cause of angina and myocardial infarction

CORONARY ARTERY STENTS: short metallic lattice-like tubes inserted into a coronary artery after a balloon angioplasty has reduced atherosclerotic blockage; help prevent recurrence of blockage of the artery; usually imbedded with medication to reduce scar formation in the area of the stent

DEFIBRILLATION: the rapid application of high energy electrical shock to the heart muscle to disrupt a fast and dangerous rapid heartbeat; can be achieved by an external device or a surgically implanted device

DEFIBRILLATOR: the device that supplies the energy to achieve defibrillation, using direct current (DC) charge

DIABETES MELLITUS: a common metabolic disease which impairs the body's use of insulin and carbohydrates, leading to high levels of blood glucose; either due to insulin deficiency (Type I) or insulin resistance (Type II); Type II strongly associated with obesity; both forms are major risk factors for atherosclerosis formation

ELECTROCARDIOGRAM (EKG): a device that converts the electrical energy of the heart into a recording; invented by Willem Einthoven in Holland in 1901

ENZYME: a protein molecule that converts one molecule into another molecule in a chain of metabolism

EPIDEMIOLOGY: a branch of medical science that examines the incidence, prevalence, distribution, and possible control of diseases and other factors relating to health

FOAM CELL: a type of white blood cell seen under the microscope in atherosclerotic plaque in arteries; they ingest lipoproteins and cholesterol, and the inside of the cell appears as if it contains foam of some kind

HYPERTENSION: high blood pressure, currently diagnosed with blood pressure of over 130 systolic over 80 diastolic; cause unknown in ninety-five percent of people; causes constriction of arteries through the circulation leading to heart, the coronary artery, kidney, brain, and eye damage if not controlled well with medication

INFLAMMATION: the response of the body to injury from trauma, infection, cancer, and atherosclerosis; mediated by antibodies made by white blood cells (B cells) and other types of white blood cells (T cells)

LEFT ATRIUM: one of the four chambers of the heart, receiving blood returning from the lungs, and filling the left ventricle with blood during the diastolic phase of the contraction of the heart when its valve, the mitral valve, opens

LEFT VENTRICLE: the largest and most important chamber of the heart; ejects blood with each heartbeat through the aortic valve, into the aorta; occlusion of its blood supply leads to myocardial infarction and acute and/or chronic dysfunction of the heart overall

LIPOPROTEINS: the complex set of molecules that carry cholesterol and fat from the intestine and the liver throughout the circulation

METABOLISM: the process by which all of the important molecules of the body, such as insulin or cholesterol, are produced by a series of chemical reactions using enzymes and generate energy for the function of cells and organs

MITRAL VALVE: valve on the left side of the heart that opens during diastole, the relaxation phase of the heart's contraction, to allow blood to flow from the left atrium into the left ventricle

MYOCARDIAL INFARCTION: permanent damage to the heart muscle due to occlusion of one or several coronary arteries; can result in rapid death or severe chronic dysfunction of the heart

NITROGLYCERIN: an explosive organic chemical first made in a laboratory; initially used as the main element of dynamite, and then in much smaller concentration as the second and most important medication for the treatment of angina pectoris

NUCLEAR CARDIAC IMAGING: the use radioactive elements to create images of cardiac function and/or the blood supply of the heart muscle

P VALUE: a statistical measure of the probability that data comparing a treatment or test with a "control group" or another treatment group is either significant or not; in medicine, a P value of less than five percent (.05) indicates that there is a ninety-five percent or greater chance that a different in two data sets is significant and is the standard used in research studies

PERIPHERAL BLOOD VESSELS: the arteries and veins of the body supplying the arms, legs, and brain

QRS COMPLEX: the portion of the EKG signal that indicates the contraction of the right and left ventricles

RADIOISOTOPE: a radioactive form of an element used in the imaging of organs

RECEPTOR MOLECULE: a molecule on the surface of a cell that binds molecules from the circulation such as adrenaline and LDL cholesterol; this binding initiates a specific metabolic process

SMOOTH MUSCLE CELLS: one of the two types of muscle cells, named so because of their appearance under the microscope; these cells make up the middle lining, the media, of blood vessels

ST SEGMENT: the portion of the EKG signal immediately after the QRS complex; elevation of this signal is seen in many acute myocardial infarctions and indicates damage to the entire layer of the muscle of the heart; depression of this segment often indicates ischemia, lack of blood supply to an area of the heart muscle and may or may not be associated with a myocardial infarction

STATINS: a class of medications that inhibit cholesterol production by the liver by inhibiting the action of a specific enzyme, HMG CoA reductase

STATISTICS: a branch of mathematics that interprets data and allows for assessment of probabilities

STRESS TEST: a diagnostic test using exercise or medication to assess the blood supply of the heart

STROKE: permanent damage to brain cells caused by occlusion of a brain blood vessel from atherosclerosis, high blood pressure, or other processes, or occlusion caused by an embolism of blood clot from the heart or the carotid arteries of the neck

THROMBOLYSIS: the administration of specific medications that break up blood clots ("clot busters")

THROMBOSIS: the formation of a blood clot in response to injury or inflammation

VENTRICLES: two of the four chambers of the heart; the right ventricle pumps blood from the veins into the lungs to obtain oxygen; the left ventricle pumps blood into the aorta to supply the organs of the body

VENTRICULAR FIBRILLATION: a life-threatening cardiac arrhythmia often due to an acute myocardial infarction, chronic severe damage to the left ventricle, types of congenital heart disease, or inherited electrical disorders of the heart

VENTRICULAR TACHYCARDIA: rapid beating of the left or right ventricle caused by structural disease of the heart of many types; will often result in fatal ventricular fibrillation if not treated promptly with medication or electrical shock

BIBLIOGRAPHY

CHAPTER 1

1. Bacon F. The advancement of learning: Jazzybee Verlag; 1951.

2. Dalen JE, Alpert JS, Goldberg RJ, Weinstein RS. The epidemic of the 20th century: coronary heart disease. The American Journal of Medicine 2014; 127:807-12.

3. Frost, N. How the US Army botched feeding its female soldiers in World War II. May 25, 2018.Atlasobscura.com/articles/what-did-women-soldiers-eat-world-war-two.

4. Hester, Jere. New York Daily News. 1997. Mother Teresa dies at 87 years old after heart fails at a convent." NYDailyNews.com/new/world/dead-87-mother-teresaheart-fails-nobelist-missionary-article/1.769700

5. History.com/topics/world-war-ii/american-women-in-world-war-ii1. American women in World War II.

6. Jemal A, Ward E, Hao Y, Thun M. Trends in the leading causes of death in the United States, 1970-2002. Journal of the American Medical Association 2005; 294:1255-9.

7. Joseph AM, Muggli M, Pearson KC, Lando H. The cigarette manufacturers' efforts to promote tobacco to the US military. Military Medicine 2005; 170:874-80.

8. Koehler FA. Special Rations for the Armed Forces: Army Operational Rations. A Historical Background. QMC Historical

Studies, Historical Branch, Office of the Quartermaster General, Washington, DC 1958.

9. Messerli FH, Messerli AW, Luscher TF. Eisenhower's billion-dollar heart attack—50 years later. New England Journal of Medicine 2005; 353:1205-7.

10. Nationalww2museum.org/students-teachers/student-resources/research-starters-us-military-numbers. Research starters: US military by the numbers.

11. New York Times January 23, 1973. Lyndon Johnson, 36th President, Is Dead; Was Architect of Great Society Program.

12. News Bbc Uk/2/hi/americas/851817stm2010 2010. Bill Clinton 'in good spirits' after heart procedure.

13. Stallones RA. The rise and fall of ischemic heart disease. Scientific American 1980; 243:53-9.

14. Sutherland JE, Persky VW, Brody JA. Proportionate mortality trends: 1950 through 1986. Journal of the American Medical Association 1990; 264:3178-84.

15. www.latimes.com/local/obituaries/la-me-clark 11/17/60 Clark Gable Dies at 59. November 17, 1960.

16. www.medicalbag.com/what-killed-em/clark-gable/article/486656/.

17. www.nbcnews.com/id/5906976/ns/heath-heart-health/clinton-leaves-hospital-after-surgery/#XAVmkxNKjAw 2004. Clinton leaves hospital after surgery.

18. www.olive-drab.com/od_rations_kphp. Military Rations: K Rations.

CHAPTER 2

1. Alberti FB. John Hunter's Heart. The Bulletin of the Royal College of Surgeons of England 2013; 95:168-9.

2. Bruetsch Wl. The earliest record of sudden death possibly due to atherosclerotic coronary occlusion. Circulation 1959; 20:438-41.

3. Edmondstone W. Cardiac chest pain: does body language help the diagnosis? British Medical Journal 1995; 311:1660-1661.

4. Fye WB. Cardiology in 1885. Circulation 1985; 72:21-6.

5. Heberden W. Commentaries on the History and Cure of Diseases: Payne and Foss; 1816.

6. Herrick JB. Thrombosis of the coronary arteries. Journal of the American Medical Association 1919; 72:387-90.

7. Herrick JB. A Short History of Cardiology. Springfield, Ill., Baltimore, MD: C. C. Thomas; 1942.

8. Herrick JB. Memories of Eighty Years. Chicago: Univ. of Chicago Press; 1949.

9. Herrick JB. Landmark article (JAMA 1912). Clinical features of sudden obstruction of the coronary arteries. By James B. Herrick. Journal of the American Medical Association 1983; 250:1757-65.

10. Herrick JB. Peculiar elongated and sickle-shaped red blood corpuscles in a case of severe anemia. Journal of the American Medical Association 2014; 312:1063.

11. Herrick JB, Nuzum FR. Angina pectoris: clinical experience with two hundred cases." Journal of the American Medical Association 1918; 70:67-70.

12. Khan IA, Mehta NJ. Initial historical descriptions of the angina pectoris. The Journal of Emergency Medicine 2002; 22:295-8.

13. Leach MA. History of angina. Res Medica 1967.

14. Levine SA. Clinical heart disease: Saunders; 1945.

15. Moore W. The Knife-Man: The Extraordinary Life and Times of John Hunter, Father of Modern Surgery. 2005.

16. Netter FH. The Ciba Collection of Medical Illustrations, Volume 5: Heart: Ciba Medical Education Division; 1972.

17. Netter FM, Roper WL. Medicine's Michelangelo: The Life & Art of Frank H. Netter, MD: Quinnipiac University Press; 2013.

18. Walker H, Hall WD, Hurst JW, editors. Clinical Methods: The History, Physical, and Laboratory Examinations: 3rd Edition: Boston Butterworths 1990 1900.

CHAPTER 3

1. Booth J. A short history of blood pressure measurement. SAGE Publications; 1977.

2. Cheng AM. The Real Death of Vitalism. Penn Ethics Journal 1(1) 2005.

3. Dudgeon RE. The sphygmograph: its history and use as an aid to diagnosis in ordinary practice: Baillière, Tindall, and Cox; 1882.

4. Fye WB. T. Lauder Brunton and amyl nitrite: A Victorian vasodilator. Circulation 1986; 74:222-9.

5. Fye WB. Nitroglycerin: a homeopathic remedy. Circulation 1986; 73:21-9.

6. greenmedicine.ie/school/images/Library. A Brief History of Organic Chemistry. online.

7. Hunting P. Sir Thomas Lauder Brunton Bt FRCP FRS (1844 -1916). Journal of Medical Biography 2016; 24:433-9.

8. Jorpes JE. Alfred Nobel. British Medical Journal 1959;1:1.

9. MacDonald GW. Historical papers on modern explosives. Chapter XXII ed: Whittaker & Company; 1912.

10. Marsh N, Marsh A. A short history of nitroglycerine and nitric oxide in pharmacology and physiology. Clinical and Experimental Pharmacology and Physiology 2000; 27:313-9.

11. Ramberg PJ. The death of vitalism and the birth of organic chemistry: Wöhler's urea synthesis and the disciplinary identity of organic chemistry. Ambix 2000; 47:170-95.

12. Tolf RW. The Russian Rockefellers: The Saga of the Nobel Family and the Russian Oil Industry: Hoover Press; 1976.

CHAPTER 4

1. Besterman E, "Creese R. Waller—pioneer of electrocardiography." British Heart Journal 1979; 42:61.

2. Burnett J. "The origins of the electrocardiograph as a clinical instrument." Medical History 1985; 29:53-76.

3. Cope Z. Augustus Desire Waller (1856-1922). Medical History 1973; 17:380-5.

4. Einthoven W. Le telecardiogramme. Archives of International Physiology 1906; 4:132-64.

5. Henderson J. Servants of Medicine: Augustus Waller—father and son physiologists. SAGE Publications Sage UK: London, England; 2005.

6. Snellen HA. Willem Einthoven (1860-1927) Father of electrocardiography: Life and work, ancestors and contemporaries: Springer Science & Business Media; 2012.

7. Waller AD. A demonstration on man of electromotive changes accompanying the heart's beat. The Journal of Physiology 1887; 8:229-34.

8. Wiggers CJ. Willem Einthoven (1860-1927) Some Facets of His Life and Work. Circulation Research 1961; 9:225-34.

CHAPTER 5

1. Anichkov N, Chalatov S. Euber experimentelle cholestetinsteattose- Ihre Bedeutung für die Enstehung einiger pathologischer Proessen. Centr F Allegem Pathologic Pathology Anatomy 1913;1:1.

2. Anitschkow N, Wolkoff K, Kikaion E, Pozharisski K. Compensatory adjustments in the structure of coronary arteries of the heart with stenotic atherosclerosis. Circulation 1964; 29:447-55.

3. Dock W. Research in arteriosclerosis—the first fifty years. Annals of Internal Medicine 1958; 49:699-705.

4. Friedman M. Medicine's 10 greatest discoveries: Yale University Press; 1998.

5. Ignatowski A. Über die Wirkung des tierischen Eiweißes auf die Aorta und die parenchymatösen Organe der Kaninchen. Virchows Archiv Für Pathologische Anatomie und Physiologie und Für Flinische Medizin 1909; 198:248-70.

6. Konstantinov IE, Mejevoi N, Anichkov NM. Nikolai N. Anichkov and his theory of atherosclerosis. Texas Heart Institute Journal 2006; 33:417.

7. Marchand F. Über arteriosklerose (atherosklerose). Verhandlungen des Kongress Für Innere Medizin; 1904.

8. Osler W. The Principles and Practice of Medicine: Designed for the Use of Practitioners and Students of Medicine: New York: D. Appleton; 1892.

9. Rokitansky K. Über Einige der Wichtigsten Krankheiten der Arterien: Aus der Kaiserlich-Königlichen Hof-und Staatsdruckerei; 1852.

10. Virchow R. Der atheromatose prozess der arterien. Wiener Medizinische Wochenschrift 1856; 6:143-52.

11. Windaus A. Über Cholesterin. Berichte der deutschen chemischen Gesellschaft 1906; 39:2008-14.

CHAPTER 6

1. Bousfield G. Angina Pectoris: Changes in electrocardiogram during paroxysm. The Lancet 1918; 192:457-8.

2. Bruce RA, DeRouen T, Peterson DR, et al. Noninvasive predictors of sudden cardiac death in men with coronary heart disease: predictive value of maximal stress testing. The American Journal of Cardiology 1977; 39:833-40.

3. Bruce RA, Hossack KF, DeRouen TA, Hofer V. Enhanced risk assessment for primary coronary heart disease events by maximal exercise testing: 10 years' experience of Seattle Heart Watch. Journal of the American College of Cardiology 1983; 2:565-73.

4. Bruce RA, Lovejoy FW, Pearson R, Yu P, Brothers GB, Velasquez T. Normal respiratory and circulatory pathways of adaptation in exercise. The Journal of Clinical Investigation 1949; 28:1423-30.

5. Bruce RA, Lovejoy FW, Yu P, Pearson R, McDowell M. Further observations on the pathological physiology of chronic pulmonary granulomatosis associated with beryllium workers 1, 2. American Review of Tuberculosis 1950: 62(1), 29-44.

6. Bruce RA, McDonough JR. Stress testing in screening for cardiovascular disease. Bulletin of the New York Academy of Medicine 1969; 45:1288.

7. Kennedy JW, Cobb LA, Samson WE. Robert Arthur Bruce, MD: 1916-2004. American Heart Association; 2005.

8. Master AM. The two-step test of myocardial function. American Heart Journal 1935; 10:495-510.

9. Master AM. Reminiscences of fifty years of cardiology at Mt. Sinai with special reference to the two-step test. Mt Sinai Journal of Medicine 1972: 486-505.

10. Master AM, Friedman R, Dack S. The electrocardiogram after standard exercise as a functional test of the heart. American Heart Journal 1942; 24:777-93.

11. *New York Times* March 2, 1973. Dr. Harold E. Pardee Dies: Electrocardiographic Pioneer.

12. *New York Times* September 5, 1973. Arthur M. Master MD.

13. *New York Times* December 19, 1990. Francis Wood, 89, Medical Educator; Helped Perfect EKG.

14. Pardee HE. An electrocardiographic sign of coronary artery obstruction. Archives of Internal Medicine 1920; 26:244-57.

15. Scherf D, Schaffer A. The electrocardiographic exercise test. American Heart Journal 1952; 43:927-46.

16. Wenger N. Arthur M. Master, 1895-1973. Clinical Cardiology 1988; 11:509-12.

17. Wolferth CC, Wood FC. The electrocardiographic diagnosis of coronary occlusion by the use of chest leads. The American Journal of the Medical Sciences 1932; 183:30-4.

18. Wood FC, Wolferth CC. Angina pectoris: The clinical and electrocardiographic phenomena of the attack and their comparison with the effects of experimental temporary coronary occlusion. Archives of Internal Medicine 1931; 47:339-65.

CHAPTER 7

1. Afshar A, Steensma DP, Kyle RA. Werner Forssmann: A Pioneer of Interventional Cardiology and Auto-Experimentation. Mayo Clinic Proceedings; 2018: Elsevier. p. e97-e8.

2. Berry D. History of cardiology: Werner Forssmann, MD. 2006.

3. Forssmann W. Die sondierung des rechten herzens. Klinische Wochenschrift 1929; 8:2085-7.

4. Forssmann W. Über Kontrastdarstellung der Höhlen des lebenden rechten Herzens und der Lungenschlagader. Münchener Medizinische Wochenschrift 1931; 78:489-92.

5. Forssmann W. Experiments on myself: St. James Press; 1974.

6. Forssmann-Falck R. Werner Forssmann: a pioneer of cardiology. The American Journal of Cardiology 1997; 79:651-60.

7. Goerig M, Agarwal K. Werner Forssmann: the typical man before his time!—self-experiment shows feasibility of cardiac catheterization. Anasthesiologic Intensivmedizin Notfallmed Schmerztherapie 2008; 43:162-5.

8. Kisslinger J, Mathewson T. Living Legacies at Columbia: Columbia University Press; 2006.

9. Meyer JA. Werner Forssmann and catheterization of the heart, 1929. The Annals of Thoracic Surgery 1990; 49:497-9.

10. Nobelprize.org/prizes/medicine/1956/forssmann/facts/ 1956. Werner Forssmann-Facts.

11. Zimmerman HA, Scott RW, Becker NO. Catheterization of the left side of the heart in man. Circulation 150; 1: 357-359.

CHAPTER 8

1. Bruenn HG. Clinical notes on the illness and death of President Franklin D. Roosevelt. Annals of Internal Medicine 1970; 72:579-91.

2. Chang K. Thomas R. Dawber, 92, Dies: First Director of Heart Study. *New York Times* December 1, 2005

3. D'Agnostino RaK, W. Epidemiologic Background and Design; The Framingham Study. Proceedings of the American Statistical Association Sesquicentennial Invited Papers Session 1989.

4. Dawber TR. The Framingham study: the epidemiology of atherosclerotic disease. Cambridge, Mass.: Harvard University Press; 1980.

5. Dawber TR, Meadors GF, Moore Jr FE. Epidemiological approaches to heart disease: the Framingham Study. American Journal of Public Health 1951; 41:279-86.

6. Dawber TR, Moore F, Mann G. Measuring the risk of coronary heart disease in adult population groups: A symposium. II. Coronary heart disease in the Framingham study. American Journal of Public Health 1957; 47.

7. https://history.nih.gov. A Short History of the National Institutes of Health.

8. Kannel WB. Contribution of the Framingham Study to preventive cardiology. Journal of the American College of Cardiology 1990; 15:206-11.

9. Kannel WB, Dawber TR, Kagan A, Revotskie N, Stokes J. Factors of risk in the development of coronary heart disease—six-year follow-up experience: the Framingham Study. Annals of Internal Medicine 1961; 55:33-50.

10. Kannel WB, McGee D, Gordon T. A general cardiovascular risk profile: the Framingham Study. The American Journal of Cardiology 1976; 38:46-51.

11. Levy RL, White PD, Stroud WD, Hillman CC. Overweight: Its prognostic significance in relation to hypertension and cardiovascular-renal diseases. Journal of the American Medical Association 1946; 131:951-3.

12. Mahmood SS, Levy D, Vasan RS, Wang TJ. The Framingham Heart Study and the epidemiology of cardiovascular disease: a historical perspective. The Lancet 2014; 383:999-1008.

13. Merrill R. Design, strategies and statistical methods in analytic epidemiology. Introduction to epidemiology Sudbury: Jones and Bartlett 2010: 186-208.

14. Oppenheimer GM. Becoming the Framingham study 1947—1950. American Journal of Public Health 2005; 95:602-10.

15. Pace E. Mary Lasker, Philanthropist for Medical Research, Dies at 93. *The New York Times* 1994.

16. Peters, John. Franklin Delano Roosevelt 'Statement of the President on the Signing of the Public Health Service Act, July 1, 1944. https://www.presidency.ucsb.edu/ws/?pid=16528.

17. Root HF, Bland EF, Gordon WH, White PD. Coronary atherosclerosis in diabetes mellitus: a postmortem study. Journal of the American Medical Association 1939; 113:27-30.

18. Snow J. Cholera, and the water supply in the south districts of London. British Medical Journal 1857;1: 864.

19. Sorlie Paul PhD. Personal communication. October 2018.

20. Vasan RS, Larson MG, Benjamin EJ, Evans JC, Levy D. Left ventricular dilatation and the risk of congestive heart failure in people without myocardial infarction. New England Journal of Medicine 1997; 336:1350-5.

21. www.epi.umn.edu: The United States National Heart Act. University of Minnesota.

22. www.presidency.ucsb.edu. Franklin Delano Roosevelt, 32nd President of the United States: 1933-1945. 49—Statement of the President on the Signing of the Public Health Service Act 1.

23. www.profilesnlmnih.gov The Mary Lasker Papers.

CHAPTER 9

1. Brown WV. From the Editor-in-Chief. Journal of Clinical Lipidology 2007;1: 97-9.

2. Gofman, John D., MD. Personal communication. September 2018

3. Gofman JW. Dietary prevention and treatment of heart disease: Putnam; 1958.

4. Gofman JW, Delalla O, Glazier F, et al. The serum lipoprotein transport system in health, metabolic disorders, atherosclerosis and coronary heart disease. Journal of Clinical Lipidology 2007;1: 104-41.

5. Gofman JW, Jones HB, Lindgren FT, Lyon TP, Elliott HA, Strisower B. Blood lipids and human atherosclerosis. Circulation 1950;2: 161-78.

6. Gofman JW, Lindgren FT, Elliott H. Ultracentrifugal studies of lipoproteins of human serum. Journal of Biological Chemistry 1949; 179:973-9.

7. Kaskel L. Who Was John Gofman? ReachMD audio interview of W Virgil Brown MD 2018.

8. Olson RE. Discovery of the lipoproteins, their role in fat transport and their significance as risk factors. The Journal of Nutrition 1998;128: 439S-43S.

9. www.epi.umn.edu/cvdep/eulogy-obit/john-gofman-1918-2007. John Gofman (1918-2007).

CHAPTER 10

1. Association MH, Minnesota U. Recent advances in cardiovascular physiology and surgery: a symposium presented by the Minnesota Heart Association and the University of Minnesota, September 14, 15, and 16, 1953: University of Minnesota; 1954.

2. Camishion RC. Remembering John H. Gibbon, Jr, MD. The Annals of Thoracic Surgery 2003; 76:S2199-S200.

3. DeBakey ME. John Gibbon and the heart-lung machine: a personal encounter and his import for cardiovascular surgery. The Annals of Thoracic Surgery 2003; 76:S2188-S94.

4. Dunn, PM. Dr. Helen Taussig (1898-1986): pioneering American paediatric cardiologist. Archives of the Diseases of Children and Fetal Neonatal Education 2008 98; F74-76.

5. Fou AA. John H. Gibbon. The first 20 years of the heart-lung machine. Texas Heart Institute Journal 1997;24: 1.

6. Gibbon JH, Dobell AR. Part II. Personal reminiscences. The Annals of Thoracic Surgery 1982; 34:342-4.

7. Gibbon JH, Hill JD. Part I. The development of the first successful heart-lung machine. The Annals of Thoracic Surgery 1982; 34:337-41.

8. Lim M. The history of extracorporeal oxygenators. Anaesthesia 2006; 61:984-95.

9. Mack MJ. Advances in the treatment of coronary artery disease. The Annals of Thoracic Surgery 2003; 76:S2240-S5.

10. Malinin TI. Remembering Alexis Carrel and Charles A. Lindbergh. Texas Heart Institute Journal 1996; 23:28.

11. Romaine-Davis A. John Gibbon and His Heart-Lung Machine. 1991.

12. Schumacher Jr HB. John Heysham Gibbon, Jr. Biographical Memoirs 1982; 53:213.

13. Wardrop D, Keeling D. The story of the discovery of heparin and warfarin. British Journal of Haematology 2008; 141:757-63.

CHAPTER 11

1. Akselrod H, Kroll MW, Orlov MV. History of defibrillation. Cardiac Bioelectric Therapy: Springer; 2009:15-40.

2. Beck CS, Pritchard WH, Feil HS. Ventricular fibrillation of long duration abolished by electric shock. Journal of the American Medical Association 1947; 135:985-6.

3. Cakulev I, Efimov IR, Waldo AL. Cardioversion: past, present, and future. Circulation 2009; 120:1623-32.

4. Cohen SI. Paul Zoll MD: The Pioneer Whose Discoveries Prevent Sudden Death: Free People Press; 2015.

5. Geddes L. The first stimulators-reviewing the history of electrical stimulation and the devices crucial to its development. IEEE Engineering in Medicine and Biology Magazine 1994; 13:532-42.

6. Gurvich N. The main principles of cardiac defibrillation. Moscow: Medicine 1975.

7. Hooker D, Kouwenhoven W, Langworthy O. The effect of alternating electrical currents on the heart. American Journal of Physiology-Legacy Content 1933; 103:444-54.

8. Hurst JW, Fye WB, Silverman ME, Fye WB. John A. MacWilliam: Scottish pioneer of cardiac electrophysiology. Clinical Cardiology 2006; 29:90.

9. Hurt R. Modern cardiopulmonary resuscitation—not so new after all. Journal of the Royal Society of Medicine 2005; 98:327-31.

10. Kermode-Scott B. Wilfred G Bigelow. BMJ: British Medical Journal 2005; 330:967.

11. Kouwenhoven W, Milnor W, Knickerbocker G, Chestnut WR. Closed chest defibrillation of the heart. Surgery 1957; 42:550-61.

12. Lown B, Neuman J, Amarasingham R, Berkovits BV. Comparison of alternating current with direct current electroshock across the closed chest. American Journal of Cardiology 1962; 10:223-33.

13. Theruvath TP, Ikonomidis JS. Historical perspectives of The American Association for Thoracic Surgery: Claude S. Beck (1894-1971). The Journal of Thoracic and Cardiovascular Surgery 2015; 149:655-60.

14. www.youtube.com/ It's Alive! Frankenstein (2/9) movie CLIP (1931) HD

15. Zoll PM. Resuscitation of the heart in ventricular standstill by external electric stimulation. New England Journal of Medicine 1952; 247:768-71.

16. Zoll PM, Linenthal AJ, Gibson W, Paul MH, Norman LR. Termination of ventricular fibrillation in man by externally applied electric countershock. New England Journal of Medicine 1956; 254:727-32.

17. Zoll PM, Linenthal AJ, Zarsky LRN. Ventricular fibrillation: treatment and prevention by external electric currents. New England Journal of Medicine 1960; 262:105-12.

CHAPTER 12

1. Braunwald E, Ross Jr J, Sonnenblick EH. Mechanisms of contraction of the normal and failing heart. New England Journal of Medicine 1967; 277:962-71.

2. Califf RM. Life and Times of Leading Cardiologists: Eugene Braunwald. https://www.medscape.com/viewarticle/834507 November 13, 2014.

3. Fisch C. William Withering: An account of the foxglove and some of its medical uses 1785-1985: Elsevier Science Pub.; 1985.

4. Katz AM. Ernest Henry Starling, his predecessors, and the "Law of the Heart". Circulation 2002; 106:2986-92.

5. Lee TH. Eugene Braunwald and the Rise of Modern Medicine: Harvard University Press; 2013.

6. Maroko PR, Kjekshus JK, Sobel BE, et al. Factors influencing infarct size following experimental coronary artery occlusions. Circulation 1971; 43:67-82.

7. Messerli FH, Messerli AW, Luscher TF. Eisenhower's billion-dollar heart attack—50 years later. N England Journal of Medicine 2005; 353:1205-7.

8. Zipes DP, Libby P, Bonow RO, Mann DL, Tomaselli GF. Braunwald's Heart Disease E-Book: A Textbook of Cardiovascular Medicine: Elsevier Health Sciences; 2018.

CHAPTER 13

1. Abrams HL. Selectivity in the study of the cardiovascular system. California Medicine 1962; 96:149.

2. Abrams HL. History of cardiac radiology. American Journal of Roentgenology 1996; 167:431-8.

3. Bruschke AV, Sheldon WC, Shirey EK, Proudfit WL. A half century of selective coronary arteriography. Journal of the American College of Cardiology 2009; 54:2139-44.

4. Judkins MP. Selective coronary arteriography: part I: a percutaneous transfemoral technique. Radiology 1967; 89:815-24.

5. Little WC, Reeves RC, Coughlan C, Rogers EW. Effect of cough on coronary perfusion pressure: Does coughing help clear the coronary arteries of angiographic contrast medium? Circulation 1982; 65:604-10.

6. Mueller RL, Sanborn TA. The history of interventional cardiology: cardiac catheterization, angioplasty, and related interventions. American Heart Journal 1995; 129:146-72.

7. Proudfit WL, Shirey EK, Sones Jr FM. Selective cine coronary arteriography: correlation with clinical findings in 1,000 patients. Circulation 1966;33:901-10.

8. Rao SV, Cohen MG, Kandzari DE, Bertrand OF, Gilchrist IC. The transradial approach to percutaneous coronary intervention: historical perspective, current concepts, and future directions. Journal of the American College of Cardiology 2010;55: 2187-95.

9. Spellberg RD, Ungar I. The percutaneous femoral artery approach to selective coronary arteriography. Circulation 1967; 36:730-3.

CHAPTER 14

1. Campbell R, Murray A, Julian DG. Ventricular arrhythmias in the first 12 hours of acute myocardial infarction. Natural history study. British Heart Journal 1981; 46:351.

2. Day HW. An intensive coronary care area. Diseases of the Chest 1963; 44:423-7.

3. Forrester JS, Diamond G, Chatterjee K, Swan H. Medical therapy of acute myocardial infarction by application of hemodynamic subsets. New England Journal of Medicine 1976; 295:1356-62.

4. Julian DG. Coronary care and the community. Annals of Internal Medicine 1968; 68:1157-.

5. Julian DG. The history of coronary care units. British Heart Journal 1987; 57:497.

6. Killip III T, Kimball JT. Treatment of myocardial infarction in a coronary care unit: a two year experience with 250 patients" American Journal of Cardiology 1967; 20:457-64.

7. Lown B, Fakhro AM, Hood WB, Thorn GW. The coronary care unit: new perspectives and directions. Journal of the American Medical Association 1967; 199:188-98.

8. Silverman ME. Desmond Gareth Julian: Pioneer in coronary care. Clinical Cardiology 2001; 24:695.

9. Swan H, Ganz W, Forrester J, Marcus H, Diamond G, Chonette D. Catheterization of the heart in man with use of a flow-directed balloon-tipped catheter. New England Journal of Medicine 1970; 283:447-51.

CHAPTER 15

1. Ahlquist RP. A study of the adrenotropic receptors. American Journal of Physiology-Legacy Content 1948; 153:586-600.

2. Barcroft H, Talbot J. Oliver and Schäfer's discovery of the cardiovascular action of suprarenal extract. Postgraduate Medical Journal 1968; 44:6.

3. Black J. Drugs from emasculated hormones: the principles of syntopic antagonism. Nobel Lecture 1988;December 8, 1988: 418-40.

4. Black JW, Crowther AF, Shanks RG, Smith LH, Dornhorst AC. A New Adrenergic Beta Receptor Antagonist. Lancet 1964;1: 1080-1.

5. Hoffman BB. My journey with adrenaline. *Huffington Post* 2013; April 10, 2013.

6. Leoutsakos B, Leoutsakos A. The adrenal glands: a brief historical perspective." Hormones 2008; 7:334-6.

7. Levine SA, Ernstene AC, Jacobson BM. The use of epinephrine as a diagnostic test for angina pectoris: With observations on the electrocardiographic changes following injections of epinephrine into normal subjects and into patients with angina pectoris. Archives of Internal Medicine 1930; 45:191-200.

8. Mansoon AH KU. Beta blockers in cardiovascular medicine. Journal of Association of Physicians of India 2009; 57 Supplement:1-6.

9. Obituary Raymond P. Ahlquist. International Journal of Cardiology 1983; 4:483-5.

10. Obituary Sir James Black, OM. The Telegraph (telegraph.co.uk 2010; May 23, 2010.

11. Quirke V. Putting theory into practice: James Black, receptor theory and the development of the beta-blockers at ICI, 1958-1978. Medical History 2006; 50:69-92.

12. Stapleton MP. Sir James Black and propranolol. The role of the basic sciences in the history of cardiovascular pharmacology. Texas Heart Institute Journal 1997; 24:336.

13. Wenger NK, Greenbaum LM. From adrenoceptor mechanisms to clinical therapeutics: Raymond Ahlquist, PhD, 1914—1983. Journal of the American College of Cardiology 1984; 3:419-21.

CHAPTER 16

1. Alderman EL, Bourassa MG, Cohen LS, et al. Ten-year follow-up of survival and myocardial infarction in the randomized Coronary Artery Surgery Study. Circulation 1990; 82:1629-46.

2. Buxton BF, Galvin SD. The history of arterial revascularization: from Kolesov to Tector and beyond. Annals of Cardiothoracic Surgery 2013; 2:419.

3. Chaitman BR, Ryan TJ, Kronmal RA, Foster ED, Frommer PL, Killip T. Coronary Artery Surgery Study (CASS): comparability of 10 year survival in randomized and randomizable patients. Journal of the American College of Cardiology 1990; 16:1071-8.

4. D'Agostino RS, Jacobs JP, Badhwar V, et al. The Society of Thoracic Surgeons adult cardiac surgery database: 2018 update on outcomes and quality. The Annals of Thoracic Surgery 2018; 105:15-23.

5. Favaloro RG. The Challenging Dream of Heart Surgery: From the Pampas to Cleveland. 1995.

6. Foundation B-F. Our Founder-Rene G. Favaloro. Fundacionfavaloro. org/doctor-rené—geronimo-favaloro/.

7. Group VACABSCS. Eleven-year survival in the Veterans Administration randomized trial of coronary bypass surgery for stable angina. New England Journal of Medicine 1984; 311:1333-9.

8. Konstantinov IE. Robert H. Goetz: the surgeon who performed the first successful clinical coronary artery bypass operation. The Annals of Thoracic Surgery 2000; 69:1966-72.

9. Konstantinov IE. Vasilii I. Kolesov: a surgeon to remember. Texas Heart Institute Journal 2004; 31:349.

10. Krauss C. Argentina Searches Its Soul Over a Suicide. *The New York Times* August 7, 2000.

11. Lipovich P. There are more questions than answers. Pagina12.com/ar/2000/00-07-31/index.htm August 31, 2000.

12. Loop FD, Cosgrove DM, Lytle BW, et al. An 11 year evolution of coronary arterial surgery (1967-1978). Annals of Surgery 1979; 190:444.

13. Mock M, Ringqvist I, Fisher L, et al. Survival of medically treated patients in the coronary artery surgery study (CASS) registry. Circulation 1982; 66:562-8.

14. Pichel R. Dr. René G. Favaloro: A Biographical Note. Profiles in Cardiology 2003.

15. René Favaloro's 96th Birthday. Doodle Archives August 12, 2019.

16. Thomas JL. The Vineberg legacy: internal mammary artery implantation from inception to obsolescence. Texas Heart Institute journal 1999; 26:107.

CHAPTER 17

1. Anderson RG, Brown MS, Goldstein JL. Role of the coated endocytic vesicle in the uptake of receptor-bound low-density lipoprotein in human fibroblasts. Cell 1977; 10:351-64.

2. Beheshti SO, Madsen CM, Varbo A, Nordestgaard BG. Worldwide prevalence of familial hypercholesterolemia: meta-analyses of 11 million subjects. Journal of the American College of Cardiology 2020; 75:2553-66.

3. Brown MS. September 2019. Personal communication.

4. Brown MS, Dana SE, Goldstein JL. Regulation of 3-hydroxy-3-methylglutaryl coenzyme A reductase activity in human fibroblasts by lipoproteins. Proceedings of the National Academy of Sciences 1973; 70:2162-6.

5. Brown MS, Goldstein JL. Scientific side trips: Six excursions from the beaten path. Journal of Biological Chemistry 2012; 287:22418-35.

6. Brown MS, Nobel Lecture. December 9, 1985. A Receptor-Mediated Pathway for Cholesterol Homestasis.

7. Goldstein JL, Anderson RG, Brown MS. Coated pits, coated vesicles, and receptor-mediated endocytosis. Nature 1979; 279:679.

8. Goldstein JL, Brown MS. Familial hypercholesterolemia: identification of a defect in the regulation of 3-hydroxy-3-methylglutaryl coenzyme A reductase activity associated with overproduction of cholesterol. Proceedings of the National Academy of Sciences 1973; 70:2804-8.

9. Goldstein JL, Brown MS. Atherosclerosis: the low-density lipoprotein receptor hypothesis. Metabolism 1977; 26:1257-75.

10. Goldstein JL, Brown MS. Progress in understanding the LDL receptor and HMG-CoA reductase, two membrane proteins that regulate the plasma cholesterol. Journal of Lipid Research 1984; 25:1450-61.

11. Goldstein JL, Brown MS. A century of cholesterol and coronaries: from plaques to genes to statins. Cell 2015; 161:161-72.

12. Heynick F. Jews and Medicine: An Epic Saga: KTAV Publishing House, Inc.; 2002. Paul Ehrlich

13. Hobbs HH, Russell DW, Brown MS, Goldstein JL. The LDL receptor locus in familial hypercholesterolemia: mutational analysis of a membrane protein. Annual review of genetics 1990; 24:133-70.

14. Khachadurian AK. The inheritance of essential familial hyperlipidemia. American Journal of Medicine 1964; 37:402-7.

15. Lindgren FT, Elliott HA, Gofman JW. The ultracentrifugal characterization and isolation of human blood lipids and lipoproteins, with applications to the study of atherosclerosis. The Journal of Physical Chemistry 1951; 55:80-93.

16. Müller C. Xanthomata, hypercholesterolemia, angina pectoris. Acta Medica Scandinavica 1938; 95:75-84.

CHAPTER 18

1. Allisy A. Henri Becquerel: the discovery of radioactivity. Radiation Protection Dosimetry 1996; 68:3-10.

2. Beller GA, Zaret BL. Contributions of nuclear cardiology to diagnosis and prognosis of patients with coronary artery disease. Circulation 2000; 101:1465-78.

3. Berger HJ, Reduto LA, Johnstone DE, et al. Global and regional left ventricular response to bicycle exercise in coronary artery disease: assessment by quantitative radionuclide angiocardiography. American Journal of Medicine 1979; 66:13-21.

4. Blumgart HL, Weiss S. Studies on the velocity of blood flow: VII. The pulmonary circulation time in normal resting individuals. Journal of Clinical Investigation 1927; 4:399-425.

5. Friedman M. Medicine's 10 greatest discoveries: Yale University Press; 1998.

6. Iskandrian AE, Garcia EV. Nuclear cardiac imaging. Japanese Society of Nuclear Cardiology; 2016.

7. Johnstone DE, Sands MJ, Berger HJ, et al. Comparison of exercise radionuclide angiocardiography and thallium-201 myocardial perfusion imaging in coronary artery disease. American Journal of Cardiology 1980; 45:1113-9.

8. Marshall RC, Berger HJ, Costin JC, et al. Assessment of cardiac performance with quantitative radionuclide angiocardiography: sequential left ventricular ejection fraction, normalized left ventricular ejection rate, and regional wall motion. Circulation 1977; 56:820-9.

9. Prinzmetal M, Corday E, Spritzler RJ, Flieg W. Radiocardiography and its clinical applications. Journal of the American Medical Association 1949; 139:617-22.

10. Ritchie JL, Trobaugh GB, Hamilton GW, et al. Myocardial imaging with thallium-201 at rest and during exercise. Comparison with coronary arteriography and resting and stress electrocardiography. Circulation 1977; 56:66-71.

11. Zaret BL. August 2019. Personal communication.

12. Zaret BL, Strauss HW, Hurley PJ, Natarajan T, Pitt B. A noninvasive scinti photographic method for detecting regional ventricular dysfunction in man. New England Journal of Medicine 1971; 284:1165-70.

13. Zaret BL, Strauss HW, Martin ND, Wells Jr HP, Flamm Jr M. Noninvasive regional myocardial perfusion with radioactive potassium: study of patients at rest, with exercise and during angina pectoris. New England Journal of Medicine 1973; 288:809-12.

CHAPTER 19

1. Casarella WJ. Andreas Roland Gruentzig, MD: 1939-1985. Radiology 1986; 159:285-.

2. Dotter CT, Judkins MP. Transluminal treatment of arteriosclerotic obstruction: description of a new technique and a preliminary report of its application. Circulation 1964; 30:654-70.

3. Eefting F, Popma J, Serruys P. Clinical trials on intracoronary stenting. Seminars in Interventional Cardiology: SIIC; 1996. p. 233-45.

4. Geddes LA, Geddes LE, Boo M. The catheter introducers: Mobium Press; 1993.

5. Grines CL, Browne KF, Marco J, et al. A Comparison of Immediate Angioplasty with Thrombolytic Therapy for Acute Myocardial Infarction. New England Journal of Medicine 1993; 328:673-9.

6. Grüntzig AR. Transluminal dilatation of coronary-artery stenosis. The Lancet (London, England) 1978; 1:263.

7. Grüntzig AR, Senning Å, Siegenthaler WE. Nonoperative dilatation of coronary-artery stenosis: percutaneous transluminal coronary angioplasty. New England Journal of Medicine 1979; 301:61-8.

8. Iqbal J, Gunn J, Serruys PW. Coronary stents: historical development, current status and future directions. British Medical Bulletin 2013; 106.

9. Keller F, Rosch J. A personal memoir of Charles Dotter [foreword]. The father of interventional radiology Charles Dotter: highlights of his life and research Tokyo: Excerpta Medica Publishers 1994: 7-9.

10. Kent KM, Bentivoglio LG, Block PC, et al. Long-term efficacy of percutaneous transluminal coronary angioplasty (PTCA): report from the National Heart, Lung, and Blood Institute PTCA Registry. American Journal of Cardiology 1984; 53:C27-C31.

11. King III SB. Angioplasty from bench to bedside to bench. Circulation 1996; 93:1621-9.

12. King III SB, Douglas JS. Coronary arteriography and angioplasty. 1985.

13. Kinney TB. Radiologic history exhibit. Charles T. Dotter: a pioneering interventional radiologist. Radiographics 1996; 16:697-707.

14. Levine GN, Bates ER, Bittl JA, et al. 2016 ACC/AHA guideline focused update on duration of dual antiplatelet therapy in patients with coronary artery disease: a report of the American College of Cardiology/American Heart Association Task Force on Clinical Practice Guidelines: an update of the 2011 ACCF/AHA/SCAI guideline for percutaneous coronary intervention, 2011 ACCF/AHA guideline for coronary artery bypass graft surgery, 2012 ACC/AHA/ACP/AATS/PCNA/SCAI/STS guideline for the diagnosis and management of patients with stable ischemic heart disease, 2013 ACCF/AHA guideline for the management of ST-elevation myocardial infarction, 2014 AHA/ACC guideline for the management of patients with non -ST-elevation acute coronary syndromes, and 2014 ACC/AHA guideline on perioperative cardiovascular evaluation and management of patients undergoing noncardiac surgery. Circulation 2016; 134:e123-e55.

15. Levy RI, Mock MB, Willman VL, Frommer PL. Percutaneous Transluminal Coronary Angioplasty. New England Journal of Medicine 1979; 301:101-3.

16. Levy RI, Mock MB, Willman VL, Passamani ER, Frommer PL. Percutaneous Transluminal Coronary Angioplasty—A Status Report. New England Journal of Medicine 1981; 305:399-400.

17. Members ATF, Steg PG, James SK, et al. ESC Guidelines for the management of acute myocardial infarction in patients presenting with ST-segment elevation: The Task Force on the management of ST-segment elevation acute myocardial infarction of the European Society of Cardiology (ESC). European Heart Journal 2012; 33:2569-619.

18. Monaghan, David. Journey Into the Heart: A Tale of the Pioneering Doctors and Their Race to Transform Cardiovascular Medicine. 2007.

19. O'Neill W, Timmis GC, Bourdillon PD, et al. " Prospective Randomized Clinical Trial of Intracoronary Streptokinase versus Coronary Angioplasty for Acute Myocardial Infarction. New England Journal of Medicine 1986; 314:812-8.

20. Payne MM. Charles Theodore Dotter: the father of intervention. Texas Heart Institute Journal 2001; 28:28.

21. Schmidt T, Abbott JD. Coronary stents: history, design, and construction. Journal of Clinical Medicine 2018; 7:126.

22. Yellayi SS, Schatz RA. Indications and use of the Palmaz-Schatz coronary stent. Cardiology Clinics 1994; 12:651-63.

CHAPTER 20

1. Campbell KD. Robert Swanson, 52, Alumnus who launched the biotechnology industry. MIT News December 8, 1999.

2. Chesebro, J. H., Knatterud, G., Roberts, R., Borer, J., Cohen, L. S., Dalen, J., Dodge, H. T., Francis, C. K., Hillis, D., Ludbrook, P., et al., Thrombolysis in Myocardial Infarction (TIMI) Trial, Phase I: A comparison between intravenous tissue plasminogen activator and intravenous streptokinase. Clinical findings through hospital discharge. Circulation. 1987; 76(1):142-54.

3. DeWood MA, Spores J, Notske R, et al. Prevalence of total coronary occlusion during the early hours of transmural myocardial infarction. New England Journal of Medicine 1980; 303:897-902.

4. Fletcher AP, Alkjaersig N, Smyrniotis FE, Sherry S. The treatment of patients suffering from early myocardial infarction with massive and prolonged streptokinase therapy. Transactions of the Association of American Physicians 1958; 71:287-96.

5. Friedman M, Van den Bovenkamp G. Role of thrombus in plaque formation in the human diseased coronary artery. British Journal of Experimental Pathology 1966; 47:550.

6. Group TS. The Thrombolysis in Myocardial Infarction (TIMI) trial: phase I findings. New England Journal of Medicine 1985; 312:932-6.

7. Hugenholtz P, Simoons M, Serruys P, van den Brand M. Intracoronary Streptokinase in Acute Myocardial Infarction A review. Acta Medica Scandinavica 1985; 218:135-41.

8. Rentrop KP. Thrombi in acute coronary syndromes: revisited and revised. Circulation 2000; 101:1619-26.

9. Rentrop KP, Blanke H, Karsch K, Kaiser H, Köstering H, Leitz K. Selective intracoronary thrombolysis in acute myocardial infarction and unstable angina pectoris. Circulation 1981; 63:307-17.

10. Russo E. Special Report: The birth of biotechnology. Nature 2003; 421:456-7.

11. Schröder R, Biamino G, Von Leitner E, et al. Intravenous short-term infusion of streptokinase in acute myocardial infarction. Circulation 1983; 67:536-48.

12. Sherry S. The origin of thrombolytic therapy. Journal of the American College of Cardiology 1989; 14:1085-92.

13. Sherry S. *Reflections and reminiscences of an academic physician*: Lea & Febiger; 1993.

14. Taylor GJ, Mikell FL, Moses HW, et al. Intravenous versus intracoronary streptokinase therapy for acute myocardial infarction in community hospitals. American Journal of Cardiology 1984; 54:256-60.

15. www.TIMI.org Thrombolysis in Myocardial Infarction study group

16. Walton-Shirly M. Dr. Lloyd Rudy and "that night" : From chicken soup and bedrest to anticlot therapy. Medscape.com February 24, 2018.

17. Werf FVd, Ludbrook PA, Bergmann SR, et al. Coronary Thrombolysis with Tissue-Type Plasminogen Activator in Patients with Evolving Myocardial Infarction. New England Journal of Medicine 1984; 310:609-13.

CHAPTER 21

1. Brown MS, Faust JR, Goldstein JL, Kaneko I, Endo A. Induction of 3-hydroxy-3-methylglutaryl coenzyme A reductase activity in human fibroblasts incubated with compactin (ML-236B), a competitive inhibitor of the reductase. Journal of Biological Chemistry 1978; 253:1121-8.

2. Cannon CP, Braunwald E, McCabe CH, et al. Intensive versus moderate lipid lowering with statins after acute coronary syndromes. New England Journal of Medicine 2004; 350:1495-504.

3. Downs JR, Clearfield M, Weis S, et al. Primary prevention of acute coronary events with lovastatin in men and women with average cholesterol levels: results of AFCAPS/TexCAPS. Journal of the American Medical Association 1998; 279:1615-22.

4. Endo A. A historical perspective on the discovery of statins. Proceedings of the Japan Academy, Series B 2010; 86:484-93.

5. Endo A, Tsujita Y, Kuroda M, TANZAWA K. Inhibition of Cholesterol Synthesis in vitro and in vivo by ML-236A and ML-236B, Competitive Inhibitors of 3-Hydroxy-3-methylglutaryl-Coenzyme A Reductase. European Journal of Biochemistry 1977; 77:31-6.

6. Fine RA. The Great Drug Deception. 1972.

7. Fong, C. Statins in therapy: Cellular transport, side effects, drug-drug interactions and cytotoxicity—the unrecognized role of lactones. [Research Report] Eigenenergy, Adelaide, Australia. 2016. ffhal-01185910v2f

8. Gauthier JM, Massicotte A. Statins and their effect on cognition: let's clear up the confusion. Canadian Pharmacists Journal/Revue des Pharmaciens du Canada 2015; 148:150-5.

9. Group SSSS. Randomised trial of cholesterol lowering in 4444 patients with coronary heart disease: the Scandinavian Simvastatin Survival Study (4S). The Lancet 1994;3 44:1383-9.

10. Grundy SM, Cleeman JI, Merz CNB, et al. A summary of implications of recent clinical trials for the National Cholesterol Education Program Adult Treatment Panel III guidelines. American Heart Association; 2004.

11. Ho K. Cataract formation by triparanol. Archives of Ophthalmology 1962; 68:486-9.

12. Kinch MS, Surovtseva Y, Hoyer D. An analysis of FDA-approved drugs for cardiovascular diseases. Drug Discovery Today 2016; 21:1-4.

13. LaRosa JC, Grundy SM, Waters DD, et al. Intensive lipid lowering with atorvastatin in patients with stable coronary disease. New England Journal of Medicine 2005; 352:1425-35.

14. *New York Times* July 3, 2018. Alfred Alberts, Unsung Father of a Cholesterol Drug, Dies at 87

15. Nielsen SF, Nordestgaard BG. Negative statin-related news stories decrease statin persistence and increase myocardial infarction and cardiovascular mortality: a nationwide prospective cohort study. European Heart Journal 2016; 37:908-16.

16. Rojas-Fernandez CH, Goldstein LB, Levey AI, Taylor BA, Bittner V. An assessment by the statin cognitive safety task force: 2014 update. Journal of Clinical Lipidology 2014; 8:S5-S16.

17. Steinberg D. Thematic review series: the pathogenesis of atherosclerosis. An interpretive history of the cholesterol controversy, part V: the discovery of the statins and the end of the controversy. Journal of Lipid Research 2006; 47:1339-51.

18. Steinberg D, Avigan J, Feigelson EB. Effects of triparanol (MER-29) on cholesterol biosynthesis and on blood sterol levels in man. Journal of Clinical Investigation 1961; 40:884-93.

19. Toth PPaB, Marciej. Statins: Then and Now. Methodist Debakey Cardiovascular Journal 2019; 15:23-31.

20. Zhang H, Plutzky J, Skentzos S, et al. Discontinuation of statins in routine care settings: a cohort study. Annals of Internal Medicine 2013; 158:526-34.

CHAPTER 22

1. Buxton AE, Lee KL, Fisher JD, Josephson ME, Prystowsky EN, Hafley G. A randomized study of the prevention of sudden death in patients with coronary artery disease. New England Journal of Medicine 1999;341:1882-90.

2. Kastor JA. Michel Mirowski and the automatic implantable defibrillator. American Journal of Cardiology 1989;63:977-82.

3. Klein HU, Inama G. Implantable defibrillators: 30 years of history. Giornale Italiano Cardiologia 2010;11:48s-52s.

4. Lown B, Axelrod P. Implanted standby defibrillators. Circulation 1972;46:637-9.

5. Mirowski M, Mower MM, Gott VL, Brawley RK. Feasibility and effectiveness of low-energy catheter defibrillation in man. Circulation 1973;47:79-85.

6. Mirowski M, Reid PR, Mower MM, et al. Termination of malignant ventricular arrhythmias with an implanted automatic defibrillator in human beings. New England Journal of Medicine 1980; 303: 322-4.

7. Moss AJ, Hall WJ, Cannon DS, et al. Improved survival with an implanted defibrillator in patients with coronary disease at high risk for ventricular arrhythmia. New England Journal of Medicine 1996;335:1933-40.

8. Moss AJ, Zareba W, Hall WJ, et al. Prophylactic implantation of a defibrillator in patients with myocardial infarction and reduced ejection fraction. New England Journal of Medicine 2002;346:877-83.

9. Winkle RA, Mead RH, Ruder MA, et al. Long-term outcome with the automatic implantable cardioverter-defibrillator. Journal of the American College of Cardiology 1989;13:1353-61.

CHAPTER 23

1. Califf R. The Life and Times of Leading Cardiologists. Medscape.com/editorial/series/1352995 November 15, 2011 2011.

2. Gopalakrishnan P RM, Tak T. Gender Differences in Coronary Artery Disease: Review of Diagnostic Challenges and Current Treatment. Postgraduate Medicine 2015; 121:60-8.

3. Gulati M, Shaw L, Bairy Marz CN. Myocardial ischemia in women: lessons from the NHLBI WISE study. Clinical Cardiology 2012; 3: 141-148.

4. Lerner DJ, Kannel WB. Patterns of coronary heart disease morbidity and mortality in the sexes: a 26-year follow-up of the Framingham population. American Heart Journal 1986; 111:383-90.

5. Levy H, BOAS EP. Coronary artery disease in women. Journal of the American Medical Association 1936; 107:97-102.

6. Mieres JH, Shaw LJ, Arai A, et al. Role of noninvasive testing in the clinical evaluation of women with suspected coronary artery disease: consensus statement from the Cardiac Imaging Committee, Council on Clinical Cardiology, and the Cardiovascular Imaging and Intervention Committee, Council on Cardiovascular Radiology and Intervention, American Heart Association. Circulation 2005; 111:682-96.

7. Oliviero H. Meet a local cardiologist who changed how we think about heart disease. Atlanta Journal Constitution December 12, 2017.

8. Pepine CJ. Ischemic heart disease in women. Journal of the American College of Cardiology 2006; 47:S1-S3.

9. Pepine CJ, Ferdinand KC, Shaw LJ, et al. Emergence of nonobstructive coronary artery disease: a woman's problem

and need for change in definition of angiography. Journal of the American College of Cardiology 2015; 66:1918-33.

10. Reynolds HR, Srichai MB, Iqbal SN, et al. Mechanisms of myocardial infarction in women without angiographically obstructive coronary artery disease. Circulation 2011; 124:1414-25.

11. Shaw LJ, Merz CNB, Pepine CJ, et al. Insights from the NHLBI-Sponsored Women's Ischemia Syndrome Evaluation (WISE) Study: Part I: gender differences in traditional and novel risk factors, symptom evaluation, and gender-optimized diagnostic strategies. Journal of the American College of Cardiology 2006; 47:S4-S20.

12. Steingart RM, Packer M, Hamm P, et al. Sex differences in the management of coronary artery disease. New England Journal of Medicine 1991; 325:226-30.

13. Wenger NK. Gender, coronary artery disease, and coronary bypass surgery. Annals of Internal Medicine 1990; 112:557-8.

14. Wenger NK, Speroff L, Packard B. Cardiovascular health and disease in women. New England Journal of Medicine 1993; 329:247-56.

CHAPTER 24

1. Albert MA, Danielson E, Rifai N, Ridker PM, Investigators P. Effect of statin therapy on C-reactive protein levels: the pravastatin inflammation/CRP evaluation (PRINCE): a randomized trial and cohort study. Journal of the American Medical Association 2001; 286:64-70.

2. Berk BC, Weintraub WS, Alexander RW. Elevation of C-reactive protein in "active" coronary artery disease. American Journal of Cardiology 1990; 65:168-72.

3. Blake GJ, Ridker PM. C-reactive protein and other inflammatory risk markers in acute coronary syndromes. Journal of the American College of Cardiology 2003; 41:S37-S42.

4. Bray C, Bell LN, Liang H, et al. Erythrocyte sedimentation rate and C-reactive protein measurements and their relevance in clinical medicine. Western Medical Journal 2016; 115:317-21.

5. Danesh J, Collins R, Appleby P, Peto R. Association of fibrinogen, C-reactive protein, albumin, or leukocyte count with coronary heart disease: meta-analyses of prospective studies. Journal of the American Medical Association 1998; 279:1477-82.

6. Danesh J, Muir J, Wong Y, Ward M, Gallimore J, Pepys MB. Risk factors for coronary heart disease and acute-phase proteins. A population-based study. European Heart Journal 1999; 20:954-9.

7. Danesh J, Wheeler JG, Hirschfield GM, et al. C-reactive protein and other circulating markers of inflammation in the prediction of coronary heart disease. New England Journal of Medicine 2004; 350:1387-97.

8. Enos W, Holmes R, Boyer J. Coronary disease among US soldiers killed in action in Korea. Preliminary report. Journal of the American Medical Association 1953; 152(12): 1090-1093.

9. Granger DN, Senchenkova E. Inflammation and the Microcirculation. Colloquium series on integrated systems physiology: from molecule to function; 2010: Morgan & Claypool Life Sciences. p. 1-87.

10. Hansson G. Mechanisms of Disease: Inflammation. Atherosclerosis, and Coronary Artery Disease. New England Journal of Medicine 2005; 352:1685-96.

11. Hansson GK, Libby P, Tabas I. Inflammation and plaque vulnerability. Journal of Internal Medicine 2015; 278:483-93.

12. Harrington RA. Targeting inflammation in coronary artery disease. New England Journal of Medicine 2017; 377:1197-8.

13. Jaffer FA, Libby P, Weissleder R. Molecular and cellular imaging of atherosclerosis: emerging applications. Journal of the American College of Cardiology 2006; 47:1328-38.

14. Lawrence HS. William Smith Tillett 1892-1974. National Academy of Sciences 1993.

15. Libby P, Hansson GK. From focal lipid storage to systemic inflammation: JACC review topic of the week. Journal of the American College of Cardiology 2019; 74:1594-607.

16. Nelson F. In memoriam: Russell Ross. American Journal of Pathology 1999; 154:1309.

17. Newby LK. Inflammation as a treatment target after acute myocardial infarction. Massachusetts Medical Society; 2019.

18. Nieto FJ. Historical Reflections on the Inflammatory Aspects of Atherosclerosis. Inflammation and Atherosclerosis: Springer; 2012:1-17.

19. Rasmussen FN. Dr. Richard Ross, former Hopkins med school dean and cardiologist, dies. The Baltimore Sun 2015;August 14, 2015

20. Ridker PM, Everett BM, Pradhan A, et al. Low-dose methotrexate for the prevention of atherosclerotic events. New England Journal of Medicine 2019; 380:752-62.

21. Ridker PM, Everett BM, Thuren T, et al. Antiinflammatory therapy with canakinumab for atherosclerotic disease. New England Journal of Medicine 2017; 377:1119-31.

22. Ridker P, MacFadyen J, Fonseca F, Genest J, Gotto A, Kastelein J. Number needed to treat with rosuvastatin to prevent first cardiovascular events and death among men and women with low

low-density lipoprotein cholesterol and elevated high-sensitivity C-reactive protein: justification for the use of statins in prevention: an intervention trial evaluating rosuvastatin (JUPITER). Circ Cardiovasc Quality Outcomes. 2009; 2 (6): 616-23. Cyber Pub du 2009;22.

23. Rinsema TJ. One hundred years of aspirin. Medical History 1999; 43:502-7.

24. Ross R, Glomset J, Harker L. Response to injury and atherogenesis. American Journal of Pathology 1977; 86:675.

25. Ross R, Glomset JA. Atherosclerosis and the arterial smooth muscle cell. Science 1973; 180:1332-9.

26. Stefanadis C, Diamantopoulos L, Vlachopoulos C, et al. Thermal heterogeneity within human atherosclerotic coronary arteries detected in vivo: a new method of detection by application of a special thermography catheter. Circulation 1999; 99:1965-71.

27. Stefanadis C, Toutouzas K, Tsiamis E, et al. Increased local temperature in human coronary atherosclerotic plaques: an independent predictor of clinical outcome in patients undergoing a percutaneous coronary intervention. Journal of the American College of Cardiology 2001; 37:1277-83.

28. Tardif J-C, Kouz S, Waters DD, et al. Efficacy and safety of low-dose colchicine after myocardial infarction. New England Journal of Medicine 2019; 381:2497-505.

29. Tillett WS, Francis T. Serological reactions in pneumonia with a non-protein somatic fraction of pneumococcus. Journal of Experimental Medicine 1930; 52:561-71.

30. Wick G, Grundtman C. Inflammation and atherosclerosis: Springer Science & Business Media; 2011.

CHAPTER 25

1. Bhatt DL, Steg PG, Miller M, et al. Cardiovascular Risk Reduced with Icosapent Ethyl for Hypertriglyceridemia. New England Journal of Medicine 2019 380: 11-22.

2. Boccara F, Kumar PN, Caramelli B, et al. Evolocumab in HIV-Infected Patients With Dyslipidemia: Primary Results of the Randomized, Double-Blind BEIJERINCK Study. Journal of the American College of Cardiology 2020; 75:2570-84.

3. Cho L, Davis M, Elgendy I, et al. Summary of Updated Recommendations for Primary Prevention of Cardiovascular Disease in Women: JACC State-of-the-Art Review. Journal of the American College of Cardiology 2020; 75:2602-18.

4. Dalen JE, Alpert JS, Goldberg RJ, Weinstein RS. The epidemic of the 20th century: coronary heart disease. American Journal of Medicine 2014; 127:807-12.

5. Group SR. A randomized trial of intensive versus standard blood-pressure control. New England Journal of Medicine 2015; 373:2103-16.

6. Jamal A, Phillips E, Gentzke AS, et al. Current cigarette smoking among adults—United States, 2016. Morbidity and Mortality Weekly Report 2018; 67:53.

7. Lopez AD, Adair T. Is the long-term decline in cardiovascular-disease mortality in high-income countries over? Evidence from national vital statistics. International Journal of Epidemiology 2019; 48:1815-23.

8. Ohira T, Iso H. Cardiovascular disease epidemiology in Asia. Circulation Journal 2013:CJ-13-0702.

9. Preston SH, Vierboom YC, Stokes A. The role of obesity in exceptionally slow US mortality improvement. Proceedings of the National Academy of Sciences 2018; 115:957-61.

10. Ray KK, Bay HE, Catapano AL, et al. Safety and Efficacy of Bempedoic Acid to Lower LDL Cholesterol. New England Journal of Medicine 2019 380: 1022-1032.

11. Ray KK, Wright RS, Kallend D, et al. "wo phase 3 trials of Inclisiran in patients with elevated LDL cholesterol. New England Journal of Medicine 2020; 382:1507-19.

12. Sinha A, Feinstein MJ. Coronary artery disease manifestations in HIV: what, how, and why. Canadian Journal of Cardiology 2019; 35:270-9.

13. Sniderman AD, Toth PP, Thanassoulis G, Pencina MJ, Furberg CD. Taking a longer term view of cardiovascular risk: the causal exposure paradigm. British Medical Journal 2014; 348:g3047.

14. Stallones RA. The rise and fall of ischemic heart disease. Scientific American 1980; 243:53-9.

15. Timmis A, Townsend N, Gale C, et al. European Society of Cardiology: cardiovascular disease statistics 2017. European Heart Journal 2018; 39:508-79.

16. www.who.int. WHO Global Health Observatory (GHO) Overweight and Obesity

INDEX

A

Abdilgaard, P. C., 143
Abel, J. J., 206
Abrams, H., 179
Acetylcholine, 207, 208
Adrenal glands, 204, 205–207, 245
Adrenaline, 18, 149, 158, 162–163, 165
   See also Beta-blockers
Ahlquist, R. P., 209
Albert and Mary Lasker Foundation, 104, 105
Alberti, F. B., 18
Alberts, A., 322, 328
American Heart Association (AHA), 120, 122, 275, 278
Amyl nitrite:
   angina pectoris, treatment of, xiv, 34–35, 69, 384
   effects of, 33–34, 35, 36, 37
   initial synthesis of, 33
   short-lived effect of, 36
   See also Lidocaine; Medications; Nitroglycerin
Aneurysms, 17, 21–22, 64, 229
Anger, H. O., 258, 260
Angina pectoris:
   amyl nitrite and, xiv, 34–35
   arterioles, contracted state of, 35
   atherosclerosis and, 9–10, 16, 23, 35, 58, 63
   blood pressure and, 20, 34–35
   case example and, 17–19
   coronary arteries and, 95
   distinct forms of, 20
   drug treatments, development of, 28–29
   early description of, 14–15, 25 (figure), 26
   electrocardiogram, use of, 50, 52, 69
   Levine's Sign/clenched fist enactment of, 23–24
   Netter's drawings and, 24–26, 25 (figure)
   nitroglycerin and, xiv, 32–33, 36–37, 159
   propranolol and, 210–212, 211 (figure)
   recognition of, xiv, 10, 14
   sudden cardiac death and, 15, 23
   therapeutic bleeding and, 34
   See also Amyl nitrite;

Coronary artery bypass
grafting (CABG);
Coronary artery bypass
surgery; Framingham
Heart Study (FHS);
Nitroglycerin; Stress tests
Angiocardiography technique, 91
Angiograms. *See* Coronary artery
angiograms
Angioplasty, 270
   acute angioplasty treatment
and, 291–293
   animal studies and, 284
   artery recoil problem and, 288
   balloon catheters,
development of, 274–275
   benefits, questions about,
287–288
   blood clots and, 285, 289–290,
291, 292, 293
   bypass grafts, blockage of, 11
   case example and, 270–271,
293–295
   chemotherapy medications,
role of, 290
   chronic stable angina, use in,
290–291
   diffuse atherosclerosis and,
285
   dual-channel catheters,
creation of, 275
   early coronary artery
angioplasty, xv, 11,
276–278
   expanded practice/
overutilization of,
283–286, 287
   inflatable balloon, dilating
arteries and, 274–275
   interventional radiology, early
development of, 272–273
   left anterior descending
coronary artery blockage
and, 270–271, 276–278,
280 (figure)
   multiple angioplasties/single
procedure and, 285
   post-heart attack angioplasty
and, 285
   restenosis, problem of, xv, 279,
286–287, 288, 289–290,
355
   risks of, 281, 287, 290, 293
   scar tissue and, 290
   steerable catheters,
development of, 281
   stents, development/use of,
288–290, 355, 360–361,
387
   televised demonstration of,
279
   widespread application of,
281–283
   See also Coronary artery
bypass grafting (CABG);
Coronary artery bypass
surgery; Coronary artery
stents
Anichkov, N., xiv, 57, 58, 60–64,
119, 153, 186, 325, 386
Animal studies:
   adrenal glands concoction and,
206
   angioplasty techniques and,
284

atherosclerosis studies and,
    55–56, 367
blood supply restriction, heart
    function and, 74
catheterization experiment
    and, 88–89
cholesterol-lowering
    compounds and, 319,
    320, 321, 322–323
coronary artery bypass
    grafting and, 222, 226
electric shock/defibrillation
    and, 142–144
heart-lung machine,
    development of, 129–130,
    131, 132
lidocaine studies and, 193–194
massive heart attacks and,
    166–167
personal defibrillators and,
    332–333, 335
radioactive heart imaging and,
    259–260
Triparanol studies, 319, 320
Anti-inflammatory medications,
    376–380
Antiarrhythmia medications, 144,
    193–194, 199
Antibiotics, 103, 237, 316–317
Anticoagulant medications, 113,
    129
Aorta, 59, 60, 63, 96
Aortic valve, 69, 95, 96, 172
Aortic valve disease, 70
Arrhythmias:
    atrial fibrillation-stroke linkage
        and, 113
    incidence of, 190

medications for, 144
See also Atrial fibrillation;
    Defibrillation;
    Electrocardiogram
    (ECG/EKG); Ventricular
    fibrillation; Ventricular
    tachycardia
Arterioles, 20, 35
Aschoff, K., 61, 62
Atherosclerosis, 55
    angina pectoris and, 9–10, 16,
        23, 35, 58, 63
    animal studies and, 55–56, 367
    anti-inflammatory
        medications, use/efficacy
        of, 376–380
    aorta, blockage of, 59, 60, 63
    arterial calcification and, 16,
        23, 366–367, 393–394
    blockages, detours around,
        21–23, 64, 227
    blockages, material in, 58, 59,
        366–367, 368, 369
    blood clots and, 16, 58, 59, 64,
        121
    C-reactive protein, marker
        for inflammation and,
        373–376
    case example and, 9–11
    causes, early work on, 57–62,
        106
    cholesterol and, xiv, 9, 16, 59–
        61, 62, 65, 66, 118–122
    cigarette smoking and, 7, 64
    coronary arteries, effect on, 63
    coronary artery angiograms
        and, 175

dietary factors in, 59, 60–61,
63, 65, 115, 116–119, 122
diseases of, 23
elastin cap over lipid buildup
and, 366
end-stage lesions, elements in,
366
fatty streak and, 366
foam cells, role of, 62, 369, 371
(figure)
genetics, influence of, 112, 113
high blood pressure/
hypertension and, 7
incidence of, 8
inflammation, immune system
response and, 365, 367,
368–371, 371 (figure)
injury response, multi-pronged
nature of, 366–368
low-density lipoprotein and,
xiv, 9, 118–122, 367–368,
370–371
mind-heart interaction and,
18–19
myocardial infarction and, 8
(figure), 23, 62, 63
plaque cover-up process and,
366, 372–373
plaque, role of, 58, 59, 60–61,
62
platelets, role of, 368, 369, 372
progressive stages of, 64–66,
65 (figure), 366–367, 368,
370–371, 371 (figure)
Q waves, evidence of blockage
and, 176, 178 (figure)
risk factors in, 7, 18–19
salt intake and, 7, 168–169
smooth muscle cells and,
366–369, 371 (figure)
translational research,
importance of, 62–64
war-time rations and, 4, 6
white blood cells and, 16, 58,
61–62, 363–365, 368
See also Cholesterol;
Coronary artery disease;
Framingham Heart
Study (FHS); Stress tests;
Widowmaker's malady
Atria, 47
Atrial fibrillation, 47, 54, 113, 144
Atrial flutter, 47
Automatic implantable cardiovert
defibrillator (AICD), 336–
343, 339 (figure), 344, 390
Autonomic nervous system,
208–209, 220

B

Bacon, F., 11
Bairey Merz, C. N., 355
Balard, A., 33
Batelli, F., 144
Beck, C. S., 146, 150
Becker, N., 95
Becquerel, A. H., 257
Belgard, A., 150
Berkovits, B., 154, 191
Bernard, C., 88
Beta-blockers, xv, 201, 307
acetylcholine, effect of, 207,
208
adrenal glands, function of,
205–207

adrenal glands, nerve plexuses
and, 204
adrenaline, double-edged
sword of, 203–204
adrenaline molecule,
separation of, 206
adrenaline, synthesization of,
206
alpha/beta receptor molecules,
role of, 209, 210–211, 211
(figure)
angina, adrenaline's effect and,
204, 208, 209
angina treatment and,
210–212, 211 (figure),
213–215
asthma attacks, adrenaline's
effects and, 207
atherosclerosis, adrenaline's
effects and, 204
autonomic nervous system,
dual functions of,
208–209
beta-receptor effects, heart
cells and, 209, 210–211,
211 (figure)
case example of, 201–202,
213–215
catecholamines, effects of,
207–209, 210
catecholamines, synthesization
of, 206
ganglionic blockers and, 210
heart rate, slowing of, 204, 212
isoprenaline, experiments
with, 210
mechanism of action of,
210–212, 211 (figure)
modern proliferation of, 213
propranolol, development of,
210–212, 211 (figure),
213, 214
radial artery blood flow
experiments and, 205–
206
receptor molecules, role of,
208, 209
sympathetic/parasympathetic
nervous systems,
function of, 208–209
transmitter molecules,
function of, 207, 209
See also Angina pectoris;
Medications
Bianchi, G., 142, 143
Bigelow, W., 147, 148
Billroth, T., 92
Birth Control Federation, 104
Black, J. W., xv, 203–204, 207–
212, 388
Blalock, A., 133
Bloch, K., 317, 318
Blockages. See Atherosclerosis;
Cardiac catheterization;
Coronary artery bypass
surgery; Coronary artery
catheterization; Heart
attacks; Widowmaker's
malady
Blood clots, xv
aspirin, effects of, 376
atherosclerosis and, 16, 58, 59,
64, 121
coronary thrombus, formation
of, 23, 299–304, 303–304
(figures), 314

heart attacks and, 121, 299–301, 304
mental outlook/stress levels and, 18–19
pulmonary embolisms and, 126
Widowmaker's malady and, 299–304, 303–304 (Figures)
See also Clot-buster medications; Heart attacks

Blood pressure:
afterload and, 163–164
angina pectoris and, 20, 34–35
cigarette smoking and, 7
definition of, 163
medications for, 112, 159
nitroglycerin, effect of, 36
normal vs. damaged heart function and, 163–165
optimal range of, 164, 395–396
preload and, 164
salt intake and, 396
sphygmographs, use of, 34, 36
therapeutic bleeding and, 34
therapeutic increase in, 163, 165, 167
See also Heart assist factors; High blood pressure; Hypertension; Low blood pressure; Stress tests

Blood tests, 10, 388
Blumgart, H., 257
Boas, E., 349, 350, 351, 354
Body-mass index (BMI), 400
Bordy, A. J., 82
Bousfield, G., 50, 69, 70, 73

Boyer, H., 311, 312, 314
Braunwald, E., 159–168, 187, 195, 313, 384, 385
Brown, M. S., xv, 237–247, 249, 250, 318, 321, 325, 388, 392
Brown-Séquard, É., 128
Brown, W. V., 122
Bruce, R. A., 80–83, 85, 388
Brunton, T. L., xiv, 34–35, 36, 384
Bundle branch block, 70
Buxton, A., 340

C

C-reactive protein (CRP), 373–376, 377, 378
CABG. *See* Coronary artery bypass grafting (CABG)
Callaghan, J., 148
Cambridge Scientific Instrument Company, Ltd., 48
Canakinumab Anti-inflammatory Outcomes Study (CANTOS), 379
Capillaries, 20, 21, 196, 220
Cardiac arrest. *See* Cardiopulmonary resuscitation; Heart attack epidemic; Heart attacks; Widowmaker's malady
Cardiac Care Units. *See* Coronary Care Units (CCUs)
Cardiac catheterization, 86–87
angiocardiography technique and, 91
animal studies and, 88–89
catheter materials/design, reworking of, 179–180

coronary arteries, exploration
of, 10, 86, 96–97
development of, recognition
for, 93–94, 97
European medical
establishment and, 93–94
internal cardiac pressure,
measurement of, 98–100
left ventricle, exploration of,
95–96
lung blood vessels, pressure
within, 99–100
medical advancements,
perspectives on, 91–92,
97
plaque, information on, 96
pulmonary function,
experiments on, 92–93
right ventricle, exploration of,
88–91
self-heart catheterization and,
xiv, 88–91
x-ray contrast dye, use of, 91,
93 (figure), 97
See also Coronary artery
bypass surgery; Coronary
artery catheterization
Cardiac surgery, 137
congenital heart disease
treatment and, 137
coronary artery disease
treatment and, 137
heart valve disease treatment
and, 137
See also Cardiac
catheterization; Coronary
artery bypass grafting
(CABG); Coronary artery

bypass surgery; Heart-
lung machines
Cardiogenic shock, 193
Cardiology Society of Leningrad,
227
Cardiology specialty:
cardiac catheterization,
importance of, 94, 96
emergence of, 48, 69, 85
National Institutes of Health,
role of, 105
See also Framingham Heart
Study (FHS)
Cardiopulmonary resuscitation,
152, 390
Cardiovascular Inflammation
Reduction Trial, 379
Carrel, A., 128
Catecholamines, 206–209, 210
Catheterization. See Angioplasty;
Cardiac catheterization;
Clot-buster medications;
Coronary artery
catheterization
Centrifuges, 114–115, 116, 117,
244
Cerebral hemorrhage, 103
Chasing the Widowmaker. See
Timeline of the Chase;
Widowmaker's end;
Widowmaker's malady
Chatalov, S., 60, 61
Chauveau, A., 88
Chemical processes. See
Adrenaline; Amyl nitrite;
Beta-blockers; Cholesterol
code; Coronary artery
disease; Heart assist factors;

Medications; Nitroglycerin;
Statins; Widowmaker's end
Cholesterol, 55
   atherosclerosis, role in, xiv, 9,
      16, 59–61, 62, 65, 66
   bounded nature of, 118
   cholesterol-lowering drugs
      and, xv, 247, 250–251,
      317–319, 394
   dietary factors and, 115–119,
      120, 121–122
   genetics, influence of, 112
   immune response and, 62
   low-density lipoprotein and,
      xiv, 9, 118–122
   metabolism of, xv, 63, 116, 119,
      239–242
   pathological processes and,
      61, 62
   xanthomas, formation of, 238
   See also Atherosclerosis;
      Cholesterol code;
      Lipoproteins; Receptor
      molecules; Statins
Cholesterol code, 234
   antibiotics, development of,
      237
   atherosclerosis, development
      of, 246
   biochemical reaction kinetics,
      rate-limiting step in,
      239–240
   case example and, 234–235,
      248–249
   cholesterol-lowering drugs
      and, xv, 247, 250–251,
      317–319, 394
   cholesterol metabolism,
      feedback regulation
      process and, 241–242,
      243, 245, 246
   cholesterol metabolism,
      fundamentals of, xv, 63,
      116, 119, 239–240
   cholesterol metabolism, steps
      in, 240–241
   "coated pits", LDL harbors and,
      245
   defective metabolic processes
      and, 246
   dietary sources of cholesterol
      and, 239, 240
   DNA, influence of, 242, 245
   endocytosis and, 244, 246
   familial hypercholesterolemia/
      hyperlipidemia, effects
      of, 238–239, 242, 243,
      244–245
   fibroblast cell walls, receptor
      molecules and, 243, 244,
      245
   fibroblast cells of skin, HMG
      CoA reductase in,
      242–243
   heart attack epidemic and, 235
   HMG CoA reductase, role of,
      239–240, 241, 242–243,
      245
   hydrophilic cholesterol
      mixture, HMG enzyme
      regulation and, 243–244
   intra-cellular cholesterol and,
      240, 243
   lipoproteins, carrier molecule
      function of, 240
   liver, metabolic factory

function of, 239–240, 241, 242
low-density lipoprotein receptors, life cycle of, 245, 246
low-density lipoprotein receptors, structure of, 246, 248 (figure)
low-density lipoproteins and, 242–243, 244, 245
organic chemistry, biological processes and, 235–237, 239
plasmapheresis treatment and, 250
receptor molecules, cell wall physiology and, 236, 237, 243
receptor molecules, malfunction of, 244–246
receptor molecules, spatial clustering of, 245
stains, cell component coloration and, 237
in vivo studies and, 245–246
xanthomas, formation of, 238
See also Cholesterol; Lipoproteins; Statins
Churchill, E. B., 126
CIBA Collection of Medical Illustrations, 24
Cigarette smoking, 4, 5, 7, 8, 64, 111, 348, 396–397
Clark, E. J., 132
Clarke, A. C., 87
Cleveland, G., 105
Clinton, W. J., 9–11
Clot-buster medications, xv, 296
angioplasty treatment and, 285, 289–290, 291, 292, 293
bacteria, protein manufacturing capability of, 311, 312
blood clots, Widowmaker's malady and, 299–304, 303–304 (figures), 309, 314
cardiac catheterization, use of, 301, 308
case example and, 296–299, 298 (figure)
coronary artery bypass grafting, use of, 300–301
emergency room protocol, efficiencies in, 310
Fogarty catheters, blood clot removal and, 302
gene manipulation and, 311–312
heart attacks, dual-process etiology of, 303
heart attacks, speedy response to, 300–301, 308–309, 310
intracoronary streptokinase infusion and, 308–309, 314
intravenous streptokinase infusion and, 309–310, 314
ischemia, bypass surgery and, 300–301
ischemia, EKG results and, 297, 298 (figure)

left anterior descending
coronary artery
blockage and, 297–304,
298 (figure), 303–304
(figures)
plasmin, clot-busting
capability of, 312
streptococci, protein
destruction property of,
305
streptokinase, development/
testing of, 305–307
streptokinase, rekindled
interest in, 307–313, 314
Thrombolysis in Myocardial
Infarction study group
and, 313–314
thrombus, occurrence of,
302–303, 303–304
(figures), 307
tissue plasminogen activator/
tPA, role of, 312–314
See also Heart attacks;
Medications
Cohen, S., 145, 311
Cohnheim, J. F., 20–21
Colchicine Cardiovascular
Outcome Trial, 379
Collateral blood vessels, 227
Computerized tomography (CT
scans), 267, 390
Congestive heart failure, 7, 41, 54,
94, 103, 165
See also Framingham Heart
Study (FHS)
Contractility, 162–163, 164
Coronary angiography. *See*
Coronary artery angiograms

Coronary arteries, 14
angina pectoris, distinct forms
of, 20
atherosclerosis and, 63
blockages, detours around,
21–22
blood vessels/arteries,
structural pattern of,
20–23
catheterization and, 10, 86,
96–97
"end-artery" assumption and,
20–21
thromboses, formation of, 23
See also Heart anatomy
Coronary artery angiograms, xiv,
219
atherosclerosis, picture of, 178
(figure)
case example and, 183–184
coronary artery bypass
grafting technique and,
223, 226–227
early angiogram and, 172–173,
174 (figure), 175
Coronary artery bypass grafting
(CABG), 216, 300–301, 389
animal studies and, 222, 226
aorta, vein bypass grafts and,
229
aspirin, efficacy of, 376
breakthrough surgical
techniques, development
of, 227–232
bypass grafts, blockage of, 11
case example and, 216–217,
232–233

collateral arteries, potential
    detours and, 227
coronary artery angiograms,
    utility of, 223, 226–227
dead heart muscle tissue,
    removal of, 229
earliest foundation of, 217–220
early human candidates for,
    222, 225, 226
early surgical advances and,
    222, 223–227
heart anatomy, features of, 220
heart-lung machines, use of,
    225, 226, 230
heart valve replacements and,
    229
internal thoracic arteries,
    utilization of, 221–222,
    223, 224, 226, 229
left anterior descending artery,
    direct grafts into, 228,
    229, 233
leg vein segments, harvesting
    of, 228–229, 230 (figure)
mammary artery-coronary
    artery graft and, 224, 226,
    230 (figure)
nuclear cardiac imaging and,
    264
oxygenated blood, diffusion
    technique and, 220–221,
    224
proof-of-concept
    demonstrations and, 222,
    225, 227
revascularization technique
    and, 224–225, 226–232,
    230 (figure)

surgical instruments, redesign
    of, 223, 226
survival rate for, 231
"third coronary artery", need
    for, 220–221, 222
See also Coronary artery
    bypass surgery
Coronary artery bypass surgery,
    177
case example and, 10–11
first bypass surgery and, xv
nuclear cardiac imaging and,
    264
stress tests, diagnostic efficacy
    of, 84–85
See also Coronary artery
    bypass grafting (CABG)
Coronary artery catheterization,
    11, 170–171
atherosclerosis, evidence of,
    175–176, 178 (figure),
    183
case example and, 181–184
catheter materials/design,
    reworking of, 179–180,
    196–198
chest pain, sources of, 175–
    176, 177
coronary artery angiograms
    and, 172–173, 174
    (figure), 175, 178 (figure),
    183–184
coronary artery disease,
    evidence of, 177
exertional chest pain and, 176
"gray areas" of clinical
    judgment and, 177

guidewire technique,
   expansion of, 179–180
guidewire technique, initial
   use of, 179
nuclear imaging, use of, 177
percutaneous entry and,
   178–179
polyurethane catheters,
   introduction of, 180
pulmonary artery, wedge
   pressure and, 196–197
Q waves, arterial blockage and,
   176
rest-related chest pain and,
   177
Swan-Ganz right heart
   catheterization,
   development of, 196–198
See also Cardiac
   catheterization; Coronary
   artery bypass surgery
Coronary artery disease, 360
   adipokines and, 371
   animal studies and, 367
   anti-inflammatory
      medications, use/efficacy
      of, 376–380
   aspirin, use/efficacy of,
      376–377
   atherosclerosis, abnormal
      cells/fatty material and,
      364–365, 366, 368, 369
   atherosclerosis, inflammatory
      disease of, 365, 368–371,
      371 (figure)
   atherosclerosis, multiple stages
      in, 366–367, 368, 369
   atherosclerosis research,
      renaissance of, 365–368
   blood clot formation and, 369,
      372
   C-reactive protein/CRP,
      inflammation marker
      and, 373–376, 377, 378,
      379
   calcification process and, 16,
      23, 366–367
   Canakinumab Anti-
      inflammatory Outcomes
      Study and, 379
   canakinumab use and, 379
   case example, 360–362,
      380–381
   cell markers, use of, 367
   Colchicine Cardiovascular
      Outcome Trial and, 379
   colchicine use and, 379
   combination medications,
      therapeutic approach of,
      378–380
   cytokine cascade and, 370–371
   electrocardiogram, use of,
      50–52
   "endarteritis deformans"
      process and, 364–365
   foam cells/macrophages, role
      of, 62, 369, 371 (figure),
      372
   heart attack/stroke risk,
      C-reactive protein levels
      and, 374–375
   heat generation, plaque lesions
      and, 368
   hydraulics/physiology
      perspective and, 362

inflammation, immune system
response and, 365, 367,
368–371, 371 (figure)
inflammation, molecular
directors of, 369–371
inflammation, risk factor of,
374–375
injury response, multi-pronged
nature of, 366–368, 372
low-density lipoprotein, role
of, 367–368, 369, 370–
371, 377, 379, 380
matrix metalloproteinases/
cysteine proteases, role
of, 372
methotrxate use and, 379
mind-heart interaction and,
18–19
molecular biology, application
of, 367, 369–370, 372, 379
plaque cover-up process and,
371–373
plaque rupture, explanation
for, 372–373
plaque vulnerabilities,
identification of, 373–376
platelets, role of, 368, 369, 372,
377
protective collagen, eroding of,
372–373
questions about, persistence
of, 362–363, 367, 376
rheumatoid arthritis, effects of,
360–362, 367, 380–381
smooth muscles cells, role of,
366–369, 371 (figure)
statins, anti-inflammatory
effect and, 377–378

T cells, role of, 370, 371
(figure), 372
vascular cell adhesion
molecules/VCAM-1, role
of, 370
white blood cells, role of,
363–365, 366, 368–369,
380–381
women's coronary artery
disease and, xv, 6, 177,
375
See also Angina pectoris;
Atherosclerosis; Cardiac
surgery; Coronary artery
bypass grafting (CABG);
Coronary artery bypass
surgery; Coronary
artery catheterization;
Electrocardiogram (ECG/
EKG); Heart attack
epidemic; Heart attacks;
Stress tests
Coronary artery stents:
bypass grafts, blockage of, 11
development/use of, 288–290
restenosis, risk of, xv, 279,
286–287, 288, 289
See also Angioplasty
Coronary Care Units (CCUs), xiv,
54, 159, 185, 307
AC vs. DC electrical charges,
defibrillation and, 191
admission criteria, changes in,
192
antiarrhythmia medications
and, 193–194
arrhythmias, incidence of, 190

assessment process,
    complexity of, 195
cardiogenic shock and, 193
case examples and, 185–186,
    190–193, 198–199,
    360–362
catheterization procedures,
    impracticalities of, 195
complete heart block,
    recognition/treatment of,
    190–191
conduction system, damage to,
    190–191
defibrillation, rapid application
    of, 187, 188, 190, 191,
    192, 198, 199
efficacy of, 189, 190, 198–199
electrical system defects and,
    190–191, 192
electrocardiograms, warning
    function of, 188
establishment of, 188–189,
    191–193
heart monitoring, role of, 186,
    187, 188, 189, 190–191,
    198, 200 (figure)
heart muscle damage, acute
    heart failure and, 192–
    193
hospital stays, reduced length
    of, 189
intense nursing care in, 189,
    191, 198
lidocaine, application of,
    193–194, 199
medications, use of, 190,
    193–194, 198

mortality rate and, 189, 190,
    192, 198
Myocardial Infarction
    Research Units,
    establishment of, 195–
    196
oscilloscope monitoring
    technology and, 190
patient typology and, 192–193
proactive/prophylactic
    treatment, practice of,
    192, 194
Swan-Ganz right heart
    catheter, development of,
    196–198
technical advances in heart
    care and, 186–187
temporary pacemakers, use
    of, 190
twenty-four/seven staffing of,
    188, 189, 191
Widowmaker lesions and,
    192–193
Widowmaker's malady,
    counterattack on,
    186–193, 198
Widowmanker's malady,
    treatment deficits and,
    187, 191
Coronary thrombosis, 24, 299–
    304, 303–304 (figures)
Cortisol, 18
Cosgrove, D., 230
Cournand, A., 92, 94, 160
Crick, F., 311

D

Daiichi Sankyo, Inc., 321, 322–323
Dakin, H. D., 206
Dale, H., 205
Dawber, T., 109, 110
Day, H., 188–189, 198
de Gallois, L., 127
DeBakey, M., 130–131
Defibrillation, xiv, 140–141, 390
    AC vs. DC electrical charges and, 152, 153–154, 191
    animal studies and, 142–144
    antiarrhythmia medications, lack of, 144
    atrial fibrillation and, 144
    biphasic shock technique and, 152–153
    case example of, 155–156
    closed chest approach to, 150, 155–156
    defibrillation technology, innovative approach to, 147–150
    early experimentation with, 143–144
    electric shock utility, rediscovery of, 145–152
    electrical charge, potential of, 141–142
    fibrillation, induction of, 144
    heart monitoring capability, development of, 150–151
    heart muscle hypersensitivity state and, 144
    myocardial infarction, treatment of, 147 (figure)
    open-heart surgery, restored heart rhythm and, 145–146
    pacemakers, development of, 148–150
    political influence, scientific research and, 152–153
    Stokes-Adams disease and, 146, 148
    ventricular fibrillation and, 146, 147, 147 (figure), 150, 151
    ventricular tachycardia and, 141, 147, 147 (figure)
    See also Pacemakers; Personal defibrillators
Demikhov, V., 226
Denning, W. E., 122
Deoxyribonucleic acid (DNA), 242, 245, 311–312
Dewood, M., xv, 299–303, 307, 314, 362, 387
Diabetes mellitus:
    cardiologist management of, 397
    cigarette smoking and, 7
    genetics, influence of, 112
    heart attack epidemic and, 7, 111
    obesity and, 7
    Type II diabetes, 7, 397
    See also Framingham Heart Study (FHS)
Diet:
    animal fat, danger of, 121
    atherosclerosis and, 59, 60–61, 63, 65, 115, 122
    cholesterol and, 116, 119, 120, 239, 240

fat molecules and, 115–116
fats, avoidance of, 392
healthy diets, impact of, 120, 121–122
low-density lipoprotein levels and, 119, 120, 121
low fat/low carbohydrate meals and, 121
salt intake and, 5, 6, 7, 168–169, 396
South Beach Diet, 9
war-time rations and, 4, 6–7
Digitalis, 144, 165
Disease. *See* Atherosclerosis; Coronary artery disease; Heart attack epidemic; Heart disease; Widowmaker's malady; Women's heart disease
Ditzen, G., 89, 90
Diuretics, 54, 100, 158, 165, 193
Dobbin, E. V., 121
Dock, W., 65
Dotter, C., 272, 273, 275, 293, 387
Drug therapies. *See* Amyl nitrite; Beta-blockers; Lidocaine; Medications; Nitroglycerin; Statins

E

Edelman and Sons, 48, 50
Effler, D., 219, 220, 222, 223, 227
Ehrlich, P., 236–237, 243
Einthoven, W., xiv, 42–44, 46–49, 52, 54, 69, 75, 84, 89, 112, 144, 386
Eisenhower, D. D., 7, 159, 167

Electrocardiogram (ECG/EKG), 40
angina pectoris and, 50, 52, 69
arrhythmias, documentation of, 47, 52–54, 69
atrial enlargement and, 47–48
bundle branch block and, 70
coronary artery disease, documentation of, 50–54, 70–71, 74–75
Coronary Care Units and, 188
diagnostic strength of, 69–72, 73
gender-based differences in, 353
heart block/dropped beats and, 47
heart rhythm, electrical signals and, 47–48, 50 (figure), 69–70
high blood pressure and, 48
inconclusive clinical presentation and, 40–41, 52–54
invention of, xiv, 42–47, 49
ischemia, EKG results and, 297, 298 (figure)
lead attachments, placement of, 47–48
Lippman's capillary electrometer and, 42, 44–45, 46
manufacturing contracts for, 48
myocardial infarction diagnosis and, 10, 49, 50, 51–52, 69, 71

normal variants, recognition of, 81–82
P waves/atrial deflections and, 47–48, 50 (figure), 75 (figure)
potential applications for, 46–49, 69–72
PR interval and, 75 (figure)
PR segment and, 75 (figure)
Q waves, arterial blockages and, 176, 297, 298 (figure)
QRS complexes/ventricular deflections and, 50 (figure), 51, 70–71
QT interval and, 75 (figure)
ST segment and, 51–52, 54
ST segment depression/ restricted blood flow and, 75 (figure), 82
ST segment elevation/Pardee's sign and, 71, 298 (figure), 309, 386
string galvanometer and, 46–47, 49
T wave abnormality/Pardee's T waves and, 71, 298 (figure)
T waves/repolarization and, 50 (figure), 51, 52, 70, 71, 75 (figure)
telecardiograms, use of, 47
tombstone sign and, 297, 298 (figure), 309
ventricular fibrillation and, 147 (figure)
ventricular tachycardia and, 147 (figure)
See also Defibrillation; Framingham Heart Study (FHS); Stress tests
Electrodyne Company, 150
Eli Lilly Corporation, 210
Empirical theory, 11–12, 42, 43–44
Endo, A., 317–322, 326, 328, 388, 392
Epidemics:
cholera outbreaks and, 102–103
heart disease/stroke and, 103–104
Public Health Service, role of, 105
scientific focus on, 102
social medicine, introduction of, 103–104
See also Epidemiology; Framingham Heart Study (FHS); Heart attack epidemic
Epidemiology, 102
cholera outbreaks and, 102–103
early practice of, 104–105
epidemiologic activism, stance of, 110
heart disease research, emerging focus on, 105–106
heart disease/stroke incidence and, 103–104
infectious disease deaths and, 106
malaria incidence and, 106
National Health Act of 1939 and, 106

natural history acquisition
process of, 107–108, 113
preventive measures,
implementation of, 106
refinement of, 106
See also Framingham Heart
Study (FHS)
Exercise, 9
ischemia, induction of, 263
See also Stress tests

F

Familial hypercholesterolemia/
hyperlipidemia (FH),
238–239, 242, 243, 244–245,
321–322
Fast food industry, 7, 9
Favaloro, R., xv, 177, 216, 217–
220, 223–224, 225, 227,
228–230, 231, 232, 233, 389
Fearon, R., 181–184
Fibrillation. *See* Arrhythmias;
Atrial fibrillation;
Defibrillation; Ventricular
fibrillation
Fiedotin, A., 171
Field, A. G., 32–33, 36
Fight or flight response, 208
Fish, P. A., 116
Fleming, A., 320
Foam cells, 62, 369, 371 (figure)
See also Atherosclerosis;
Coronary artery disease;
White blood cells
Fogarty catheters, 302
Fogarty, T., 302
Food intake. *See* Diet

Forssmann, W., xiv, 87–91, 93–94,
96, 131, 148, 160, 172, 198,
263, 386
Framingham Heart Study (FHS),
xiv, 101–102
atrial fibrillation-stroke linkage
and, 113
cholesterol levels and, 111
cigarette smoking, danger of,
111
clustered risk factors, additive
nature of, 110–111
diabetes, danger of, 111
dropout rate for, 109
electrocardiogram, use of,
111–112
epidemics, robust scientific
focus on, 102–104, 106
epidemiologic activism, stance
of, 110
epidemiology, practice of,
104–105, 106, 113
ethnic/racial groups, study of,
113
Framingham Risk Score model
and, 110–111, 394
Framingham, "typical" town
status of, 107
genetics, influence of, 112, 113
heart attack incidence findings
and, 111
heart disease research,
emerging focus on,
105–106, 108
hypertension-atherosclerosis
linkage and, 109
hypertension-stroke linkage
and, 110

hypertension, targeted
    treatment of, 110, 112
life style choices, impact of,
    111
local buy-in for, 107
multi-year data collection and,
    109–110, 113
"normal"-level indicators,
    misleading nature of, 112
participant enrollment in,
    108–109
prevention goal of, 108, 109,
    110, 112, 113
research focus/purpose and,
    108, 109, 113
research methodology for,
    107–108
results, realizations from,
    110–113
risk factors in heart disease
    and, 108, 110–111, 112,
    391
sample characteristics and,
    108, 109
social medicine, introduction
    of, 103–104
systolic pressure, significance
    of, 111
women/elderly participants
    and, 109, 111, 350, 351
Frank-Starling relationship, 164
Frydman, M., 331
Fundación Favaloro, 231
Furchgott, R., 37

G

Gable, C., 7
Gage, S. H., 116

Galvani, L., 42
Ganz, W., 100, 197–198, 274, 299
Genentech, 312
Genetics:
    gene manipulation, clot-
        busting medications and,
        311–312
    heart disease and, 7, 112, 113
    medication development and,
        393
Gibbon, J. H., xiv, 125–137, 263
Goetz, R., 224, 225, 226, 228
Gofman, J., xiv, 116–122, 186, 239,
    325, 386, 391
Goldstein, J. L., xv, 238–247, 249,
    250, 318, 321, 325, 388, 392
Goldstein, S., 122
Gottschalk, A., 258
Grass Stimulator Company, 148,
    149
Grines, C., 292, 387
Grüntzig, A., xv, 270, 271, 272,
    273–282, 279 (figure), 286,
    288, 293, 295, 386, 387
Grüntzig, J., 271
Gurvich, N. L., 152, 153
Guthrie, F., 33

H

Hahnemann, S., 31
Harken, D., 145, 148, 224
Harrison, D., 193
Hartmann, D., 276
Hartzler, G., 283–286, 291
Harvey, W., 14, 65
Heart anatomy:
    angina pectoris, early
        description of, 14–15

aorta, 59, 60, 63, 96
aortic valve and, 69, 70, 95
arterioles and, 20, 35
atria, 47
blockages, detours around,
  21–23
blood vessels/arteries,
  structural pattern of,
  20–23
capillaries and, 20, 21, 220
circulation, early description
  of, 14, 20–21
coronary arteries and, 14,
  96–97
coronary artery angiograms
  and, xiv, 172–173, 174
  (figure), 175
"end-artery" assumption and,
  20–21
general anatomical features,
  220
left atrium, 48
left ventricle, 48, 95–96, 112
mitral valve, 48, 172
Netter's drawings and, 24–26,
  25 (figure)
right ventricle, 88–91
sinusoids and, 220
ventricles, 47, 48, 88–91,
  95–96
venules and, 20
See also Heart assist factors;
  Widowmaker's malady
Heart assist factors, 157
actin/myosin, function of, 162,
  164
adenosine triphosphate
  molecule and, 162

adrenaline/noradrenaline, role
  of, 162–163, 167
afterload, arterial blood flow
  and, 163–164, 165
animal studies, massive heart
  attacks and, 166–167
blood pressure, normal vs.
  damaged heart function
  and, 163–165
blood pressure, optimal range
  of, 164
blood pressure, therapeutic
  increase in, 163, 165, 167
cardiac blood output, drivers
  of, 162
chronotropy/inotropy,
  encouragement of, 162,
  163, 165
congestive heart failure,
  medications for, 165
contractility, role of, 162–163,
  164
digitalis and, 165
diseased hearts, study of,
  161–163
diuretics and, 158, 165
fluid retention/edema, effects
  of, 164–165, 167, 169
Frank-Starling relationship
  and, 164
heart attack injury, response
  to, 159–160, 163–168
heart attacks, surviving heart
  cells and, 163, 165, 166
heart function/circulatory
  system, information on,
  161–162, 163

heart rate, role of, 162, 163, 165, 167
massive heart attacks, treatment of, 166–168
medications, uses of, 163, 164, 165, 166–167
preload, venous blood flow and, 164, 165
propranolol, reduced heart muscle damage and, 167
salt consumption, avoidance of, 168–169
short-term rescue and, 157–159, 166–167
wall tension, oxygen demands and, 164–165
x-ray images, heart anatomy and, 160
See also Heart attack epidemic; Heart attacks; Widowmaker's malady
Heart attack epidemic, 2, 3, 235
atherosclerosis, development of, 7–8
case example and, 9–11
cigarette smoking and, 4, 5, 7, 8
coronary artery disease incidence and, 6
diabetes mellitus and, 7
fast food industry and, 7, 9
modern society, habits of, 4–5, 6–8
mortality rate and, 6, 7–8, 19, 159
obesity and, 7
prevention, factors in, 5
salt intake and, 5, 6, 7
treatments, development of, 11–12
war-time rations and, 4, 6–7
See also Atherosclerosis; Cholesterol code; Coronary artery disease; Framingham Heart Study (FHS); Heart assist factors; Heart attacks; Heart disease; Widowmaker's malady; Women's heart disease
Heart attacks:
advance warning of, 10, 23
angina pectoris and, 9–10, 15–16
blockage of blood flow and, 8 (figure)
blockages, detours around, 21–23
case examples and, 1–2, 9–11
coronary thrombosis and, 23, 24
deaths from, xii, xiii, 10, 20
early exploration/chronicling of, 19–26
early treatment of, xiii, xiv
heart muscle damage, prevention of, 307
heart muscle hypersensitivity state and, 144
increasing incidence of, 19
massive heart attacks, treatment of, 166–168
Netter's drawings and, 24–26, 25 (figure)
prevention of, xiii, xv, 2

silent heart attacks and, 111, 112, 351
speed of response to, 300–301
temperament and, 17–19
thromboses, formation of, 23, 24
Timeline of the Chase and, xiv–xv
transmural damage and, 303, 309
treatments, development of, 11–12
See also Angina pectoris; Atherosclerosis; Blood clots; Cholesterol; Clot-buster medications; Coronary artery disease; Framingham Heart Study (FHS); Heart assist factors; Heart attack epidemic; Heart disease; Lipoproteins; Myocardial infarction; Widowmaker's malady

Heart disease:
arteries, diseased condition of, xii
cigarette smoking and, 7, 111
deaths from, xii, xiii, 6
low-density lipoproteins and, 118–122
rheumatic fever and, 48
risk factors in, 108, 110, 111
Timeline of the Chase and, xiv–xv
See also Angina pectoris; Atherosclerosis; Coronary artery disease; Electrocardiogram (ECG/EKG); Framingham Heart Study (FHS); Heart attack epidemic; Medications; Myocardial infarction (MI); Widowmaker's end; Widowmaker's malady; Women's heart disease

Heart Epidemiology Study. *See* Framingham Heart Study (FHS)

Heart-lung machines, xiv, 124
anemia, damaged red blood cell walls and, 130–131
animal studies for, 129–130, 131, 132
anticoagulant medication, development of, 129
atrial septal defect, surgery on, 133–134
blood coagulation, problem of, 128–129
blood oxygenation process and, 127–128, 129–130
case example and, 133–134
conceptualization of, 126–127
coronary artery bypass surgeries and, 225, 226, 230
heart stop/restart procedure and, 132, 134
hemolysis, problem of, 130–131
human patients, open-heart surgery on, 133–139
IBM involvement with, 132
mortality rates and, 132, 133, 134, 135–136

need for, 124–127
on-bypass surgical techniques,
    development of, 132
oxygenator machines,
    development of, 128,
    130–131, 132
patent application for, 135
    (figure)
roller pump solution and, 131
technological refinement of,
    131, 136
See also Cardiac surgery
Heart transplant surgery, 231
Heberden, W., xiv, 14, 16, 17, 19,
    20, 26, 69, 71, 79, 351, 390
Heilman, S., 335
Henry, W., 44
Hering, C., 31–32
Herrick, J. B., 19–20, 21, 22–23,
    64, 79
High blood pressure:
    cigarette smoking and, 7, 111
    electrocardiogram tracings
        and, 48
    genetics, influence of, 112
    left ventricular hypertrophy
        and, 48, 112
    systolic pressure, significance
        of, 111
    women/elderly, susceptibility
        of, 111
    See also Blood pressure;
        Framingham Heart Study
        (FHS); Hypertension;
        Low blood pressure
High-density lipoproteins (HDL),
    118, 120 (figure)
    See also Cholesterol;
        Lipoproteins; Low-
        density lipoprotein (LDL)
Hipps, J., 148
History taking skill, 24
Holter, N., 337
Home, E., 17
Homeopathy, 31, 32
Honeywell International Inc., 335
Hopff, H., 274–275
Horecker, B., 318
Howell, W. H., 129
Humphrey, H. H., 153
Hunter, J., 16–19, 21–22, 64
Hypertension:
    cigarette smoking and, 7
    electrocardiogram tracings
        and, 48
    management of, 396
    prevalence of, 395
    See also Blood pressure;
        Framingham Heart
        Study (FHS); High blood
        pressure

I

Ignarro, L., 37
Ignatowski, A., 59
Imaging. *See* Coronary
    artery angiograms;
    Electrocardiogram (ECG/
    EKG); Nuclear cardiac
    imaging; Radioactive heart
    imaging; Radioisotopes;
    Widowmaker's end
Immune response. *See*
    Atherosclerosis; Coronary
    artery disease; Inflammation;
    White blood cells

Imperial Chemical Industries
    (ICI), 209–210, 211, 212
Inflammation:
    aspirin, efficacy of, 376–377
    atherosclerosis, development
        of, 365, 367, 368–371, 371
        (figure)
    C-reactive protein and,
        373–376, 377, 378
    fat cells, role of, 400
    injury response, multi-pronged
        nature of, 366–368
    molecular directors of,
        369–371
    statins, efficacy of, 377–378
    See also Atherosclerosis;
        Coronary artery disease
International Business Machines
    (IBM), 132
Ischemia, 75 (figure), 79, 261–262,
    263, 297, 298 (figure), 300

J

Jenner, E., 16, 17
Johnson, L. B., 7
Judkins, M., 179–180, 182
Julian, D., 187, 188, 190–191, 198
Justification for the Use of
    Statins in Prevention: An
    Intervention Trial Using
    Rosuvastatin (JUPITER
    trial), 377–378

K

Kannel, W., 110, 111, 112, 113
Kerry, J., 9
Keys, A., 3

Khrushchev, N. S., 153
King, S. B.,,, III, 275, 280
Kirklin, J., 136, 137
Kite, C., 143
Kolesov, V. I., 225–226, 227, 228
Kouwenhoven, W., 152, 390
Kowey, P., 337
Kritchevsky, D., 56

L

Lasker, A. D., 104
Lasker Foundation, 104, 105
Lasker, M. W., 104–105
Lasker Prize, 105
Lavoisier, A., 65
Lawrence, E. O., 117, 258
Left atrium, 48
Left ventricle, 48, 95–96, 112
Left ventricular ejection fraction
    (LVEF), 255, 260–261, 261
    (figure), 262, 340–343
Leiden jar, 142–143
Leon, M., 287
Lettsom, J. C., 17
Levant, O., 91
Levine, S., 23–24, 348
Levine's Sign, 24
Levy, H., 349, 350, 351, 354
Lewis, T., 48, 70, 75
Libby, P., 370–371
Lidocaine, xiv, 193–194, 199
    See also Amyl nitrite;
        Medications;
        Nitroglycerin
Lindbergh, C., 128
Lindbergh-Carrel perfusion
    pump, 128
Lindgren, F., 117

Lipoproteins:
    atherosclerosis, development of, 118–122
    carrier molecule function of, 240
    centrifuge, use of, 114–118
    cholesterol metabolism, fundamentals of, 239–240
    classes of, differentiation of, 118
    dietary sources and, 116, 119, 120
    discovery/early study of, 116, 117–119
    healthy diets, effect of, 120, 121–122
    heart disease, influence on, 118–122
    high-density lipoproteins and, 118, 120 (figure)
    hydrophilic nature of, 240
    low-density lipoproteins and, 118–122, 120 (figure)
    molecule layering, molecular weight/density and, 117–118, 120 (figure)
    plaque, buildup of, 118–119
    salt in blood samples, effect of, 118
    Svedberg units and, 118
    very-low-density lipoproteins and, 118, 120 (figure)
    See also Cholesterol; Cholesterol code; Statins
Lippman, G., 44–45, 46
Lippman's capillary electrometer, 42, 44–45, 46
Livingston, M. S., 258
Loop, F., 230
Lorenz, H. A., 48
Low blood pressure:
    angina pectoris and, 20, 35
    See also Blood pressure; High blood pressure
Low-density lipoprotein (LDL), xiv, 9, 118–122, 120 (figure), 175, 242–243
    See also Atherosclerosis; Cholesterol; Cholesterol code; Lipoproteins
Lown, B., 153, 154, 186, 191, 333, 334, 335, 348
Lynen, F., 317–318
Lytle, B., 230

M

MacWilliam, J. A., 143, 144
Magnetic resonance imaging (MRI), 390
Malmros, G., 132
Marchand, F., 59
Marey, E. -J., 88
Maroko, P., 166, 167
Master, A. M., 75–80, 85
Master Two-Step Test, xiv, 77–79
McClurken, J., 233
McLean, J., 129
McMichael, J., 94
Meadors, G., 106, 107, 108
Mechnikov, I., 363–364, 365
Medical advancements:
    Albert and Mary Lasker Foundation and, 104
    antibiotics, development of, 103

anticoagulant medication and, 113, 129
cardiac catheterization and, 91–92, 97
gene function, understanding of, 103
heart disease/cancer, research in, 105
Lasker Prize and, 105
National Health Act of 1939 and, 106
National Heart Act of 1948 and, 105
National Heart, Blood Vessel, Lung and Blood Act of 1972 and, 105
protein structure, understanding of, 103
Public Health Act of 1944 and, 104–105
Public Health Service, establishment of, 104, 105, 106
social medicine, introduction of, 103–104
See also Cardiac catheterization; Cardiology specialty; Coronary artery bypass surgery; Coronary artery catheterization; Defibrillation; Electrocardiogram (ECG/EKG); Epidemiology; Framingham Heart Study (FHS); Heart-lung machines; Stress tests; Widowmaker's end

Medications:
anti-inflammatory medications and, 376–380
antiarrhythmia medications and, 144, 193–194, 199
antibiotics and, 103, 237
anticoagulants and, 113, 129
aspirin and, 376–377, 389
blood pressure medications and, 112, 159
chemotherapy drugs, coronary artery stents and, 290
chemotherapy drugs, heart valve effects of, 264
cholesterol-lowering drugs, xv, 247, 250–251, 317–319
congestive heart failure and, 165
diabetes management and, 397
digitalis and, 144, 165
digoxin and, 54
diuretics and, 54, 100, 158, 165, 193
early research into, 29
effectiveness, prediction of, 31, 37
heart muscle damage, reduction in, 167
heart rate medications and, 159
homeopathic practice and, 31, 32
inclisiran clinical trials and, 393
lidocaine and, xiv, 193–194, 199
morphine, use of, 54, 158, 159, 186, 297

organic chemistry, role of,
    29–30, 31, 33
penicillin and, 316–317, 318,
    323
pharmacology discipline,
    inception of, 37
propranolol and, 167, 210–
    214, 211 (figure), 398
proving trials for, 31–32,
    36–37
streptomycin and, 317
syphilis, Salvarsen and, 237
treatment/medication effects,
    correlation of, 37
Vitalism, concept of, 29
See also Amyl nitrite; Beta-
    blockers; Clot-buster
    medications; Heart assist
    factors; Nitroglycerin;
    Statins
Medrad Inc., 335
Merck & Co., Inc.
    pharmaceuticals, 319–320,
    322, 324, 325, 328, 392
Meshkov, S., 3–5
Metabolism of cholesterol:
    feedback regulation process
        and, 241–242
    fundamentals of, xv, 63, 116,
        119, 239–240
    steps in, 240–241
    See also Cholesterol code
Metchnikov, I., 363–364, 366
Mind-heart interaction, 18–19
Mirowski, M., 331–339, 341, 343,
    390
Mischief of the heart, 14, 16, 20,
    69

See also Heberden, W.
Mitral valve, 48, 172, 346
Moran, N. C., 210
Morphine, 54, 158, 159, 186, 297
Moss, A., 340, 341
Mother Teresa, 8
Mountin, J. W., 106
Mower, M., 332, 333–338
Mukherjee, S., xii
Müller, C., 238
Multicenter Automatic
    Defibrillator Implantation
    Trial II (MADIT II), 341
Multicenter Automatic
    Defibrillator Implantation
    Trial (MADIT), 340
Multicenter Unsustained
    Ventricular Tachycardia Trial
    (MUUST), 340–341
Murad, F., 37
Murrell, W., xiv, 36–37, 384
Myler, R., 275, 278
Myocardial infarction (MI), xi, 2, 7
    atherosclerosis and, 8 (figure),
        23, 62, 63
    blood tests and, 10, 388
    cell types after, 165
    coronary arteries and, 95
    death from, 20
    diagnosis of, 10
    electrocardiogram, use of, 10,
        49, 50, 51–52, 69, 71
    nitroglycerin, use of, 37
    Q waves, arterial blockage and,
        176
    See also Framingham Heart
        Study (FHS); Heart assist
        factors; Heart attack

epidemic; Heart attacks;
Widowmaker's malady
Myocardial Infarction Research
Units, 196
Myocardial ischemia, 75 (figure),
79

N

National Health Act of 1939, 106
National Heart Act of 1948, 105
National Heart, Blood and Lung
Institute, 352, 355
National Heart, Blood Vessel,
Lung and Blood Act of 1972,
105
National Institutes of Health
(NIH), 105, 122, 153, 162,
163, 196, 238
Netter, F., 24–26, 25 (figure)
Nichols, A., 121
Nicolai, D. F., 50
Nitroglycerin:
angina pectoris, treatment of,
xiv, 32–33, 36–37, 159,
384
chemical formula for, 31
commercial availability of, xiv,
30, 31
dynamite, patenting of, 31
efficacy experimentation and,
31–33, 36–37
explosive power of, 31, 36
glonoine compound,
experimentation with,
31–32
glycerol, experimentation with,
30–31

industrial applications of, 30,
31
initial synthesis of, xiv, 29–31
isosorbide dinitrate and, 37
nitric oxide, effect of, 37
proving trials for, 31–33,
36–37
pyroglycerin, development of,
30–31
treatment regimen,
development of, 36–37,
39
See also Amyl nitrite;
Lidocaine; Medications
Nobel, A., 30–31, 38
Noradrenaline, 158, 162–163
Nuclear cardiac imaging:
blood flow imaging, xv, 177,
217, 265–266, 266
(figure)
bypass surgery success,
assessment of, 264
cardiac muscle function
imaging, xv, 177, 264
left ventricle ejection fraction,
measurement of, 340
nuclear cardiology specialty,
expansion of, 265–267
nuclear stress testing and, 265,
266 (figure), 267–269
women patients,
electrocardiogram
uncertainty and, 353
See also Radioactive heart
imaging

O

Obesity epidemic, 7, 111, 352, 399, 400–401
Oliver, G., 205–206
O'Neill, W., 292, 387
Oppenheimer, B., 75, 85
Organic chemistry. *See* Coronary artery disease; Medications; Statins; Widowmaker's end
Osler, W., 58

P

P waves, 48, 50 (figure), 75 (figure)
  See also Electrocardiogram (ECG/EKG)
Pacemakers, 147, 148–150
  AC vs. DC electrical charges and, 152, 153–154
  automatic rhythm regulation and, 151, 154
  closed chest approach and, 150
  early disadvantages of, 149–150
  efficacy rate, early pacemakers and, 151–152
  heart monitoring capability, development of, 150–151
  initial human applications of, 149
  public interest in, 149–150
  stimulators, use of, 148, 149, 151
  temporary pacemakers, Coronary Care Units and, 190
  transthoracic pacing and, 148, 149–150
  transvenous pacing and, 148
  See also Defibrillation; Personal defibrillators
Palmaz, J., 288–290, 387
Palmaz-Schatz stent, 289–290
Pardee, H., 50–51, 70, 71, 73, 75
Pasteur, L., 218, 236, 237
Pavlov, I., 58, 153
Pelouze, T. -J., 30
Penicillin, 316–317, 318, 323
Pepine, C., 355
Peripheral blood vessels, 179, 274
Perkins, M. E., 210
Personal defibrillators, 169, 329
  abnormal cardiac rhythm, detection of, 334, 337, 342
  ambulatory heart rhythm monitoring, role of, 337
  animal studies of, 332–333, 335
  automatic implantable cardiovert defibrillator/ AICD and, 336–343, 339 (figure), 344
  bad vs. good hearts, determination of, 339–340
  battery technology design for, 335, 337, 338
  case example and, 329–330, 341, 343–344
  charge, size of, 332, 333
  complications with, 338, 341–342
  coronary artery atherosclerosis treatment, advances in, 330

electrode implantation and, 335–336, 338, 339 (figure)
engineering challenges of, 332–335
ethical issues with, 333, 342
heart muscle damage risk and, 334
high-risk patients, identification of, 337
human candidates for, 335–337, 338, 339–340, 341
human trials of, 333–334, 335, 340–342
iatrogenic heart attacks/arrhythmias, risk of, 333, 335
intravascular catheter/right ventricle electrode and, 335–336, 339 (figure)
left ventricle ejection fraction, role of, 340, 343
mortality rates and, 338, 341
Multicenter Automatic Defibrillator Implantation Trial/MADIT and, 340
Multicenter Automatic Defibrillator Implantation Trial II/MADIT II and, 341
Multicenter Unsustained Ventricular Tachycardia Trial/MUUST and, 340–341
normal heart rhythm, restoration of, 331, 334, 336
post-operative ventricular fibrillation, correction of, 334
sudden cardiac death and, 330, 340, 341, 342–343, 344
See also Defibrillation; Pacemakers
Personality factors, 18–19
Pettigrew, T., 18
Pharmacology, 37, 384
Physicians' Health Study (PHS), 374–375, 376
Pitt, B., 259
Placebo effect, 224
Planned Parenthood Federation, 104
Plaques, 58–59, 60–61, 62, 96, 118–119, 175, 300
See also Angioplasty; Atherosclerosis; Cardiac catheterization; Coronary artery catheterization; Coronary artery disease
Plasmapheresis treatment, 250
Pooled Cohort Equation, 394
PR interval, 75 (figure)
Prévost, J.-L., 144
Prinzmetal, M., 257
Propranolol, 167, 210–212, 211 (figure), 213, 214, 398
Protein molecules. See Lipoproteins
Public Health Act of 1944, 104–105
Public Health Service, 104, 105, 106
Pulmonary circulation, 92–93, 126, 196–197, 310

Q

Q waves, 176, 298 (figure)
QRS complexes, 50 (figure), 51, 70–71, 297
　See also Electrocardiogram (ECG/EKG)
QT interval, 75 (figure)

R

Racial inequities, 347, 348, 359
Radioactive heart imaging, 252
　animal studies for, 259–260
　atherosclerosis, diagnostic instruments for, 254–255, 261–262, 263, 264, 265
　blood flow measurement and, 257, 258, 260, 262, 263, 264, 265–266, 266 (figure)
　bypass surgery success, assessment of, 264
　case example and, 252–253, 267–269
　chemotherapy drugs, heart valve effects of, 264
　"cold spots", imaging of, 263, 265
　computer technology applications and, 265
　diagnostic questions, answers to, 264
　"gamma" camera imaging, use of, 258, 260
　heart blood supply, comprehensive image of, 259–260
　heart valve disorders, replacement surgery and, 264
　image accuracy, improvements in, 265
　ischemia, imaging of, 261–262, 263
　left ventricular ejection fraction and, 255, 260–261, 261 (figure), 262, 265
　nuclear stress testing and, 265, 266 (figure), 267–269
　radioactive elements in use, increased numbers of, 265
　radioactive potassium, blockage imaging and, 263–264
　radioisotope imaging, utility of, 255, 257–258
　red blood cells, labeling of, 258, 260
　technetium 99m, improved imaging with, 258, 262, 265
　thallium, use of, 265
　x-ray imaging, development/ utility of, 255–256
　See also Nuclear cardiac imaging
Radioisotopes, 255, 257–258
Receptor molecules:
　alpha/beta receptors and, 209
　blood vessel constriction/ dilation and, 209
　cell wall physiology and, 236, 243

cholesterol metabolism and, xv
molecular effects, blocking of, 208
See also Cholesterol code
Rentrop, K. P., 308–309, 314, 362
Restenosis risk, xv, 279, 286–287, 288, 289, 355
Resuscitation. *See* Defibrillation
Rheumatic fever, 48
Rhoads, J. E., 27–28, 38–39, 384
Richards, D. W., 92, 94
Richman, I., 1–2
Ricketts, H., 179
Ridker, P., 374, 376, 377–378
Right ventricle, 88
Ritchie, J., 265
Roentgen, W., 255, 256, 257
Roosevelt, F. D., 7, 103, 105, 395
Ross, R., 365–368, 372
Rutherford-Merrell Chemical Company, 319, 320
Rutstein, D., 106, 107

S

Salt intake, 5, 6, 7, 168–169, 396
Sankyo, Inc., 321, 322–323
Scandinavian Simvaststin Survival Study (4S study), 324–325, 328
Schatz, R. A., 287, 290, 387
Schlesinger, M., 145
Schneider, R., 89, 90, 91
Schwartz, A., 10
Scientific method, 11, 35, 42, 43, 245
Scott, R. W., 95
Seaborg, G. T., 117

Seattle Heart Watch study, 83
Seldinger, S. I., 179, 180, 182, 387
Self-heart catheterization, xiv, 88–91
Seneca, 14
Sharpey-Schafer, E. A., 206
Shaw, L., 355
Shelley, M., 142
Sherry, S., 299, 304–307, 309, 314, 387
Shirey, E., 175
Shumaker, H., 136
Silent heart attacks, 111, 112, 351
Simmons, A., 50
Simpson, J., 276
Sinusoids, 220
Smith, C. R., 10
SmithKline & French (SKF) pharmaceutical company, 212
Smooth muscle cells:
Snow, J., 102, 103, 108
Sobrero, A., xiv, 29, 30, 31, 36, 391
Social medicine, 103–104
Sones, F. M., Jr., xiv, 97, 171, 172–177, 180, 181, 219, 220, 222, 223, 231, 278, 386
Sorlie, P., 113
Sphygmograph, 34, 36
ST segment, 51–52, 54, 71, 82, 297, 298 (figure), 309, 386
See also Electrocardiogram (ECG/EKG)
Statins, 315
animal studies and, 319, 320, 321, 323
blood cholesterol, optimal levels of, 326

blood cholesterol, reduction of, 325
cancer side effect of, 322–323
case example and, 316–317
cholesterol-lowering drugs, conceptualization of, 317–319
cholesterol metabolism, limited final step of, 319
cholesterol metabolism, rate-limiting step in, 318
compactin, development/study of, 321–323
demosterol conversion, slowing of, 319
familial hyperlipidemia patient, compactin study in, 321–322, 323
global efficacy of, 328
guidelines for widespread use of, 327
heart attack/death, reduction of, 325–326, 328, 389
heart attack prevention goal and, 325–326, 328
inflammatory process, reduction of, 377–378
Internet-based misinformation about, 327
JUPITER trial and, 377–378
liver side effects risk of, 325
lovastatin/Mevacor, development/marketing of, 322–323, 324, 325
microorganisms, interrupted lipid metabolism and, 320–321
muscle breakdown risk of, 325
noncompliance issue and, 327–328
rosuvastatin, anti-inflammatory effects and, 377–378
Scandinavian Simvastatin Survival Study and, 324–325, 328
simvastatin, efficacy study of, 324–325
statin drug trials, large-number perspective and, 323–326
Triparanol, potential of, 319–320, 323
See also Cholesterol; Lipoproteins
Statistics:
Stein, H., 68, 84–85
Stents. See Angioplasty; Coronary artery stents; Widowmaker's end
Stokes-Adams disease, 146, 148, 149
Stolz, F., 206
Storkes:
Strauss, W., 259–260, 263
Stress, 18
Stress tests, xiv, 67–68
abnormality, revised criteria for, 82–83
angina pectoris, diagnosis of, 72–73, 74, 76, 79
animal studies, restricted blood supply and, 74
cardiac blood supply restriction, effects of, 74

chest pain/heart rate/blood pressure, correlation among, 76, 80
computer-aided analysis of, 83
electrocardiograms, utility of, 69–72, 75–80
exercise/cardiac blood volume requirement, linkage between, 79, 83
hypothesis generating results of, 74
ischemia, proof of, 79
lung disease, exercise tolerance and, 81
Master Two-Step Test, xiv, 77–79, 80
normal variants, recognition of, 81–82
nuclear stress testing and, 265, 266 (figure), 267–269
population characteristics, abnormality incidence and, 82–83
predictive value of, 73, 74, 78–79, 80, 82–83, 84
Seattle Heart Watch study and, 83
standardized normal heart function and, 76–77, 78, 79
treadmill, development/use of, 81, 83–84
Stroke, 103, 104
anticoagulants, use of, 113
atrial fibrillation, linkage with, 113
C-reactive protein levels and, 374–375
hypertension and, 110, 395
incidence of, 103–104
See also Framingham Heart Study (FHS); High blood pressure; Hypertension
Sudden death. *See* Angina pectoris; Myocardial infarction; Personal defibrillators; Widowmaker's malady
Surgeon General position, 105
Surgery. *See* Cardiac catheterization; Cardiac surgery; Cardiopulmonary bypass; Coronary artery bypass grafting (CABG); Coronary artery bypass surgery; Heart transplant surgery
Svedberg, T., 118
Svedberg units (Sf), 118
Swan-Ganz right heart catheter, 196–198
Swan, H. J. C., 100, 196–198, 274, 299
Swanson, R., 311, 312, 314

T

T waves, 50 (figure), 51, 52, 70, 71, 75 (figure)
See also Electrocardiogram (ECG/EKG)
Takamin, J., 206
Taussig, H., 133
Templeton, J. Y., 135, 137
Thomas, V., 133
Thornton, M. A., 282, 286

Thrombolysis in Myocardial Infarction study group, 313–314
Thrombolytic therapy. *See* Angioplasty; Cardiac catheterization; Clot-buster medications; Coronary artery bypass grafting (CABG); Coronary artery bypass surgery; Coronary artery stents; Thrombolysis in Myocardial Infarction study group
Thrombus, 23, 24, 299–304, 303–304 (figures)
Tillett, W., 304, 305, 373
Timeline of the Chase, xiv–xv
Tobacco industry, 4, 5, 7
Transplants. *See* Heart transplant surgery
Treadmills, 81, 83–84
Two-step stress test, xiv, 77–79
Type A personality, 18
Type I/II diabetes. *See* Diabetes mellitus

U

US Food and Drug Administration (FDA), xv, 289, 319, 320, 323, 325, 337

V

Vagelos, P. R., 322, 323, 328
Van Decker, B., 216–217
Vascular cell adhesion molecules (VCAM-1), 370
Ventricles, 47, 48
Ventricular fibrillation, 47, 88, 140–141, 146, 147, 147 (figure), 150, 151, 186, 191, 199
Ventricular hypertrophy, 48, 112, 158
Ventricular tachycardia, 141, 147, 147 (figure), 186, 190, 191, 199
Venules, 20
Very-low-density lipoproteins (VLDL), 118, 120 (figure)
See also Cholesterol; Lipoproteins
Vineberg, A., 220–224, 227
Virchow, R., 21, 58–59, 115, 364–365, 366, 368
Vitalism concept, 29
von Rokitansky, C., 59

W

Waller, A. D., 42, 43, 44, 45–46, 48
Watson, J., 311
Watson, T., 132
Wellens, H., 194
Wenger, N., xv, 346–349, 351–353, 355, 356, 357 (figure)
Wharton, T., 204
White blood cells, 363
  atherosclerosis and, 16, 58, 61–62, 364–365, 368–371, 371 (figure)
  cholesterol plaque and, 62
  foam cells and, 62, 369, 371 (figure)
  immune response, role in, 61, 62, 364

phagocytes/macrophages and, 61–62
rheumatoid arthritis and, 380–381
White, P. D., 106, 107
Widowmaker's end, 382–383
  age, risk factor of, 394–395
  angina, drug treatments for, 389, 390–391
  angiography, blockage extent/location and, 388
  angioplasty procedure and, 387, 389, 402
  aspirin, utility of, 389
  automatic implantable cardioverter defibrillator and, 390
  blood clot danger, neutralization of, 387
  blood pressure optimization and, 395–396
  blood tests, biomarkers and, 388
  cardiac catheterization process and, 386–387, 388
  cardiac problems, scoring systems for, 394
  cholesterol levels, lowering of, 392, 394–395
  cigarette smoking and, 396–397
  combination medications and, 391
  coronary artery bypass graft procedure and, 389
  coronary calcium scans and, 393–394
  Coronary Care Units, responsibilities of, 387–388
  defibrillators, access to, 390
  diabetes mellitus, management of, 395, 397
  dietary fats, avoidance of, 392
  early diagnosis, importance of, 390
  electrocardiogram, preliminary data and, 386, 387, 390
  financial roadblocks and, 390, 393
  future atherosclerosis, identification of, 393–394
  genetic manipulation science, drug development and, 393
  high blood pressure/diabetes, long-term management of, 395
  HIV patients, cardiac disease risk and, 399–400
  hypertension, prevalence of, 395
  imaging technologies and, 390
  inclisiran, clinical trials for, 393
  left ventricle ejection factor, crucial number of, 388
  low-density lipoprotein particle and, 386–387
  low-density lipoprotein receptors, shortened life of, 393
  medications, applications of, 388–389, 392–393, 394–395

modern-era routine life-saving practices and, 401–403
non-statin medications and, 392–393
noninvasive tests, role for, 390
obesity epidemic, atherosclerosis incidence and, 400–401
organic molecules, power/promise of, 383–385
PCSK9 inhibitors, low-density lipoprotein removal and, 392–393
pharmacology, impact of, 384–385
pregnancy-related problems and, 399
prevention focus and, 391–394
rapid/skilled care, reduced mortality and, 385, 386–391
risk scoring systems and, 394
statins, utility of, 389, 392, 394
stents, use of, 387
stress tests, use of, 388, 390
sudden death, prevention of, 389–390
treatment techniques, proliferation of, 385
triglycerides, treatment of, 393
wearable AI and, 386
western lifestyle patterns, deleterious effect of, 398–399
See also Medical advancements; Widowmaker's malady
Widowmaker's malady, xi, 3, 137
angina pectoris, distinct forms of, 20
atherosclerosis and, 17–19
blood clots, role of, 299–304, 303–304 (figures)
blood vessels/arteries, structural pattern of, 20–23
cardiogenic shock and, 193
case examples and, 9–11, 17–19, 21–22
chasing of, xii, xiv–xv, 2, 11, 19
coronary artery angiograms and, 183–184
early exploration/chronicling of, 19–26
empirical theory and, 11–12
heart anatomy and, 20–23
heart attack, factors in, 6–7, 17–19
heart attack incidence and, 7–8, 19
heart muscle hypersensitivity, state of, 144
historic recognition of, 13–16
left anterior descending coronary artery blockage and, 270–271, 276–278, 280 (figure), 297–299, 298 (figure)
left anterior descending coronary artery, direct grafts into, 228, 229, 233
male victims of, 177
mind-heart interaction and, 18–19
myocardial infarction and, xi, 2, 7, 8 (figure)

Netter's drawings and, 24–26, 25 (figure)
sudden death and, 187, 389–390
survival from, 7, 8, 235
temperament and, 17–19
thromboses, formation of, 23
treatment deficits for, 187
urban civilization and, 19–20
women's heart disease and, 13
See also Angina pectoris; Cholesterol; Cholesterol code; Coronary artery bypass grafting (CABG); Coronary artery bypass surgery; Coronary artery disease; Coronary Care Units (CCUs); Electrocardiogram (ECG/EKG); Heart attack epidemic; Heart attacks; Heart disease; Lipoprotein; Medications; Stress tests; Widowmaker's end
Windaus, A., 59
Winkle, R., 336–338
Withering, W., 165
Wöhler, F., 29
Wolferth, C., xiv, 72, 78, 85
Women's Health Initiative (WHI), 375, 376
Women's heart disease, xv, 345
age, risk factor of, 111, 120, 351–352, 376
angina pectoris and, 32–33, 354, 355–356
angioplasty, restenosis problem and, 287, 354–355
bias, elimination of, 351–357
biased perspective and, 15, 26, 177, 235, 346–351
C-reactive protein levels, heart attack risk and, 375
case example and, 345–346, 357–359
chest pain, evaluation of, 353, 355, 356
cigarette smoking and, 348, 352
coronary artery disease, incidence of, 6, 177, 348–349
data review efforts and, 352–355
diagnosis methods and, 352
electrocardiograms, gender-based differences in, 353
Framingham Heart Study participation and, 109, 111, 350, 351
generalizations, utility of, 349
heart attack incidence and, xi, 111, 120
high blood pressure and, 111
lactic acid, cardiac buildup of, 356
low-density lipoproteins, increased levels of, 120
menopause, role of, 111, 120, 352, 375
metabolic syndrome and, 353
mortality statistics and, 352, 354

myocardial infarction risk and, 351
nuclear cardiac imaging, need for, 353
outpatient cardiac rehabilitation and, 355
prevention strategies and, 352
prodrome symptoms, experience of, 354
racial inequities and, 347, 348, 359
research on, xv, 32–33, 36, 375
rheumatoid arthritis, effects of, 360–362
risk factors, recognition of, 352–353
silent heart attacks, incidence of, 351
statin drugs, efficacy studies of, 324, 328
symptoms, gender-based differences in, 350–351, 354
Syndrome X, cardiac lactic acid buildup and, 356
treatment delays, heart damage and, 354
treatment efficacy and, 352, 354
war-time rations and, 6–7
Widowmaker's malady and, 13, 351, 353
women practitioners, bias against, 347, 359
Women's Health Initiative/ WHI and, 375, 376
Women's Ischemia Syndrome Evaluation/WISE study and, 355–356
Women's Ischemia Syndrome Evaluation (WISE) study, 355–356
Wood, F. C., xiv, 72, 78, 85
Wood, H. C., Jr., 35
World Health Organization (WHO), 400

X

X-ray imaging, 80, 90, 91, 93 (figure), 98, 160, 173, 179, 184, 255–257, 263

Y

Yamamoto, A., 321
Yu, P., 81

Z

Zaret, B., 254–255, 259–264, 388
Zimmerman, H., 95
Zoll/Belgard heart monitors, 150–151, 186, 187
Zoll, P., xiv, 145–152, 187, 191

ACKNOWLEDGMENTS

The writing of this book has been a labor of love for almost three years. From the early days of just trying to do research online and put together a concept, I have had people who have encouraged and helped me endlessly.

Firstly, I need to acknowledge the guidance of my dearest and oldest friend Bruce Alan Kehr MD, a distinguished psychiatrist and author, who first led me to believe that this was something I could accomplish but with some help. He steered to the wonderful Mary Loverde who, along with her friend Samantha Horn, guided me on the path to becoming a much better writer and storyteller.

Mary Loverde then collaborated with Kym Croft Miller MFA, and they both became my muses and editors for the last two years. I am incredibly indebted for their help. Without them, this book never would have taken form. Kym especially helped me to the "finish line."

Highest on my list of people to thank are the patients and friends who have so graciously allowed me to include their stories in this book. These include Ed Chacker, Herschel Elias, Hubiert Gramberg, Carla Jenkins, Harold Stein MD, and Joan Winkowski.

I have spoken to so many people who have advised me over these last few years, and I am especially indebted to my remarkable professor from my Yale days, Barry Zaret MD, as well as Michael Brown MD, the Nobel Prize winner from Texas. Along the way, I have received great help from the staff of the National Library of Medicine in Bethesda, Maryland, who helped me find wonderful older books and documents that were not available online and add so much to the text of this book.

It has been my great fortune to work with Janet Shapiro of SmithPublicity and John Koehler of Koehlerbooks, who have steered me through the uncharted waters of publicity and publication. Their help has been crucial. My gratitude is also boundless to my graphic artist who made sure the images all looked great—Meredith Dawson.

Many of my friends and colleagues have read portions of my book at various stages, and their comments and suggestions are greatly appreciated. These include my wonderful wife Norma, Richard Barasch, Alan and Wendy Bruck, Charles Cutler MD, Gerald Eisman PhD, Ira Garr, Natalie Ledesma, T. Sloan Guy MD, Peter Kowey MD, Richard Oller, Arthur Seidner, Daniel Seltzer, and Gary Tabas MD. It is one of life's great joys to have so many great friends you can count on.

August 2020

ABOUT THE AUTHOR

Arnold Bruce Meshkov MD grew up in suburban Philadelphia, Pennsylvania, and attended the University of Pennsylvania for his undergraduate and medical degrees. This is his first book. He did his residency in internal medicine at Temple University School of Medicine in Philadelphia, and his cardiology fellowship at the Yale University School of Medicine in New Haven, Connecticut.

He started his own private practice in 1981, a practice that grew to six cardiologists. He returned to academic life at Temple University in 1998 and became a Clinical Professor of Medicine before returning to private practice in Abington, Pennsylvania, in 2015, where he maintains a practice today.

Dr. Meshkov lectured extensively when he was at Temple University and has published in peer-reviewed journals. He is a Fellow of American College of Cardiology and board-certified in internal medicine, cardiovascular medicine, and echocardiography.

Dr. Meshkov lives in Abington, Pennsylvania, with his wife Norma of fifty years, close to his two children and four grandchildren. He loves his family and friends, science and medicine, as well as history, sailing, photography, skiing, his faith, Long Beach Island in New Jersey, and his local sports teams, especially the Philadelphia Eagles and Seventy-Sixers. If he is reincarnated, he wishes to come back as 6'9" tall, able to use both hands on the basketball court and learn the Euro Step.

CPSIA information can be obtained
at www.ICGtesting.com
Printed in the USA
LVHW091332300321
682964LV00001B/4